A Space of Their Own: The Archaeology of Nineteenth Century Lunatic Asylums in Britain, South Australia and Tasmania

CONTRIBUTIONS TO GLOBAL HISTORICAL ARCHAEOLOGY
Series Editor:
Charles E. Orser, Jr., *Illinois State University, Normal Illinois*

A SPACE OF THEIR OWN: Lunatic Asylums in Britain, South Australia, and Tasmania
Susan Piddock

AN ARCHAEOLOGICAL STUDY OF RURAL CAPITALISM AND MATERIAL LIFE: The Gibbs Farmstead in Southern Appalachia, 1790–1920
Mark D. Groover

ARCHAEOLOGY AND CREATED MEMORY: Public History in a National Park
Paul A. Schackel

AN ARCHAEOLOGY OF HISTORY AND TRADITION: Moments of Danger in the Annapolis Landscape
Christopher N. Matthews

AN ARCHAEOLOGY OF MANNERS: The Polite World of the Merchant Elite of Colonial Massachusetts
Lorinda B.R. Goodwin

AN ARCHAEOLOGY OF SOCIAL SPACE: Analyzing Coffee Plantations in Jamaica's Blue Mountains
James A. Delle

DOMESTIC ARCHITECTURE AND POWER: The Historical Archaeology of Colonial Ecuador
Ross W. Jamieson

HISTORICAL ARCHAEOLOGIES OF CAPITALISM
Edited by Mark P. Leone and Parker B. Potter, Jr.

THE HISTORICAL ARCHAEOLOGIES OF BUENOS AIRES: A City at the End of the World
Daniel Schavelzon

A HISTORICAL ARCHAEOLOGY OF THE OTTOMAN EMPIRE: Breaking New Ground
Edited by Uzi Baram and Lynda Carroll

MEANING AND IDEOLOGY IN HISTORICAL ARCHAEOLGY: Style, Social Identity, and Capitalism in an Australian
Heather Burke

RACE AND AFFLUENCE: An Archaeology of African America and Consumer Culture
Paul R. Mullins

RURAL SOCIETY IN THE AGE OF REASON: An Archaeology of the Emergence of Modern Life in the Southern Scottish Highlands
Chris Dalglish

A Continuation Order Plan is available for this series. A continuation order will bring delivery of each new volume immediately upon publication. Volumes are billed only upon actual shipment. For further information please contact the publisher.

A Space of Their Own: The Archaeology of Nineteenth Century Lunatic Asylums in Britain, South Australia and Tasmania

Susan Piddock
Flinders University, South Australia

Springer

Susan Piddock
Department of Archaeology
Flinders University
GPO Box 2100
Adelaide
5001 South Australia
spiddock@ozemail.com.au

ISBN-13: 978-0-387-73385-2   e-ISBN-13: 978-0-387-73386-9

Library of Congress Control Number: 2007932328

© 2007 Springer Science+Business Media, LLC
All rights reserved. This work may not be translated or copied in whole or in part without the written permission of the publisher (Springer Science+Business Media, LLC, 233 Spring Street, New York, NY 10013, USA), except for brief excerpts in connection with reviews or scholarly analysis. Use in connection with any form of information storage and retrieval, electronic adaptation, computer software, or by similar or dissimilar methodology now known or hereafter developed is forbidden.
The use in this publication of trade names, trademarks, service marks, and similar terms, even if they are not identified as such, is not to be taken as an expression of opinion as to whether or not they are subject to proprietary rights.

Printed on acid-free paper.

9 8 7 6 5 4 3 2 1

springer.com

Preface

This book draws largely on my unpublished Doctoral Thesis: *A Space of Their Own: Nineteenth Century Lunatic Asylums in England, South Australia and Tasmania*, and l am happy to send information on South Australia and Tasmania not included in this book to interested readers.

I would like to dedicate this book to my family who have lived for many years with my passion for lunatic asylums, and in particular my mother, Margaret Piddock, manuscript reader extraordinary.

I would like to thank Professor Vincent Megaw for introducing me to the Destitute Asylum excavation and for starting me on the path of institutional archaeology, and for his and Ruth Megaw's support through my student years, and Claire Smith and Heather Burke for helping turn research into a thesis.

I would like to thank James Gibb for preparing illustrations from my tracings and Dr. Elizabeth Heath, for her support over the years and for reading of this book in its various stages.

Glossary

Acute/manic/furious/frantic - these words were used to describe the behaviour of the insane while they were experiencing the initial on set of mental illness or a further period of mental illness when their actions were uncontrolled and the person could not be reasoned with. Patients in this state were often physically restless, sometimes violent, and difficult to reason with.

Refractory - this is used in a similar manner. Refractory patients were unable to control their behaviour and their thoughts. These patients could not be left on their own, may be violent, and required constant supervision.

Moderate/Orderly - the insane in this class were able to control their behaviour even if their mental illness continued as before, and were capable of following instructions and behaving in an appropriate manner towards staff and other patients.

Convalescent - these persons were recovering from their bout of mental illness. They were aware of their surroundings and showed the ability to distinguish reality from illusions or paranoid thoughts caused by their illness. The ability to reason was a fundamental characteristic of a sane mind. The ability to behave in a way considered appropriate by Victorian standards was essential if one was to be released from the asylum. Although convalescent patients may still be mentally ill they were able to control themselves within the company of others outside of the asylum.

Chronic - these patients were those considered to be incurable. Often after a number of years they showed little signs of recovery. In modern terms these included patients with senile dementia and similar organic degenerative diseases, the mentally retarded, the epileptic, and a range of mental illnesses that are now considered to arise from problems with brain chemistry such as schizophrenia.

Moral Treatment - encompassed ideas about the treatment of the insane, which should be characterised by humanity, kindness and reason. Moral treatment focused on using the finer feelings of the afflicted to bring them back to sanity, by focusing on the will and powers of self-restraint. The treating doctor had a pivotal role as he used all of the means at his disposal, including reasoning and talking to the patient, to bring them back to sanity by addressing the particular ideas of the individual.

Non-Restraint - Focussed on the removal of mechanical restraints and sought to improve the living conditions of the insane. Restraints were to be replaced by classification, opportunities to exercise, the employment of the patients, religious consolation and amusements. The wards should be clean, a good diet should be provided, and patients treated with all kindness. These changes led to significant improvements in the behaviour of patients and supported their return to sanity.

Classification - this was the basis of the asylum world. Patients were classed on the basis of their mental state. Spaces were designed in each ward to suit the requirements of each class of patient. Refractory patients required single rooms to limit disturbances on the wards and more observation. Convalescent patients who were quieter could be placed in dormitories and required less observation. Movement through the various wards could be a punishment for inappropriate behaviour and access to a quieter, more nicely furnished ward a reward.

Panopticon - originally advocated by Jeremy Bentham, this building design consisted of a series of arms radiating out from a central hub. This hub housed the staff and allowed all the arms to be observed at one time. The design was intended to funnel any noise to the staff rounds, giving the inmates no privacy.

Lavatory - in the world of lunatic asylums this room contained wash basins and places for hair brushes and combs. The later rooms were provide with running water. These places were intended to allow patients to freshen up through out the day.

Organic Asylums - these were asylums that grew through a series of additions to the original buildings without an overall coherent plan.

Ha-Ha - this was a sunken trench which placed before a wall allowed that wall to be placed lower. This in turn allowed a view over the top of a wall while preventing escape.

Table of Contents

Preface v

Glossary vii

CHAPTER 1. A Space of Their Own 1

    Book Outline 6

CHAPTER 2. The Archaeology of Institutions 7

    Testing History 9
    Paternalism, Domination and Resistance 10
    Reform and Symbolism 14
    Institutions and Space 16

CHAPTER 3. The Archaeology of Lunatic Asylums 19

    Research Design 19
    A Theoretical Approach to the Archaeology
    of Lunatic Asylums 22
    Practicalities: Methodology and Limitations 29
    Sources of Information: The Ideal Asylum 29
    Sources of Information: Built Asylums in England 31
    The Case Studies: South Australia and Tasmania 33
    Original Documentation 34

CHAPTER 4. The Changing Face of Insanity
            and Rise of the Institution 37

    Moral Treatment and the Asylum 38
    The Non-Restraint Movement 40

The Rise of the Lunatic Asylum	44
Discussion	46

CHAPTER 5. Constructing the 'Ideal' 49

The 'Ideal' Lunatic Asylum: Early Experiments 1807–1809	50
The Moral Environment: Tuke, Hill and Browne 1813–1838	52
The 'Ideal' Asylum Detailed: Jacobi and Conolly 1841–47	57
Further Ideas About The 'ideal' Asylum: Sankey and Arlidge	64
Variations on a Theme: Pavilion and Cottage Asylums 1860–1865	70
Conclusion	75

CHAPTER 6. The British Lunatic Asylum: Ideals and Realities 77

Variety and Experimentation: Charity Hospitals and Early Lunatic Asylums 1800–1844	78
The 'Ideal' Asylum of Browne - 1837	81
Uniformity: The County Asylums - 1845 to 1869	83
Discussion	88
Later County Asylums - 1870 to 1880	93
The 'Ideal' Asylums of Jacobi, Sankey and Robertson	94
Discussion	96
Life within the Asylum	97
A Gendered World	101
Conclusion	105

CHAPTER 7. South Australia and the 'Ideal' Lunatic Asylum ... 107

A Brief History of the Adelaide and Parkside Lunatic Asylums	108
The South Australian Asylums and the 'Ideal' Asylum Model of John Conolly	126
The 'Ideal' Asylums of Browne, Jacobi, Sankey and Robertson	133
Life in the Asylums	138
A Gendered Experience	144
Discussion	146

Contents

CHAPTER 8. Tasmania and the 'Ideal' Asylum 149

    A Convict Colony 149
    A Brief History of the New Norfolk Hospital for the Insane,
    Port Arthur and Cascades Lunatic Asylums 150
    Methodological Issues 164
    Port Arthur and Cascades Asylums and the 'Ideal' Models. . 165
    New Norfolk and the 'Ideal' Asylum of John Conolly....... 167
    New Norfolk and the Models of Browne, Jacobi, Sankey
    and Robertson 174
    Life in the Hospital 175
    Discussion....................................... 182

CHAPTER 9. The 'Ideal' Asylum: A World of Difference 183

    British Asylums and Australian Institutions:
    Commonalities or Differences? 184
    South Australia and Tasmania: Similarities
    and Differences................................... 189
    Factors Influencing the Built Provisions
    of British Asylums 191
    Factors Influencing the Built Provisions of the Adelaide
    and Parkside Asylums 194
    Economic Constraints 194
    Knowledge of the Overseas Treatment of the Insane....... 196
    Social Perceptions of the Insane 199
    Treatment Regimes 200
    Discussion....................................... 202
    Factors Influencing the Built Provisions of New Norfolk.... 203
    Economic Constraints 203
    Social Perceptions of the Insane: The Presence
    of Convicts...................................... 205
    Knowledge of the Overseas Treatment of the Insane....... 208
    Treatment Regimes 209
    Discussion....................................... 211
    Conclusion 212

CHAPTER 10. Conclusion: Archaeology and Lunatic Asylums ... 215

    Archaeology and Institutions......................... 215
    Life within the Asylum 218

	A Gendered Experience	221
	An Artificial World	222
	The Twentieth Century	223

Appendices

1.	The Location of Illustrations of Lunatic Asylums discussed in Chapter 6	225
2.	Treatment Regimes in South Australia	227
3.	Treatment Regimes in Tasmania	235

Abbreviations ... 241

References ... 245

Index ... 257

A Space of Their Own | 1

What comes to mind when you read the words lunatic asylum? The idea of imprisonment? Of being locked away from the world, cut off from all contact? The popular media images, whether in films, television, or in books about lunatic asylums tend towards bleak views of imprisonment, harsh uncaring attendants, and patients wondering around in a dazed, detached state, wearing straight jackets or having frenzied psychotic fits. Wards are portrayed as prison-like and undecorated. Is this an accurate portrayal of the reality of the experience of the mentally ill in the past?

In this book the world of nineteenth century lunatic asylums in Britain, South Australia and Tasmania (Figure 1.1) will be explored using the theoretical approaches of historical archaeology and a new methodology will be explored that allows us to understand lunatic asylums where excavation is not possible.

In the nineteenth century the primary means of caring for the mentally ill, or the insane as they were called, was to place them in a lunatic asylum. As this study will reveal this stay in a lunatic asylum was intended to be curative. The lunatic asylum was not intended to be a place where the mentally ill remained for life, rather after a short time in the asylum they would be returned to sanity and released back into society. More importantly the lunatic asylum was not simply a collection of buildings. Its shape, the arrangement of its parts, the rooms and spaces provided, were determined by specific factors that related to the care and cure of the insane person. In the asylum the insane were removed from the stresses and causes of insanity found in the external world, and under the care of the medical superintendent would be brought back to sanity (Hill 1838: 38–39; Browne 1837: 156).

In the mid to late eighteenth century there was a fundamental shift in the understanding of insanity. Skultans (1979: 56) has characterized this shift as: "the emergence of therapeutic optimism and

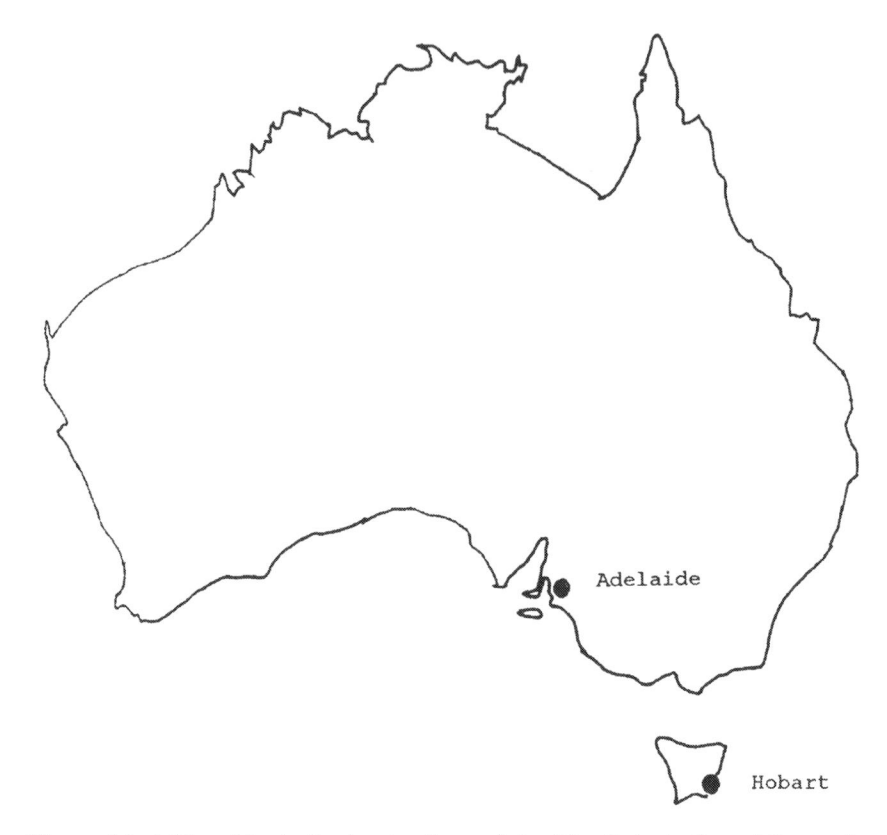

Figure 1.1. A Map of Australia showing the capitals of South Australia and Tasmania.

faith in the possibility of cure". This shift saw new modes of treatment being considered that were to dominate the early to mid-nineteenth century vision of the insane and insanity. These modes, in particular, addressed the mind of the afflicted person, and sought to re-educate them, allowing them to return to society. This was the basis of the new 'moral' therapy, which was characterized by an individual knowledge of the patient, and treatment based on kindness, humanity and reason. The insane person was to be returned to sanity by focusing on the will and the patient's powers of self-restraint (Pinel 1806: 221). This could only be achieved in a 'curative' environment as embodied in new buildings designed for the care of the insane. As the nineteenth century progressed those interested in the new treatments of non-restraint and moral therapy, which are discussed in more detail in Chapter Four, provided more and more detailed descriptions of

1. A Space of Their Own

what lunatic asylums *should be* if the insane were to be cured and returned to society. The building of lunatic asylums over the nineteenth century, in turn, allowed these authors to respond to the reality of managing the insane within these new asylums, and importantly to suggest modifications of the original ideas about lunatic asylum design in response to this reality. In this study these descriptions are turned into testable models which are tested against the reality of built lunatic asylums in England and in two English colonies, South Australia (Figure 1.2) and Tasmania (Figure 1.3).

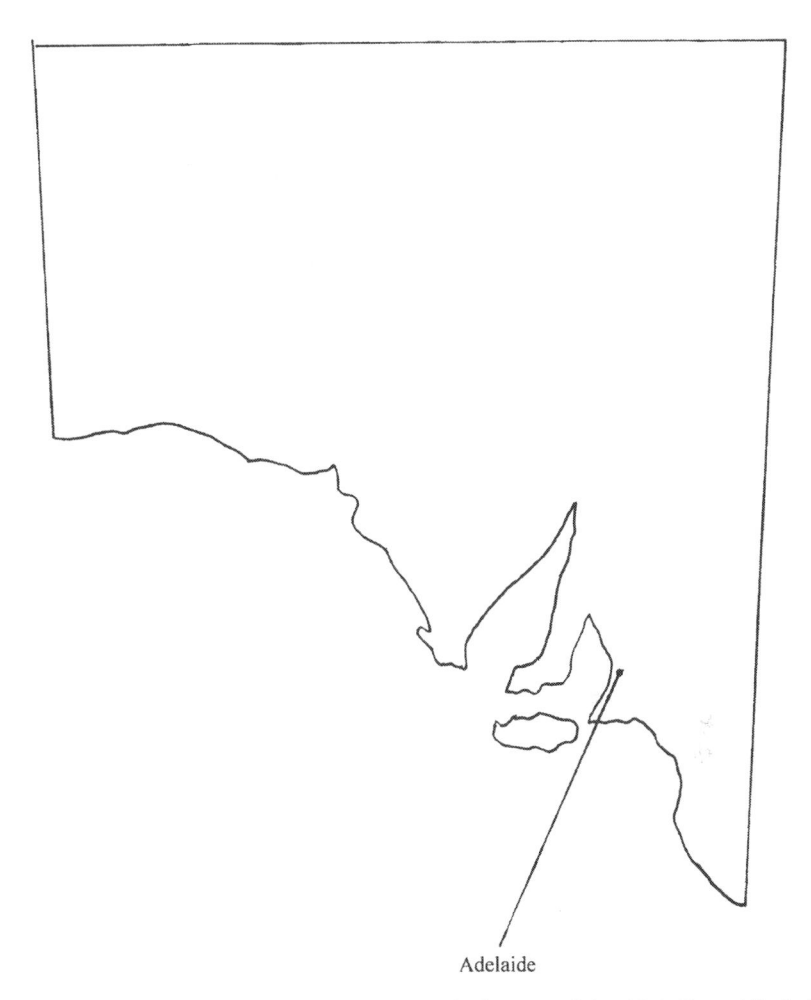

Figure 1.2. A Map of South Australia showing the location of the Adelaide and Parkside Asylums which are discussed in this book.

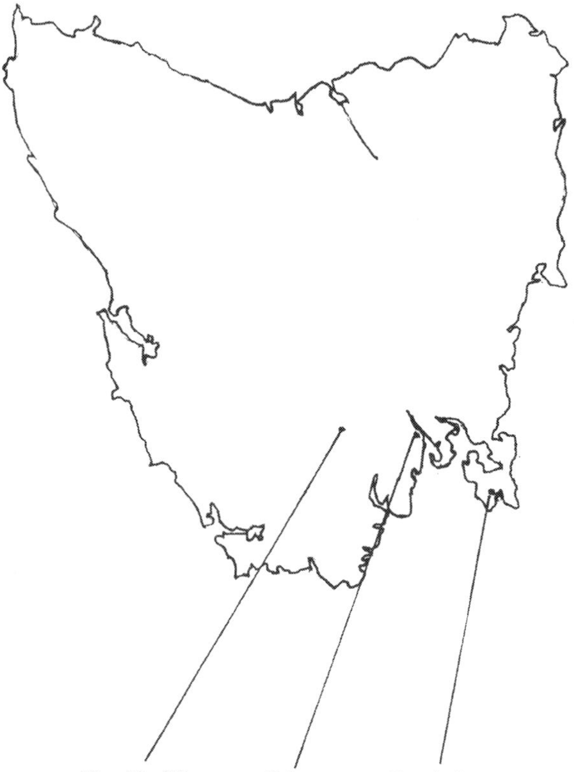

Figure 1.3. A Map of Tasmania showing the location of the New Norfolk for the Insane and Port Arthur Asylum which are discussed in this book.

This comparison was directed by several questions:

- How influential were the books and articles describing the new asylum designs on the actual provisions made for the care of the insane in nineteenth century England?
- To what extent was the nineteenth century concept of the 'ideal' lunatic asylum embodied in the lunatic asylums that remain visible on the landscape today as mental hospitals?
- Was the realization of the 'ideal' asylum model responsive to different social, cultural and economic circumstances?
- And finally, did those charged with the care of the insane in Australia during the same period use these books and articles

1. A Space of Their Own

from England as a guide when building their own asylums, or alternatively did they draw on or copy existing lunatic asylums plan for their designs?

Through the comparison of English and Australian asylums this book seeks to explore the role of the asylum environment in the care of the insane and to determine the factors influencing the type of asylum environment provided. It will be argued in this book, that while there was a range of reformist nineteenth century works describing the 'ideal' lunatic asylum; the actually constructed lunatic asylums exhibit a wide range of forms and configurations, which in turn were influenced by a knowledge of reforms in the treatment of the insane, the treatment regime applied in the institution, and various social and economic factors. In fact, the reality of the lunatic asylums was far more complex than their extant and visible remains on the landscape would suggest. Lunatic asylums represent the complex interaction between the world of ideas, the physical reality of the asylum environment, and the lived experience of that environment.

Historical archaeology is very much about the relationship between documents and material culture in all its forms. In fact, historical archaeologists are in the unique position of being able to both test hypotheses against historical documents and to test the veracity of historical documents against the reality of material culture. They are, in effect, able to contrast the rhetoric of the documents, which described what should be done, with the reality of what actually occurred. Through a consideration of the gap between the social duty of providing for the insane through the provision of lunatic asylums and the reality of lived experience within the walls of these asylums, it is possible to identify the forces at work within society that directly impacted on the care of the insane. Through material culture, in this case lunatic asylums, the rooms and spaces provided and the activities that took place within, it is possible to understand how the lives of the inmates were controlled and what limits were placed on the possibility of their being cured and subsequently returned to the outside world. Further it allows us to access ideas about insanity held by those responsible for the insane, many of whom were not part of the emerging medical profession specializing in the care of the insane. It will be argued that buildings (i.e. the physical spaces that were or were not provided) are a form of communication that can be understood as expressive of beliefs and ideas that are not necessarily expressed explicitly in documents. This book then crosses the boundaries of history and archaeology to bring to life a coherent picture of the lunatic asylum (its physical reality) and its role in the treatment of insanity.

BOOK OUTLINE

This book can be divided into a number of parts. The first part deals with the emerging ideas about insanity and the vision of the new lunatic asylum. The second part focuses on the British asylums. The third part considers the lunatic asylums provided in South Australia and Tasmania. While the fourth and final part provides the comparative study of the British and Australian asylums.

Chapter Two will look at themes within institutional archaeology while Chapter Three explores the archaeology of lunatic asylums and considers the approaches we can take in understanding these buildings.

In Chapter Four the rise of the lunatic asylum is discussed, illustrating the ideas of the new treatment regimes of moral management and non-restraint, which both focused on the lunatic asylum environment as a part of the curative and management process. This chapter also briefly considers the rise of the county lunatic asylum system in Britain. In Chapter Five the predominantly British nineteenth century books and articles that described what the lunatic asylum should be are considered and a number of models for an 'ideal' asylum are developed. In Chapter Six these models are tested chronologically against a collection of British lunatic asylum plans, with the purpose of seeing how far the 'ideal' models were realised in the county asylums actually built in Britain. This chapter further seeks to determine any patterns in the layouts of the buildings and the arrangement of rooms and spaces in the actually constructed asylums. This, then, forms a second data set against which the colonial lunatic asylums of Australia are considered in the following chapters. In Chapter Seven the South Australian lunatic asylums are considered in relation to both the 'ideal' asylum models and the built asylums in Britain. This is followed by a discussion of the effects of the built environment on life within the asylums. Chapter Eight follows the same format to consider the Tasmanian institutions. In Chapter Nine a discussion of the influence of books on what the asylum should be are considered. Using building histories, information about treatment regimes in each asylum and the results of the comparison of the built asylums against the various models as evidence, a range of factors are identified that affected the designs, room designations and uses. The factors that influenced the adoption and non-adoption of the 'ideal' asylum ideas in South Australian and Tasmania are then compared, including the effects of the presence or absence of convicts on the world of the asylum.

The Archaeology of Institutions | 2

The nineteenth century landscape in Europe, America and Australia was to become home to almshouses, workhouses, lunatic asylums, female factories, prisons, leper colonies, orphanages, Magadelen Asylums and industrial schools.[1] These places ranged from large scale institutions managed by local authorities or governmental bodies to the smaller private institution, and were expressive of the belief that environments designed to certain specifications would control an individual's behaviour, whether they were a criminal, a prostitute, victim of insanity or simply poor. These environments can be seen as 'moral' environments where the understood moral values would be impressed upon the inmate by the regime imposed, leading to their reformation and acceptance back into society in their appropriate place. These institutions fell in two broad groupings, those that were 'total' institutions, where inmates were physically separated from society to enable them to be reformed, and those that sought to reform through daily attendance (Spencer-Wood and Baugher 2001: 9). Total institutions were those that sought to completely control inmates' lives through the use of architecture and material culture (Spencer-Wood and Baugher 2001: 9). Within the walls of the institution the inmates' lives were physically controlled by the spaces provided for their use, and by: "highly routinized and tightly scheduled activities established to fulfil institutional aims" (De Cunzo 2006: 167). All types of institutions

---

[1] Some useful books that explore the role of these institutions include: Francis Finnegan (2001) *Do Penance or Perish. A study of Magdalen Asylums in Ireland*; A. Salt, A. (1984) *These Outcast Women. The Parramatta Female Factory 1821–1848*; M. A. Crowther (1981). *The Workhouse System 1834–1929* and Felix Driver (1993) *Power and Pauperism. The Workhouse System 1834–1884*. Norval Morris and David Rothman (1998) *The Oxford History of Prisons*.

sought to reinforce particular agendas as determined by groups within society, and to improve the recipient group to some perceived ideal, whether of behaviour, or moral standards. Increasingly the attention of archaeologists is being drawn to these institutions (for an overview see Du Cunzo 2006).

As institutional archaeology is an emerging field within historical archaeology, there is no established framework that can be used to shape questions or particular approaches to investigate these institutions. Many of the most recent studies have arisen from the research interests of feminist archaeologists (see Spencer-Wood 2001), and while this study is not a purely feminist one, it does follow on from such studies by going beyond the stereotyped views of the insane and lunatic asylums to understand the purpose of the built environment of the asylum and the reality of life within that environment. Importantly women's experiences of institutions were different from those of men, being based on gendered beliefs about the work and activities suitable for men and women (Piddock 1999). The studies undertaken of institutions further draw on a range of theories to explore the functioning of these places, including those of domination and resistance, paternalism, and anthropological concepts of ritual.

The unvoiced nature of those living within the walls of these various institutions has become more important because of what can be considered the dominant voice of those controlling the institutions (Spencer-Wood 2001: 103). These individuals, most frequently men, produced a range of documentation that provides an understanding of the operation of the particular institution, life within it as seen by the officers, visitors and governing bodies, and often views of the inmates written by those dominant voices and informed by the guiding philosophy of the institution. Frequently, there is no record of the institution and life within it written by those most actively involved in its daily life: the various inmates. Historical archaeology with its capacity to draw upon a wide range of analytical techniques and theoretical viewpoints can provide access to life within the walls, which may or may not provide us with a voice for these inmates. As this study will demonstrate excavation is not always necessary for us to hear these voices. By understanding the purposes and uses of buildings and the spaces they enclose it is possible to gain a better understanding of what life was like for those living within these institutions. As Lu Ann De Cunzo (2001a: 23) argues, it is possible to use all available forms of evidence to understand the role the material world played in supporting the institution's purpose and its role in negotiating the relationships of all those using the institution.

Institutions allow us to ask new questions that can challenge established theories: how institutions functioned and how the inmates experienced the internal world of the institution and responded to it. These new questions form some of the themes in institutional archaeology: testing history, paternalism, dominance and resistance, the function of symbolism in reform, and spatial patterning.

TESTING HISTORY

In her article "Visible Charity: The Archaeology, Material Culture, and Landscape Design of New York City's Municipal Almshouse Complex, 1736–1797", Sherene Baugher takes one possible approach to institutional archaeology, that of testing historical arguments or conclusions. Two contradictory arguments have been put forward by historians as to the nature of life within almshouses in the eighteenth century: firstly, that social structures of the almshouses were based on the family, with the inmates being treated as family members, or secondly, that the social structure was institutionalized and non-familial (Baugher 2001: 176). Baugher was given the opportunity to test these arguments by looking at the material world of the eighteenth century New York Almshouse, which lies beneath City Hall, the City Hall Park and Tweed Courthouse.

Plans indicated the Almshouse followed the European model for such places, which were usually arranged in a rectilinear pattern around a open area with the outbuildings forming the sides of the square and the almshouse one end (Baugher 2001: 181). The excavation of a section of the Almshouse Complex revealed part of the foundations of an outbuilding allowing the investigators to establish the orientation of the almshouse. Recovered material included architectural artifacts (building remains and associated material), food preparation and service vessels, bottles, kitchen utensils, clay smoking pipes, toys, coins and buttons (Baugher 2001: 179). An analysis of the ceramics revealed a diverse range of fashionable pieces associated more with middle and upper class households rather than the expected plainer ceramics of an almshouse. A little over half the ceramics fell into this class and included teaset pieces. However, these pieces did not form matched sets. In seeking an answer Baugher faces one of the biggest problems in institutional archaeology: determining who was using particular items in the artifact assemblage - the officers, general staff, or the inmates?

The possibilities offered by Baugher to explain this lack of sets include: that the ceramics belonged to the residents who retained them on entering the almshouse and used them while there; that they may have been donated by more affluent members of society; that they belonged to or were used by the Superintendent and his family; or were purchased as needed by the almshouse governing board (Baugher 2001: 186–7). Other artifacts recovered included part of a decorative glass decanter, brass buckles and a pewter spoon, again higher status items whose owners it was not possible to accurately identify.

The faunal assemblage at this site was dominated by fish and chicken remains, with some pig, cattle, and sheep/goat remains. The faunal evidence combined with documentary evidence reveals a modest diet. The almshouse milk herd and vegetable gardens combined with the fish, fowl and meat, however, seemed to provide a diverse diet (Baugher 2001: 188). A range of buttons, button blanks, and straight pins suggests the making of clothes, along with the documented evidence of spinning and oakum picking. The evidence of marbles, classified as toys, and the clay pipes suggests time for leisure activities (Baugher 2001: 189–191).

Baugher concludes from the documentary and archaeological evidence that those who built the almshouse had relatively benevolent intentions and did not support the oppressive view of the almshouse as an institution. This would support the argument for a more benevolent social structure where the inmates were treated as family members. Importantly, this was an institution for the "deserving poor" not the undeserving who had brought their misfortune on themselves and who were accommodated in the "Bridewell", or workhouse, where a more punitive or regimented life might be expected (Baugher 2001: 196, 197). The almshouse was designed to look like a home and its landscaped pastoral setting would have been familiar to the inmates. However the almshouse was on the main route into New York and faced onto the city's port and industrial areas, reinforcing the work ethic for the inmates (Baugher 2001: 193).

The possibility of the retention of personal possessions such as ceramic wares, Baugher believes, indicates that inmates were allowed to maintain their individuality, something that was not possible in the many institutions of the nineteenth century. This is further reflected in the absence of uniforms for inmates (Baugher 2001: 198–99). Baugher's study, more than anything, reflects a necessity for the study of individual institutions, rather than treating them as a monolithic body. Lois Feister in her discussion of the toys found in the archaeological deposits of the Daughters of Charity Schuyler Mansion Orphanage, Albany, New York, similarly concludes that popular perceptions of orphanages as operating in similar ways can be challenged by looking at the material culture (Feister 1991: 35).

PATERNALISM, DOMINATION AND RESISTANCE

Institutions are often perceived as being paternal or paternalistic and are sometimes seen as extensions of the family structure, with the father figure replaced by a male Superintendent. The inmates of the institution

Paternalism, Domination and Resistance 11

are cared for and all their physical and mental needs are provided for, however the price they pay is freedom of action and behavior. This loss of freedom is considered acceptable and justified by society if it is seen as being in the best interests of the individual concerned (Prangnell 1999: 3). The paternalistic model can be applied to various institutions such as orphanages, benevolent asylums, and lunatic asylums. The person or group/committee placed in control effectively controls the actions of the inmates and the material world of the institution. As in a family inappropriate behavior can be punished. In a paternalistic relationship the 'father' figure dictates all the behaviors and significant life decisions of his 'children' within a moral framework which gives him: "an unassailable understanding of the needs and best interests of his children" (Jackman 1994: 10). Paternalism may be seen as benevolent in the context of institutions, particularly medical ones such as lazarets provided for lepers and lunatic asylums where the illness of the individual, in the eyes of society, reduces their capacity to care for themselves or to act in their own best interests. Paternalism, however, is still about control. Inmates of paternalistic institutions may be effectively left with no control over their lives and even the material world around them, as Jon Prangnell's study (1999) of the Peel Island Lazaret illustrates.

Prangnell's study considers the physical isolation of those suffering from Hanson's Disease (leprosy) in the Lazaret on Peel Island off the Queensland coast of Australia. Opened in 1907, it was to operate for 52 years and housed white and colored men and women. Capable of housing up to 90 patients, the Lazaret was composed of a white male, white female and colored persons compounds' as well as various officer's quarters (Prangnell 1999: 3). The Lazaret sought to physically separate people believed to have become 'unclean' through suffering a disease that causes physical changes to the body (Prangnell 1999: 20). While on Peel Island the inmates were housed in wooden buildings, the design of which reflected whether one was white or colored (the latter had poorer housing), and were clothed, fed, and given a supply of alcohol, tobacco, art materials, garden implements, medicines, and wireless radios and batteries. The material world of the Lazaret was limited to those items supplied by those governing it, and this in turn affected the range of activities and employments available to those housed on the island (Prangnell 1999: 6). The behavior of the inmates, staff and visitors was further controlled by detailed regulations (Prangnell 1999: Chapter 3).

The paternalistic nature of the Lazaret that sought to control and determine what was best for the inmates was reinforced by the physical layout of the compounds. The Lazaret was designed as a panopticon with the surgery and superintendent's house centrally located with patient compounds on three sides (Prangnell 1999: 346). This design supported observation and surveillance of the inmates. Rules determined who could access particular areas. Patients were not allowed to have locks on their doors, although one female patient did obtain a barrel lock, giving her both control over her internal space and privacy. However this was one of only a few acts of resistance, the artifact assemblage from the excavations reflecting a life with few material items beyond those supplied by the Government, all of which were plain and limited in number. There appears to have been little internal or external trade to enrich the inmates' lives, and they were effectively isolated from the world (Prangnell 1999: 117, 130, 340 & 382).

While theory may predict resistance to authoritative control this is not always easily detected in the archaeological record. While paternalism may be seen as beneficial, it can come close to dominance in institutions where life within is intended to reform the character or modify the behavior of the inmates. Thus, institutions such as the workhouse, prison, and female factories, sought through their regimes to mould the inmates into fit citizens as determined by society. This was often to be achieved through work or the imposition of ideology through sermons, lectures and classes which the inmates were forced to attend. Release from an institution may only come when the inmate was seen to have reformed or modified their behavior sufficiently (Piddock 1996).

Eleanor Casella's study "To Watch or Restrain: Female Convict Prisons in 19th-Century Tasmania" (2001; see also 1996 for excavation details) uses documents, architectural plans and excavated evidence to build a picture of the world of the factory, and women's resistance to the imposed regimes and the built spaces they inhabited. Female factories were built in New South Wales and Tasmania as a means of controlling women convicts and as places where recalcitrant or criminal behavior could be punished (Salt 1984: 44). In the factory a woman's character would be improved through "morally acceptable and economically productive labor" (Casella 2001: 48). Reflecting the punitive aspects of its role, the female factory buildings were designed to control the behavior of the inmates. The Launceston Female Factory, constructed in 1832, was designed as a radial building with four arms. Three arms housed the dormitories with the central space housing the chapel and guardhouse. This design, as Casella indicates, supported direct observation and indirect supervision by channeling noises towards the central guard post (Casella 2001: 51).

The Ross Female Factory constructed in 1847 offered a different design. Rectilinear in shape, most emphasis was placed on separation of the classes (criminal and hiring), the prevention of interaction between classes, and the restriction of access between the internal world of the Factory and the outside world. This was supported by the placement of the staff quarters near the entrance of the Factory grounds and the use of internal fences and yards (Casella 2001: 54–55). Casella believes the placement of the staff quarters also sought to affect the importation into the Factory of material goods not sanctioned by the governing officers (Casella 2001: 56). However Casella found on excavating the solitary cells that women were using material culture as a means of resisting the imposed disciplinary regime of the Factory.

The solitary cells, as revealed by excavation, were approximately 1.3 meters by 2 meters (6ft by 4ft). The stratigraphy and lack of architectural evidence for a doorway indicated an apparent difference between the floor level and the entrance level of over half a meter. The women descended into the cells, which Casella believes was a metaphor for their descent into a place of punishment and atonement before ascending to rejoin the community. Women could spend up to three weeks in these cold, dank, small spaces with stone walls and compacted earth floors (Casella 2001: 58–9). While these cells were intended to physically isolate the women, the excavation revealed that women may have maintained contact with the world beyond the cells by protecting their caches of "currency". The excavated material found in the solitary cells and the crime [sic] class dormitory included olive-glass bottle fragments, kaolin clay tobacco pipes, British currency, decorative buttons and beads (Casella 2001: 56). Casella notes that tokens and currency were used by the women to illegally obtain tea, meat, sugar and tobacco from sympathetic guards. Women appear to have been either placed in the cells without being searched, or had access to one another through the guards, as a small pit dug in the dirt floor of one cell contained "a square ferrous container, faunal bone deposits, one kaolin clay pipe stem fragment, and an olive glass bottle base" (Casella 2001: 61, 64).

Casella interprets this material culture as the means by which the women manipulated their cultural landscape, improved their physical condition by importing luxuries such as tobacco, alcohol and food, and "rebel[ed] against their "separate treatment" (Casella 2001: 60, 64). This resistance also appears to have taken the form of setting fire to the solitary cells as evidenced by archaeological remains. Casella has subsequently identified through documents the use of arson and vandalism by women as an indication of insubordination and as unifying acts (Casella 2001: 62–63). Similar responses of resistance were identified at the Rhode Island state penitentiary (De Cunzo 2006: 172).

Casella's descriptions of the varying designs of the female factories in Tasmania and the use of the building placement or layout to control the behaviour of the inmates reflects a recurring theme within institutional care: that of the search for the 'ideal' design for a particular institution whose buildings would serve the purposes of the institution at that period of time, whether surveillance, moral reformation through labour, or physical isolation which reinforced self contemplation. At the base of this was the belief in the power of the built environment to modify and shape behaviour. This power was enhanced through prescribed work or activities and verbal communications by those given authority within the institution.

REFORM AND SYMBOLISM

So far, the studies discussed have been based largely on archaeological evidence detectable through excavation. As indicated above, however, institutions are not always amenable to excavation or else the evidence recovered from them is not extensive. This, however, does not preclude the possibility of constructing what Lu Ann De Cunzo has called the "material world" of an institution through artefacts, photographs, historical documents, plans and comparative studies that describe the material world of the period (De Cunzo 2001a: 23).

In her study, 'Reform, Respite, Ritual: An Archaeology of Institutions; The Magdalen Society of Philadelphia, 1800–1850' (1995), De Cunzo uses a limited range of excavated material as the basis for a holistic study of the asylum. Drawing upon feminist theory, anthropological studies of ritual, archaeological data, historical documents, contemporary nineteenth century literature and twentieth century academic studies, De Cunzo builds a picture that relates the Magdalen Asylum to the world outside and at the same time creates a picture of the world inside. She, in effect, recreates the material world of the asylum and explores how this material world was used to serve the purposes of the Magdalen Society.

The Magdalen Society had established the asylum with the purpose of providing an enclosed world to allow "unhappy females who have been seduced from the paths of virtue" to return to a "life of rectitude" (De Cunzo 1995: 17–18). De Cunzo found that the asylum building itself, the landscape around it, the furnishings, ceramics and glassware, and the uniforms provided for the Magdalens, all formed a complex set of signals/symbols that created a ritual world. It was intended that passage through this new world would separate the women from their original life and transform them into respectable women, suitable for marriage and trained in the domestic arts (De Cunzo 1995: 120; 2001a: 29, 32).

Buildings themselves are expressive of ideologies. They form a visual form of communication to the outside world, but more importantly they form a means of controlling the behavior of those living within them. As De Cunzo indicates, the doors, passages, and rooms themselves, their location within the buildings, and the asylum gardens, formed both modifiers of behavior and had symbolic roles imposed by those managing/controlling the building and its surroundings. It was anticipated that those using the buildings and gardens, the 'inmates', would understand the symbolism. The classic use of space and buildings to control the behavior of the inmates was the prison, where segregation in cells and small yards, discipline and labor sought to reform the criminal by punishing "inappropriate behavior" such as lateness, talking, and indecent behavior (Foucault 1979: 128, 178). In the Magdalen Asylum the front rooms of the building formed the link between the outside world and the interior world of the Magdalens. These rooms served as parlors where Society members would receive visitors, and along with the Magdalens participate in religious services and prayer meetings (De Cunzo 2001a: 27). Behind these rooms were the staff rooms and kitchen. In the early asylum the Magdalens lived in the three storeys above. Later additions allowed for the creation of a work room and further accommodation at the rear of the asylum where the newly arrived Magdalens were housed.

In residential houses "the private spaces of the home [were] removed from the city's corrupting influences, [and] protected working wives, mothers and servants" (De Cunzo 1995: 107). The same pattern was being followed at the asylum. This isolation from the world was reinforced initially by fences then by a 13ft wall that enclosed the garden and asylum as the formerly rural setting became part of a landscape of middle-class residences and institutions (De Cunzo 1995: 118; 2001a: 40). The asylum followed the Christian tradition of a cloistered life. Consequently, its architecture was expressive of enclosure, separation, and observation, while the garden provided a place for reflection and retreat (De Cunzo 1995: 106). De Cunzo further notes that this moral architecture had become linked firstly with discipline and subsequently with reform. She has further concluded that the arrangement of the passages and doors supported the physical isolation of the newly admitted women from their old life and formed part of the ritual life of the asylum (De Cunzo 1995: 118–119; 2001a: 26). Above all the Magdalen Asylum was not an institution in the manner of a workhouse or prison. Rather it espoused reform in the setting of a domestic house:

> The spatial organization, architectural embellishment, and furnishing of the ideal home structured and controlled social interaction and moral retreat through carefully segregating activities and establishing strict codes of behavior (De Cunzo 2001a: 27).

This, in many ways, was the home setting in which the Magdalens would be employed. As with other institutions an element of paternalism, or a system of well-meaning supervision and/or regulation, presumably played a part, with the matron fulfilling a motherly role guiding the young women along the right path.

The ritualized and symbolic use of space and seclusion from the outside world, which De Cunzo identified, is very similar to that used within the lunatic asylum. Ritualized movement through space was to form the basis of the new curative environment of the lunatic asylum, where the location of wards within the buildings, their furnishings, and the classifications they indicated, became rewards or punishments for appropriate or inappropriate behavior, as the patient sought to control their thinking and return to sanity (Hill 1838: 38–39).

INSTITUTIONS AND SPACE

A further theme within institutional archaeology is that of spatial studies. In his chapter "The Archaeology of the Workhouse: the changing uses of the workhouse buildings at St. Mary's, Southampton" (1999), Gavin Lucas considers the changing uses of rooms and their relationships to each other in St. Mary's workhouse school which was located in a former townhouse. Beginning with a consideration of the townhouse room arrangements, Lucas goes on to consider the re-arrangement of these spaces for the purposes of the school, particularly in relation to staff and pupil accommodation. He then considers the placement of the various classes of inmates within the workhouse proper, which was located a short distance away. Lucas found that the private/public axis within the townhouse had been lost in the school, but the separation of work and non-work activities remained, although separated onto different floors (Lucas 1999: 129–130). However this segregation was partially negated by the placement of the teachers' sitting rooms on the same floor as the children's bedrooms, meaning that they were not entirely separated from their work - the children (Lucas 1999: 130). Within the workhouse the classification of space was based on the ability of the individual to work or be productive, with those incapable of work being placed further back in the workhouse and those able-bodied being placed near the entrance (Lucas 1999: 134). Unfortunately Lucas does not go on to offer any further conclusions about the different uses of space within the townhouse, workhouse school, and workhouse, rather it seems to be only a set of observations.

In seeking the organizing principles that determined the layout of the Destitute Asylum of South Australia, I sought to define the features of a workhouse as found in England and to understand the principles that determined the layout of the building complexes. I found that the organizing principles of the workhouse and the rooms provided were distinct enough that it could be used as a template against which other complexes of buildings could be tested to identify their possible function as workhouses (Piddock 1996). A crucial aspect which the study highlighted was that room and space use were extremely complex and flexible and a reliance on plans to identify buildings has inherent problems (Piddock 2001: 93).

Institutions in the early to mid-nineteenth centuries were fundamentally about the use of the physical environment to reform the inmate, who was either a willing or unwilling participant. Buildings were not simply buildings. The placement of the individual parts served to allow supervision, controlled movement and limited contact between the various classes within the institution. These classes could be based on gender, age, medical condition or some arbitrary classification based on the guiding philosophy. The buildings provided work areas which both supported the economic viability of the institution and served the purpose of training the inmates in skills; as well as providing punishment spaces. The landscape also had a role providing gardens or views which were invested with symbolic meaning (Browne 1837: 182–3; Baugher 2001: 194–5; De Cunzo 1995: 80). This use of the built environment and landscape played a role in all of the institutions mentioned above. As will be seen in this study the lunatic asylum built environment was invested with just as much meaning and was essential to the perceived purpose of the asylum: the cure of the insane.

A further theme within these studies is the use of excavated remains as a launch pad for questions that seek to provide a holistic picture of the role played by the buildings, landscape and material culture at the site in question (Casella 2001: 65; Baugher 2001: 191). The material culture cannot be seen in isolation from its ideological context. But it is not just institutional space that is communicative of ideologies, for the layout of buildings, their furnishings and the activities which were carried out within them (such as providing morning or afternoon tea) can convey messages about social status, self-image and gender roles and ideals (De Cunzo 1995: 121–122; Leone 1984; Burke 1999). As will be discussed buildings are highly communicative and the symbolic meanings they convey are likely to have been understood by the viewer and participants using the building. Institutional archaeology requires the integration of documentary sources and material cultural analysis if we are to understand the symbolic roles played by material culture in all its forms.

As is demonstrated in the following chapters, the lunatic asylum buildings and spaces were intimately connected with the intended purpose of the asylum as a curative institution. The building designs supported the paternalistic relationships between the insane and the medical superintendent, who was the central pivot in the curative regime, while the treatment regime contained elements of ritual, and the rooms, spaces and activities played a role in the process that would bring the inmates back to sanity. This study thus draws on the four principal themes in institutional analysis: testing history, paternalism, the symbolic and ritual use of space, and the organization of spaces within institutions that make them fundamentally different from households. The fundamental difference between previous institutional studies above and this one, is that the material culture is the standing structures of the asylums themselves rather than excavated material and in this it most closely parallels Lu Ann De Cunzo's (1995) work.

The modern use of the nineteenth century lunatic asylum buildings and the preference for solid, not wooden floors, would potentially limit the possibilities of identifying artifacts associated within the lives of inmates through excavations. In addition the absence of a reasonable body of documents written by former asylum patients effectively means these possible sources of information about the lives of inmates are not accessible. This, however, does not preclude us from understanding the lives and experiences of the inmates.

To the observer, lunatic asylums offered a visual confirmation of society's responsibility for the mentally ill and an acceptance of a duty to provide for them. As Anderson and Moore argue in their study of the Ashton Villa, the built environment is a form of "explicit, conscious expression of communication in the "visual mode," (Anderson and Moore 1988: 402; see also Burke 1999). In this context the external view of the asylum, which was the public face of society's acceptance of its social responsibility to care for the unfortunate insane, was expressed in the use of formal or grand architecture, and the choice of building materials. The interior of the asylum, the reality of the rooms and spaces provided and the overall size of the institution can provide a different picture of attitudes towards the insane and what was thought necessary in an asylum environment. The subtle difference between what we say we are doing by providing a new lunatic asylum with its impressive architecture and physical presence on the landscape, and what life was really like within the asylum walls is accessible through an analysis of the rooms and spaces provided and omitted, and by an analysis of documents that indicate changing room and space use over time as will be explored in the next chapter.

The archaeology of institutions then allows us to test the gap between rhetoric and the reality of the built environment and life within it for the inmate whatever the type of institution.

3
The Archaeology of Lunatic Asylums

RESEARCH DESIGN

This project initially grew out of a series of questions sparked by a consideration of the plans for the Adelaide Lunatic Asylum in South Australia which I found while doing research on the Destitute Asylum of Adelaide. My research on the Destitute Asylum revealed that the rooms and spaces provided within the asylum compound were determined by a range of factors; the most important being the role of the institution and the nature of the people to be housed there. The Adelaide Destitute Asylum had been based on the English workhouse in its allocation of spaces and rooms, and followed similar principles of work and the separation of family members along gender lines (Piddock 1996 and 2001). Using this work, and the lunatic asylum plans as a basis, a set of initial questions were developed:

1) Was there a common design for lunatic asylums?
2) How did ideas about the environment provided by the asylum change over time?
3) What factors affected which rooms and spaces were provided and how they were used?
4) What sources of information were available to those charged with designing and constructing a lunatic asylum?

A review of modern studies and nineteenth century literature on insanity and lunatic asylums revealed that the asylum was a central part of the new treatment regimes of moral therapy and non-restraint that appeared in the late eighteenth and early nineteenth centuries. Books and articles were to appear throughout the nineteenth century that described all facets of lunatic asylum design and management often accompanied by chapters on the treatment of the insane (these will be discussed in more detail in chapters four and five). Importantly as the nineteenth century progresses these works changed from providing general guidelines to specifically detailed descriptions of the built environment, including building materials, window and room size, the height of windows, heating and ventilation systems, type of rooms to be provided and furnishings. Every detail of the asylum building and grounds were mentioned as the authors described what a lunatic asylum *should be* and how these features *supported the cure and management* of the insane. These books then described the material culture of the lunatic asylum. When combined with the study of actually built lunatic asylums the possibility exists to answer archaeologically based questions.

Prior to the nineteenth century the insane had been cared for in a series of madhouses and a handful of asylums and charity hospitals, such as Bethlem Hospital in London, the famous Bedlam as portrayed by many such as William Hogarth in his engravings of *The Rake's Progress* in 1735. Early treatments were characterised by a belief that the insane had lost the ability to reason, and were subsequently reduced to the level of animals (Porter 1987: 40–41; Scull 1981: 108). As animals, they had been increasingly viewed as insensate. Consequently treatment was often based purely on restraint, and sometimes on medical treatments such as vomitives and purges to balance the humours.[1] Living conditions were basic, reflecting the supposed nature of the lunatic who did not feel the cold or appreciate their surroundings. The new modes of treatment of the late eighteenth and early- to mid-nineteenth centuries returned rationality to the insane. In the face of revelations before a series of English Parliamentary Select Committees in 1807, 1815, and 1827 which revealed the environments in which the insane were being kept -often in cells with no provision for heating, ventilation or sanitation, or furnishings – the focusing drive was given, leading to the provision of new lunatic asylums under a new centralised system based around county asylums (see Chapter Four). These asylums would embody the new ideas and treatments practices being advocated by reformers. So, the parallel forces of those advocating the new treatments of the insane and those seeking to provide appropriate living conditions came together. But what was the new asylum environment to be like? How did it support the new treatment regimes? It was in response to this need that the lunacy reformers sought to describe what the lunatic asylum should be.

Reading these works by lunacy reformers led to a second higher level of questions being developed; these were designed to use the techniques of archaeology to find the answers:

---

[1] For a discussion of early treatment of the insane see Roy Porter's *Mind Forg'd Manacles*.

Research Design

1) Was it possible to identify an 'ideal' lunatic asylum model, that encompassed the ideas about the building arrangements, rooms and spaces as described by these writers, and which was testable archaeologically?
2) How far were these ideas about the 'ideal' asylum actually realised in built lunatic asylums in England?
3) What was life like in the asylums of the nineteenth century?
4) What effect did the presence or absence of the 'ideal' asylum features have on life within an asylum?

The various descriptions of the 'ideal' asylum were often written by English authors and focused on the lunatic asylums that were being provided under the British County Asylum system. As this study was undertaken from Australia a number of further questions were asked:

1) When called upon to provide for the insane in the new colonies of Australia, where did the colonists derive their ideas about the sort of buildings to be provided?
2) How widely did the ideas about the 'ideal' asylum, and all that it implied about the design of the lunatic asylum and the treatment of the insane, spread from England?
3) Did the different compositions of the Australian colonies affect the provisions made for the insane?

While most people are aware that Australia has a convict heritage, not many people outside of South Australia realise that the colony of South Australia was established as a free colony with a specific provision in its founding Act, that it would receive no convicts (Pike 1967). In light of the different origin of South Australia compared to the other Australian colonies, it was decided to consider both the provisions made for free people and for convicts. The most ready contrast was provided by Van Diemen's Land (to be renamed Tasmania in 1856), which received a large number of convicts for over twenty years. It is often assumed that the nature of convicts as prisoners led to harsher physical conditions being imposed on them through the buildings provided for their use.[2] In considering the provisions made for the insane in these two colonies it is possible to address the question of whether perceptions of the social class of the inmates being accommodated in the lunatic asylums affected the type of provisions made for them.

---

[2] For a discussion of the design of buildings provided for convicts in Australia see James Semple Kerr (1984) *Design for convicts: an account of design for convict establishments in the Australian colonies during the transportation era* Library of Australian History in association with The National Trust of Australia (NSW) and the Australian Society for Historical Archaeology, Sydney.

A THEORETICAL APPROACH TO THE ARCHAEOLOGY OF LUNATIC ASYLUMS

Today many nineteenth century lunatic asylums are still in use as mental hospitals (for example Parkside in South Australia), while others are serving different functions such as University campuses (for example the University of Sydney's Gladesville campus and the University of New South Wales's Rydalmere campus in Australia). Consequently, they are not readily open to analysis based on excavation and detailed surveys of the physical fabric. Historical archaeology, however, can provide alternative forms of analysis.

Excavation is not an essential part of archaeological practice. The questions that come to mind when considering the remains of buildings in the ground are little different from those arising from a consideration of plans or photographs. Only the context is different. As Beaudry notes (1996: 479) the cry "That's not archaeology" or "That's not archaeological enough" is often heard, particularly when the difference between historical archaeological research and historical research is not realised. The fundamental point of difference between the two lies in the questions being asked.

Lunatic asylums as buildings have not been the focus of research to any degree among historians writing about insanity and the insane. Markus in his book *Buildings and Power: freedom and control and the origin of model building types* (1993) suggests that well known writers on lunacy such as Andrew Scull and Michel Foucault, cannot see lunatic asylums as "formative objects; they are merely outcomes" (Markus 1993: 130). Thus the role of the lunatic asylum built environment is not considered as part of the overall changing and developing world of the treatment of lunacy. Scull, for example, in his chapter on the curative asylum in the book *Museums of Madness. The Social Organization of Insanity in Nineteenth-Century England* devotes fewer than three pages to the ideal asylum, of which one and a half pages are a lengthy extract from Browne's 1837 work *What Asylums Were, Are and Ought to be* (Scull 1979: 104–106). Scull's focus, in these pages, remains on the blinding failure of those advocating the lunatic asylum to see it as anything but a failed cause.

The negation of the importance of the asylum buildings themselves has been partly a response or reaction to what Skultans (1979: 1–2) has called a rose coloured view of lunacy treatment and management by those interested in the history of psychiatry. In general, this focus on the social role of the lunatic asylum or economic influences has led researchers to place little focus of the lunatic asylum itself, its buildings and the role played by its environment, despite the emphasis placed on

A Theoretical Approach to the Archaeology of Lunatic Asylums 23

it by reformist writers in the nineteenth century.[3] In many publications, the illustrations, photographs, and plans of lunatic asylums form adjuncts to the text without them being discussed within the content of the book or article (Digby 1985, Andrews et. al. 1997, Hunter and MacAlpine 1973).[4]

As Robert Schuyler (1988: 38) has noted: "Historians focus on humans, either, as with narrative and chronicle history, as individuals,

---

[3] Within the growing body of English lunacy studies it is possible to identify several threads or themes including:

- a consideration of the economic basis for the rise of the lunatic asylum system and the move towards the institutionalisation of perceived problem groups within English society (Scull 1976, 1979, 1993);
- considerations of the nature of who was being confined within the county asylums (Mackenzie 1988, Saunders 1988, Showalter 1981, Walton 1981 and 1985, Ripa 1990);
- the relationship between the administrators and administration of the county lunatic asylums and the Poor Law authorities and the workhouses (Bartlett 1999, Forsythe et al. 1999);
- developments in treatment regimes (Skultans 1975, Scull 1981, Bynum 1981, Porter 1981–2, Cooter 1981, Marland 1999);
- the creation of a new body of medical doctors who specialised in the treatment of insanity (Russell 1988, Scull 1981, Scull et. al. 1996);
- Gender and class in relation to asylum admissions and stays.

[4] A few other disciplines have considered the role of lunatic asylum buildings. The historical geographer Chris Philo, in his article "Enough to drive one mad": the organisation of space in 19th century lunatic asylums" (1989), discusses asylum design. Philo discusses the application of the panopticon design, first proposed by Jeremy Bentham, in relation to lunatic asylums and its ultimate rejection, and follows this by briefly touching on a range of alternative arrangements for ward and day space to support surveillance of patients.

From the view point of architectural studies a few books discuss the lunatic asylum. Markus (1993) provides a disjointed account of the physical space of the lunatic asylum. He suggests that the use of cells for sleeping accommodation was derived from prison design, while the use of wards in hospitals was transformed into the gallery opposite these sleeping cells (Markus 1993: 130–1). The focus is on changes in treatment, but these are not strongly linked to changes in the physical environment. Although some asylums are described briefly there is no indication of why these particular asylums are chosen for discussion (Markus 1993: 131–2, 134–5, 135–6). Rosenau in her *Social Purpose in Architecture* (1970) briefly touches on lunatic asylums as well, but, despite the inclusion of a number of plans, they are not discussed beyond some reference to open wards and shape (Rosenau 1970: 69, 75). Jeremy Taylor (1991) integrates the discussion of hospital, workhouse infirmaries and lunatic asylums in his *Hospital and Asylum Architecture in England 1840–1914*. His work covers the development of architectural practice in the period including the development of the competition system and the move towards design guides, journals, reports, general design elements, siting of the asylum, and funding. Taylor, while providing a good background does not provide any analysis of the designs of lunatic asylums, nor does he discuss the sources of these designs.

or, as with social history, as groups," rather than on the roles played by the buildings they used. Historical archaeologists, however, focus on the material remains left by people, including buildings, and from this proceed to interpret how this relates to human lives, society and social history.

As Beaudry has argued, historical archaeologists are further distinguished from historians by their approach to documents. She believes historical archaeologists use an ethnographic approach to documents that seeks to address cultural questions alongside historical ones. Certainly she is right when she notes that documents as texts are read by us as much for what they say inadvertently as for what they say openly (Beaudry 1996: 482). As will be demonstrated in this study what is omitted in the documents relating to lunatic asylums is of particular interest, as it reflects both the adoption of ideas about the care and cure of the insane, and local influencing factors that affected the provisions for the insane.

In fact, buildings form an untapped source of information that can be accessed by firstly looking at plans and illustrations, and by asking questions of these and any still standing structures or ruins, before looking to histories and themes in nineteenth century writings on lunacy. This follows on from the approach recommended by Charles Cleland in his review article of the state of the discipline "Historical Archaeology Adrift?" Cleland (2001: 2) argues that historical archaeology has become focussed too much on events (that created the archaeological deposits) and not on wider cultural questions. Cleland argues that historical archaeology should be addressing social process. Studies that have addressed class structure, consumerism, urban organisation, and plantation systems are examples of research agendas that go beyond the event to social process (Cleland 2001: 5). Cleland argues that each piece of research in historical archaeology should address larger problems and look to expand our knowledge of cultural practice, rather than simply be descriptions of the artefacts found at the site and what events they indicate went on there (Cleland 2001: 5).

To return to these wider cultural questions he argues for a three part structure to the research questions we ask when considering a site or part of the archaeological record. Each set of questions builds on the previous level with increasing complexity of theorisation. The lower level, he advocates, is based on questions about site formation processes or explanations of how events led to specific archaeological configurations, and can be derived from documents or formed of general descriptive hypotheses. The middle level uses middle range theory to ask questions derived from the artefacts and looks at dynamic processes. The upper level asks

A Theoretical Approach to the Archaeology of Lunatic Asylums 25

questions: "concerning the regularities of more complex and inclusive culture (sic) behaviour which are situated in more expansive realms of time." (Cleland 2001: 7). These questions can be asked or posed from documents and tested with artefacts. Thus the questions begin at the event level and build the archaeological data sets, progress to the second level which looks at the behaviour that created these data sets, and ultimately ascends to the third level which uses site studies to consider the larger questions, such as changing patterns of consumer behaviour, class relationships, and so forth over longer periods of time than represented by a single site. Further Cleland (2001: 6) argues that documents and artefacts should not be used simply as subjective confirmation of each other but as a means to objectively test propositions formulated from each opposing set.

In this study the research questions at the site formation level were focussed on the buildings themselves: What was a lunatic asylum? What rooms and spaces did it have? When were they built and where? These questions were answerable from examining the buildings themselves, from photographs, plans and relevant nineteenth century documents. The second level of research is based on the 'why' questions: Why was this particular design chosen for a lunatic asylum? How did ideas about the asylum environment change over time? These can be directly asked of the lunatic asylums through a comparative process by looking at how the asylum space and rooms were used over time, and by comparing what authors said the asylum should be like with the reality of the built asylum. This research uses the documents about lunatic asylums and the asylums themselves (the artefacts) as opposing sets to generate new questions. These questions form Cleland's third level and ask: what forces at work within society led to the lunatic asylums being built the way they were? What role did economic change play in the provisions made as indicated by the material culture of the asylum? Did attitudes towards the insane directly affect the built provisions made for them? and, as this study concerns Britain and Australia, what can the lunatic asylums tell us about the spread of ideas from Britain in the northern hemisphere to its colonies in the southern hemisphere? As Cleland indicates, the third level of questions can be theorised from documents and tested against the reality of the artefacts; in this case the lunatic asylums, where choices are recorded in the form of the buildings at the time of their construction and as they were added to or modified over time.

The fundamental point of this book is that lunatic asylums are artefacts. They are not simply buildings in a particular architectural style. The rooms, spaces, layouts and designs all have a meaning beyond their physical fabric. They represent a complex set of ideas about the treatment of the insane. Lunatic asylums were subject to a range of social forces beginning with the buildings themselves. As James Deetz has argued "Every aspect of the environment that people have purposely shaped according to cultural plans comprises material culture" (Deetz paraphrased by De Cunzo 2001b: 16).

Cleland (2001: 5), while arguing for a focus on cultural practice, seems to offer a limited view of historical archaeology in his assertion that many practitioners present studies which do not involve excavation or even artefacts and consequently, are not about historical archaeology. Articles in response to Cleland's comments by Lu Ann Cunzo, Douglas Armstrong, Gregory Waselkov and Roberta Greenwood (all 2001), pick up various strands of his arguments and, while all support the idea of focusing on culture, they all argue for a wider interpretation of what is historical archaeology.

Armstrong (2001: 11) argues for an historical archaeology with a strengthened set of analytical techniques that looks for both Cleland's regularities of behaviour and considers the irregular or variations as a way of understanding culture. For Armstrong, and for many of us in historical archaeology, its power lies in our ability to use documents and a detailed analysis of material culture to understand the past. The "daily lives and cultural patterns of the invisible men and women of the past" are the key to what archaeology is about (Orser quoted by Armstrong 2001: 10).

In this and in tackling topics on the periphery such as "ethnicity, class, status, social structures, gender dynamics and age" (Armstrong 2001: 11), we can make a significant contribution to 'grey' areas (see for example Scott 1991, the articles in Scott 1994; Spencer-Wood 1994). It is generally recognised that documents are not an unbiased record of the past, rather "they represented subjective, intentional, self conscious, ideal or at least prescriptive statements" (De Cunzo 2001b: 16). People write for a wide range of reasons; whether the documents are public or private they all serve a particular purpose and reflect a wide range of ideas, beliefs and intentions. These may be intentional or subjective, may arise from the beliefs and experiences of the writer, or reflect the intended function of the document whether letter, diary, official report etc. Rhys Isaac, for example, has successfully shown that the diary entries of Colonel Landon Carter, and their internal imagery, reflected the intellectual and natural philosophies of the eighteenth century (Isaac 1992: 403–406).

As this study demonstrates, while many documents exist there are few descriptions of life within the lunatic asylums of the nineteenth century by those directly experiencing it - the inmates and the lower orders of staff.[5] These descriptions are in documents intended to highlight the problems of the asylum life in an effort to bring about change, such as in Minutes of Evidence of the Parliamentary Select Committees and Commissions in Britain and Australia, or in newspapers and pamphlets. To draw questions only from these documents would provide a skewed approach. Rather than use the documents in opposition to the material culture as suggested by Cleland, they both need to be treated as separate but equal data sets which can be used like the pieces of a jigsaw puzzle to build a picture of what life was like in the asylum. In this case the focus is on the living spaces and the organisation of the parts of the buildings and grounds and how they were used. Through understanding these it is possible to gain a better understanding of what life was like in the asylum.

The relationship between documents and material culture is never an easy one. The existence of documents relating to a site may limit the questions asked, especially if they are the only source of questions asked of the material remains we discover, an approach which has been defined as the handmaiden approach relegating archaeology to a sub-discipline of history (Hardesty 2001: 23). Other approaches to the relationship between documents and the archaeological record are possible. As Leone and Potter indicate, two commonly used methods linking the documentary record and archaeological finds - excavating and using the documents to identify the finds, and beginning with a history based on documents then excavating to fill in the gaps - places any discrepancies between the documents and the material culture to one side and labels them as exceptions (Leone and Potter 1988: 12, 14). Equally the person using the material culture was not necessarily the person who wrote the documents; and to link the two would create a link that did not exist in the past (see also Leone and Crosby 1987: 399).

Leone and Potter offer an alternative approach of using middle range theory in a historical archaeological context. They suggest drawing on four parts of middle range theory: the independence of the archaeological and documentary records; the concept of ambiguity; the use of descriptive grids; and the idea of organizational behaviour

---

[5] Many of the Accounts of life within asylums are provided by American writers, see for example Geller and Harris book *Women of the Asylum. Voices from behind the walls, 1840–1945*. Mary Elene Wood in her Ph.D thesis *The writing on the wall: Autobiographies by women in American Mental institutions, 1868–1890* looks at the context and reasons behind such writings. The use of these works to understand asylums in other countries are fraught with difficulties because of the different system and stages and types of treatment regimes in other countries.

(Leone and Potter 1988: 13–14). This approach uses documents as a descriptive framework from which to derive expectations of the archaeological record, and uses the deviations from these expectations, which Binford called ambiguities, as the basis for new questions about the archaeological and documentary records (Leone and Potter 1988: 14, 18; Leone and Crosby 1987: 398). As Leone and Crosby argue the goal of this approach is not to explain away exceptions, but to create a greater understanding of the archaeological record through seeking to understand the reasons for the differences (Leone and Crosby 1987: 408, 409).

This study follows this approach in using what I have called the 'ideal' asylum model (the ideal design for a curative lunatic asylum as written about by nineteenth century lunacy reformers) as the descriptive framework against which the material culture of the lunatic asylums is tested, and the discrepancies between the model and the reality of the built asylum are used as the basis for new questions that seek to understand the processes affecting the provisions made for the insane and the use of the buildings.

Narrow views of historical archaeology have also been challenged by Beaudry and others, who have argued archaeology is an approach to the study of culture rather than a specific activity (Beaudry 1996: 480). Historical archaeology is by nature multi-disciplinary. It draws on a wide range of techniques, theories, and sources of information to answer questions that are founded ultimately in questions about material culture and the ideas, beliefs, and practices associated with it.

Today's historical archaeologists are studying culture in its widest definition, as "grounded in systems of meaning for which material culture serves as expression, medium, sign or symbol" (Beaudry 1996: 480). This meaning is active and not static. The lunatic asylum as a form of material culture was, and still is, expressive of constantly changing meanings determined by those using the buildings - the patients, visitors and staff - as well as the viewer and beyond them by society as a whole. For those involved in lunacy reform in the early nineteenth century the physical presence of the new lunatic asylums on the landscape was expressive of the possibility of a cure for insanity; for those suffering insanity it may have represented safety and/or the possibility of cure, or it may have been an embodiment of imprisonment and the cutting of family links. For society and the governing body the asylum represented the acceptance of society's duty to provide for the mentally ill, a physical embodiment of this care that could be viewed with awe and pride. Any analysis of an institution has to be aware of these complexities of meaning. Using middle range theory all sets of data are given equivalent value as we seek to understand the various levels of meaning attributed to material culture. Documentary evidence of meaning is not given more weight than the meaning experienced by those who are unvoiced and using the material culture in question.

PRACTICALITIES: METHODOLOGY AND LIMITATIONS

As indicated previously the continued use of many nineteenth century asylums as modern psychiatric hospitals means they are not usually accessible via the usual methods of historical archaeology as the privacy of patients must be protected. While this could have proved a serious limitation, in fact, their inaccessibility stimulated the development of a new research methodology which sought alternative means to access information about life within the lunatic asylum. To answer the questions posed in the research design a descriptive framework was constructed which described the 'ideal' asylum as written about by nineteenth century writers. This framework could then be tested against the lunatic asylums actually built. The descriptive framework used includes details such as site location, the layout of buildings, and the provision of particular rooms (this will be discussed in more detail in Chapter Five). This was compared to data sets on each asylum which were drawn from plans, photographs, and building histories compiled by the author with a specific focus on building chronologies, room descriptions and changes to the buildings. In turn the disparities between what was recommended and described in the framework and what actually occurred in the building and use of lunatic asylums forms the basis of new questions that allow us to understand factors affecting the realisation of the 'ideal' lunatic asylum and to build a picture of life within an asylum.

Sources of Information: The Ideal Asylum

The nineteenth century writers wrote on all aspects of the lunatic asylum and its management, and the available pool of information about lunatic asylums themselves was reasonably large and tended to fall into date clusters. The earlier works, such as William Stark's 1807 *Remarks on the Construction of Public Hospitals for the Cure of Mental Derangement*, which included a plan for the Glasgow Lunatic Asylum, and the *Observations on the Structure of Hospitals for the Treatment of Lunatics* (1809) which included Robert Reid's plan for the Edinburgh Asylum, were primarily descriptions of the planned buildings. Browne's 1837 book, *What Asylums Were, Are and Ought to Be*, included some details about the built environment required in a lunatic asylum. However it was not until Jacobi's *On the Construction and Management of Hospitals for the Insane*, published in English in 1841, and John Conolly's *The Construction and Government of Lunatic Asylums and Hospitals for the Insane* published in 1847 appeared that specific details were provided as to the design requirements of a lunatic asylum. These four books provided a range of information about what the lunatic asylum should be, with the minimum being a plan of the asylum often combined with descriptions of treatment regimes and management practices.

The period 1858–1867 saw a cluster of works appear, including Sankey's 1856 article 'Do the Public Asylums of England, as presently constructed, afford the greatest facilities for the care and treatment of the Insane?'; Arlidge's article 'On the Construction of Public Lunatic Asylums'(1858), and his book, *On the State of Lunacy and the Legal Provision for the Insane, with Observations on the Construction and Organisation of Asylums* (1859); the anonymous article 'Description of a Proposed New Lunatic Asylum for 650 Patients on the Separate-Block System, for the County of Surrey' which appeared in *The Journal of Mental Science* (1862); Toller's 'Suggestions for a Cottage Asylum'(1865); and Lockhardt Robertson's 'Pavilion Asylums'(1867). These works reflected the experience gained in the operation of the English County Lunatic Asylum system that had seen a number of lunatic asylums built compulsorily after 1845 (discussed in more detail in the next chapter), and focused on different options for the layout of the asylum buildings and the rooms to be provided.

Later articles including Clouston's 'An Asylum, or Hospital-Home, for Two Hundred Patients: constructed on the principle of adaptation of various parts of the needs and mental states of inhabitants; with Plans, &c.' (1879), and Greene's 'A Public Asylum, Designed for 414 Beds, capable of Extension to 600' (1880), focussed on the flexibility of the asylum to meet the needs of the now recognised groups that were to form the mainstay of the lunatic asylum population, and the need for the asylum to be expandable. At the turn of the century two further works appeared: Henry Burdett's *Hospitals and Asylums of the World: Their Origin, History, Construction, Administration, Management, and Legislation,* which appeared in several volumes over 1891 to 1893 and included the best designs for lunatic asylums, and George Hine's 'Asylums and Asylum Planning'(1901). These surveyed existing lunatic asylums and reflected the changing ideas about asylum designs and layouts.

Of these books and articles John Conolly's book on the construction of lunatic asylums was identified as the most valuable. It described in considerable detail what a lunatic asylum should be, including such fine-grained details about window size and placement, floor and wall materials, systems of sanitation, furnishings, rooms to be provided and arrangement of these rooms. Of these details only those that were testable from an archaeological point of view could be added to the descriptive framework of the 'ideal' asylum model. For example details about furnishings and interior decoration are not available for testing due to the continued use of the buildings today and their later modification in the twentieth century to meet modern standards; while accessibility issues limited the possibilities of measuring windows and their placement on the walls. Conolly's 'ideal' asylum model, as it developed, came to include: location factors; layout features of the buildings; rooms required and the arrangement of these rooms in relation to each other; and sanitation provisions. These features could be observed visually in the extant buildings themselves, or identified through the documentary record and from plans and photographs.

Conolly's 'ideal' asylum model became the core model for this study, but as indicated above ideas about the 'ideal' asylum changed over time both in terms of the building designs and in the treatment and management regimes recommended. Consequently I decided to construct a series of 'ideal' asylum models covering the period of 1830 to 1880 using those works that provided the most testable data like Conolly's did. I decided to use the arbitrary cut off point of 1880, as the period 1830–1880 most closely fitted the construction and modification dates of the Australian lunatic asylums used as later case studies.

The 'ideal' asylum models then form a descriptive framework of various features against which the rooms and spaces provided in the built asylums could be compared. The presence of matches or non-matches could then be used as a way of accessing information about life in the asylums, and as a force for generating new questions as to why the asylums did or did not reach the 'ideal'.

Sources of Information: Built Asylums in England

As indicated above, data sets about the actually built asylums needed to be compiled to allow the questions posed in the research design to be answered. The first data sets were built around the asylums of Britain. As this study began with a consideration of Australian asylums, this pool of information about British asylums served two purposes within the research design. Along with the descriptions of the 'ideal' asylum, the evidence provided by a consideration of whether the built asylums matched the ideal descriptions, formed a second part of the descriptive framework against which the South Australian and Tasmanian lunatic asylums could be tested. In particular, the question of trends in the design and layouts of the built asylums was considered important, for if the British lunatic asylums did not meet the ideal, was there a common design being used? Were ward arrangements and the rooms provided consistent over several asylums? The descriptive framework then had two parts against which the Australian asylums could be tested: the 'ideal' asylum and any patterns identified in the British lunatic asylums built which differed from the 'ideal'.

This section on British lunatic asylums had to be based solely on plans obtained from books and journals as there was not sufficient time and funding to go to England and collect original data for all the county asylums

These plans and illustrations came primarily from the architectural journal *The Builder*, the leading voice in its field in the nineteenth century, which published illustrations and plans of lunatic asylums as well as descriptions and editorials throughout the nineteenth century.[6] Plans of the asylums were identified through references in Taylor (1991), and through a consideration of indices of *The Builder*. Other sources of plans included histories of lunatic asylums, such as Crammer's *Asylum History. Buckinghamshire County Pauper Lunatic Asylum-St. John's* (1990), and Frederick Norton Manning's *Report on Lunatic Asylums* for the New South Wales Legislative Assembly (1868–9).

The methods used for this part of the study were limited primarily by the question of access to original lunatic asylums and access to overseas material from Australia. In fact, this part of the research clearly indicated the limitations of an approach based only on plans and illustrations. The primary limitation is that these plans were static snapshots of lunatic asylums as they were on being opened. If they did not meet the 'ideal' asylum model then there was no indication of whether they were later added to or modified to bring them closer to the 'ideal'. Similarly, if they met the model, did their actual day to day use transform the rooms and spaces provided for other purposes and shift them away from the 'ideal' model? To address these issues, two separate colonies of Australia were chosen to answer these questions. The assumption behind this was that the factors influencing the adoption or non-adoption of the 'ideal' asylum features would then become identifiable, and the realities of room and space use, and its effects on life within the asylum, would become clearer.

The value of the British material, while slightly lessened by the limitations discussed above, remained important as the 'ideal' model

---

[6] *The Builder* was subsequently identified in evidence given before the Commission appointed to inquire into and report on the Management etc. of the Lunatic Asylum and Hospital by the South Australian Parliament in 1864 as an important source of information to the architects in the colony (S.A S.C. 1864 Q. 910).

Practicalities: Methodology and Limitations 33

had been primarily discussed by English reformers, and it was anticipated that their ideas would have the most impact in Britain. The British asylum plans offered an opportunity to test this in a limited way, forming a predictive guide to how the lunatic asylums in Australia might be arranged and the rooms and spaces included in the design. Importantly the plans from *The Builder* would be available to the colonists of Australia and formed a second source of information which they could draw upon in planning new lunatic asylums, along with the literature about lunatic asylums.

The Case Studies: South Australia and Tasmania

The lunatic asylums of South Australia and Tasmania were chosen as case studies because of the different origins of these Australian colonies as indicated previously. South Australia, established in 1836, was a free colony which did not receive convicts, while Tasmania, established in 1803, began its existence as a convict colony and received transported convicts until 1853. It was anticipated that the provisions made would reflect the composition of each society, and that provisions made for free colonists would vary from those made for convicts. Further, by using two colonies it was possible to more accurately determine what variables were affecting the design of the lunatic asylums in Australia.

Lunacy in South Australia has received only limited attention. Evelyn Shlomowitz's Ph.D. Thesis, *The Treatment of Mental Illness in South Australia, 1852–1884. From Care to Custody* (1990), looks at the treatment of the insane following the American model of the shift from care to custody. While Shlomowitz did briefly consider the lunatic asylums of South Australia in terms of the expenditure on asylums as a part of the overall decline in services, she did not provide a history of the asylums. Marian Quartly in 1966 wrote an article entitled 'South Australian Lunatics and Their Custodians' and Bostock's *The Dawn of Australian Psychiatry* (1968), which focused primarily on New South Wales, has a few pages on the treatment of lunatics in South Australia up to 1850. A less formal study is H. T. Kay's pictorial guide to celebrate Parkside Lunatic Asylum's centenary in 1970.

Similarly in Tasmania there have been only limited studies of the asylums there. R. W. Gowlland's *Troubled Asylum* (1981) does provide a history of the New Norfolk Asylum; however the book is largely composed of directly quoted material from the Tasmanian Archives, Parliamentary Papers and newspapers. Often whole letters are quoted but the book offers no analysis of the material. Effectively Gowlland included most, if not all, of the material on New Norfolk and the Cascades Asylum. Consequently rather than reiterating Gowlland's work, this study seeks to identify a history of the buildings provided for the insane and look for evidence of the treatment regime practised in the colony which Gowlland does not discuss. The other main piece on lunacy in Tasmania is W. T. Southwood's 1973 article on Bishop Willson and his work to improve conditions for the insane in New South Wales, Victoria and Tasmania. Unfortunately the plans and blueprints of lunatic asylums mentioned by Southwood as being among the Bishop's papers have proved to be un-locatable by the archivist of the Catholic Archives of Tasmania where there are meant to be held (pers. comm. Archivist, Catholic Archives, 2000).

As existing studies were so limited I decided to initially build a range of data sets which included histories of the lunatic asylums in both colonies with a particular focus on information about the design of the original asylum buildings, information about changes and additions made to the buildings over time, and information about room and space use, and the problems associated with their use. This data was derived from original documentation, plans and photographs, and observations of extant buildings. These data sets about the buildings were supplemented by a further data set comprised of information about the treatment regimes within the study period, as these can be directly linked to choices made about rooms provided, their arrangement and the activities undertaken within. For instance it would be illogical to assume that an environment existed apart from the contextual ideas about the treatment of the insane from which they grew. These data sets formed the 'material culture' of the study.

Original Documentation

To build these data sets it was necessary to consult as much original nineteenth documentary material as possible (including plans etc.). State archives and libraries were searched in both South Australia and Tasmania for material relating to the institutions. The available material in South Australia included: Parliamentary Papers, including several Select Committees and Commissions into the management of the lunatic asylums and treatment of the insane in the colony; Annual Reports of the Medical Superintendent to the Asylums which were published most years in the *Government Gazette* (these were available in the State Library of South Australia); Letters to the Colonial Secretary; the Official Visitors to the South Australian Lunatic Asylums Books; and the Colonial Architect's Record Books. These formed the official voice about the asylums. The only other available voice was that of the *South Australian Register*, which was searched but provided very few comments on the lunatic asylums and treatment within them. There were no voices of the inmates, except when they testified before the Parliamentary inquiries, and here they spoke mainly of treatment by the attendants rather than the physical environment in response to the questions asked. These documents provided a range of details about the gross environment of the buildings and some information on room use; there was little detail about the physical environment of the asylums in terms of furnishings, wall treatments etc. A number of plans were found at the South Australian State Archives which provided both evidence about the design of the original asylums and showed, in the case of the Adelaide Lunatic Asylum, evidence about building additions and their placement in the grounds.

From the South Australian histories and surviving plans it was possible to identify the original rooms, spaces and buildings provided, changes to the rooms used, buildings added and, importantly, requests for rooms and other additions. The histories also provided the evidence to answer the third level of questions concerning the effects of social and economic variables on the adoption of the 'ideal' asylum features.

As with the South Australian material the primary documentation available in Tasmania was official in nature and included: Colonial Secretary's Letters; the New Norfolk Hospital Correspondence Book; the New Norfolk Commissioner's Minute Book; Annual Reports of the New Norfolk Commissioners; and the Parliamentary Papers of the Legislative Council of Tasmania which included Commission and Committee Reports into New Norfolk. An alternative voice was provided by Bishop Willson's letters to the Colonial Secretary published in the Parliamentary Papers.

The primary limitation in the data used in this study was a significant difference in the survival of original documentation in South Australia and Tasmania. While South Australia was reasonably rich in this material, Tasmania was not. Only two plans survived of the New Norfolk Hospital for the Insane, one of which showed what the New Norfolk Commissioners wished to do to the Hospital if and when funding was available. Architects' records appear not to have survived and the only indications of what work was done were the Annual Reports of the New Norfolk Commissioners. The Parliamentary Papers also survived sporadically. Thus, while a Committee Report might survive, the Minutes of Evidence, which would have allowed ideas about the Hospital and knowledge about the treatment of the insane and asylum design to be accessed, did not (pers. comm. State Library Of Tasmania 2000). Similarly while photographs existed of the Adelaide asylums, there is one photograph of New Norfolk dating to the early twentieth century. The remaining building at New Norfolk, which is still in use today as a mental hospital, comprises only of the original building that was the Invalid Barracks before becoming part of the Hospital. Due to these limitations it was harder to form these data sets and this particular case study had to rely more on historical data than a multi-faceted analysis.

The limits of the study were determined by the nature of the available material. As indicated above, there were limits to the information available within the documents and the voices they offered. The records which survived in South Australia and Tasmania were different and consequently direct comparison was not always possible and the building chronologies varied in their level of detail. Similarly the available government documents reflected different management structures and the survival of the original papers. The choice of a cut off point of 1890 for the research in Tasmania and South Australia was arbitrary and reflected the survival of plans and the time frame for the construction of the institutions. The sample size of three lunatic institutions in total for both colonies meant that statistical methods of analysis were not viable and the conclusions derived cannot be seen as reflective of all Australian colonies.

The two case studies then offered the opportunity, through surviving plans to identify the original rooms and buildings provided, and these were then compared to the 'ideal' asylum models. The histories of each institution allowed room changes, building additions and requests for additions and their nature to be identified. This effectively allowed each asylum to be compared to the different models which appeared over time. Importantly, the 'ideal' was not static but changed over time, with the Australian asylums being compared to the models that most closely related to them in time. Following this the asylums were compared to the British built asylum designs to answer the questions posed earlier relating to the spread of ideas from England to the colonies about the design of lunatic asylums. But before looking at these case studies l will firstly look at the treatment regimes and movements that lead to the re-appraisal of lunatic asylum design.

The Changing Face of Insanity and Rise of the Institution | 4

While lunatic asylums, hospitals for the insane and madhouses had existed prior to the nineteenth century, it was not until this century that these new emerging treatment regimes bought attention to the physical design of these places and what life was like within them. This attention was to lead to the systematic construction of new lunatic asylums.

As indicated in Chapter One, the lunatic asylum of the nineteenth century was not simply a collection of buildings. It was intended to be a curative institution supporting the treatment of the insane person, who would be returned to sanity and re-introduced into society, and this was to influence both the overall design of the lunatic asylum and the types of rooms and spaces provided. The emergence of the idea of the lunatic asylum as a curative environment and as an appropriate place for the care of the insane is fundamentally linked to two emerging movements in the late eighteenth and early nineteenth centuries in England and Europe: moral treatment and non-restraint. Moral treatment focused on the removal of the insane from their homes to an appropriate environment where, under the direct influence of the treating doctor[1], the insane would be brought back to sanity. The non-restraint regime sought to replace chains and appalling living conditions with a new system of management that structured the lives of patients and used the attendant and treating doctor in such a way that restraints were no longer required (Hill 1838; Conolly 1856). These two treatment regimes required similar rooms and spaces and similar arrangements of the parts

---

[1] In this context the term 'doctor' does not necessarily refer to a medical doctor. In the eighteenth and nineteenth centuries those who made a career of treating the insane did not have medical training. Hence the term only reflects common usage. See Scull 1979 Chapter Four and the articles in Scull 1981.

of the lunatic asylum to facilitate their operation. Moral treatment offered the hope of a cure in an appropriate environment away from the exciting causes of the home environment (Hill 1838: 6), while non-restraint, which also emphasized the appropriate environment, sought to make life within the asylum more bearable and humane. These two treatment regimes formed part of the background against which the concept of what I have called the 'ideal' lunatic asylum appeared.

The second contributing factor to the development of the concept of the 'ideal' asylum was a growing trend towards the provision of centrally administered lunatic asylums by the English government. This change occurred in response to revelations about the unacceptable treatment of the insane in existing madhouses and lunatic asylums (for an overview see Jones 1993; Scull 1979). The 'ideal' asylum sought to embody features that would support the cure of the insane person. It provided a comfortable environment in which the insane could be managed without the need for physical restraints, such as leg-locks, and chains securing patients to walls, chairs and troughs. The 'ideal' asylum was not a static concept, but rather a changeable one adapted to reflect the reality of the built lunatic asylums and the day-to-day management of the patients within them.

MORAL TREATMENT AND THE ASYLUM

The two seminal works that focused attention on the new moral treatment regime were Phillipe Pinel's *Treatise on Insanity* (*Traité médico-philosophique sur l'aleniation mentale; ou la manie* published in 1801 translated into English by D.D. Davis in 1806) and Samuel Tuke's *Description of the Retreat* (1813). Pinel's *Treatise* was to combine elements of previous ideas about insanity with a new regime that focused on the management of the insane. The most important aspect of Pinel's work was its focus on the moral treatment of patients. It is difficult to precisely define 'moral' in this context. It encompassed ideas about the treatment of the insane - which should be characterized by humanity, kindness and reason - and about the nature of the individual. Moral treatment focused on using the finer feelings of the afflicted to bring them back to sanity, by focusing on the will and powers of self-restraint. The treating doctor had a pivotal role as he used all of the means at his disposal, including reasoning and talking to the patient, to bring them back to sanity by addressing the particular ideas of the individual (Pinel 1806: 221–224). The keys to moral treatment as practiced by Pinel were:

- The kind treatment of the patient.
- No patient should be unnecessarily restrained or struck.

- The removal of all things that may irritate the patient.
- The classification of the patients was to be based on their illness and stage of recovery.
- Treatment should be specifically suited to the patient.
- Patients should be provided with some kind of work to occupy their mind during their convalescence and allowed freedoms such as walking in the gardens.
- A reasonable diet should be provided.

Classification allowed the violent and furious to be separated from the convalescent who needed quiet. Similarly it was thought that the distressing sights of dementia, idiotism, and epilepsy should be kept from other lunatics with separate areas in the hospital for each (Pinel 1806: 176 & 204). This regime could only be supported in the asylum environment, not the patient's home. The asylum environment then had to support this regime, but Pinel did not, however, describe the features of the environment himself. Later lunacy reformers were to take on this task and develop his ideas.

Pinel's ideas formed a new basis for the treatment of the insane in the last decades of the eighteenth century and the early decades of the nineteenth. This new treatment was to find its first concrete expression in The Retreat, a Quaker asylum that became the model for the means of putting ideas of moral treatment into practice in a uniform way. Interestingly, it appears that the founders of the Retreat were not aware of Pinel's work but followed a similar path based on their own beliefs, which were founded in Quakerism (Digby 1985: 32). In some way the new ideas of the treatment of the insane may have been a part of more subtle changes in society as a whole that Porter (1981–2: 15) has characterized as the new belief in the limitless possibilities of improvement in human knowledge and conduct. Thus Pinel's work, based on the individual treatment of the insane and the focus on a more humane daily life, can be seen as part of this more general philosophical change.

The Retreat was founded in Yorkshire, England at the instigation of William Tuke in 1792 and opened in 1796. In 1813 Samuel Tuke published a book entitled *A Description of The Retreat*, which detailed the operation of the therapeutic system of treatment and the management of the patients' lives and movements through The Retreat. As with Pinel's work, the therapeutic regime was based on reasoning and conversations with the patients that sought to allow their own nature and self-will to return them to sanity (Skultans 1979: 58). In practice a cure was brought about through therapeutic discussion combined with a system of rewards and punishments, a regime of daily activities, classification and the provision of an appropriate environment (Tuke 1813 Chapter 5).

Classification formed part of the system of rewards and punishments at The Retreat. Patients were divided into various classes based on their behavior - 'disorderly and disruptive' and 'clean and tranquil' were two such groups. These groups were housed in different parts of the house. If a patient was well behaved they were moved into the better furnished rooms and allowed access to the gardens, if not, they were demoted to the lesser rooms occupied by the noisier patients and allowed fewer privileges. Access to outside areas could also be withheld, or a patient could be restricted to a room and not allowed to participate in communal activities (Digby 1985: 67–69, 74). All patients were expected to take part in some activity to distract their minds. This activity reinforced moral discipline through the need for self control and through the responsibility to act appropriately during the activity (Digby 1985: 42, 45 & 63). Importantly, fear and restraint still played a part in the moral regime of The Retreat (Skultans 1979: 58). As can be seen The Retreat buildings and the structured life within them were a fundamental part of the treatment which could not be provided if the individual remained at home. The buildings and grounds of The Retreat were designed to allow the separation of patients. There had to be grounds to allow outdoor activities such as gardening, and some aspects of the landscape had to include pleasing scenery which meant access to them could be used as a reward. The Retreat buildings were designed in such a way, using windows without obvious bars, muffled locks and a domestic form of architecture, that the patients did not feel imprisoned (Tuke 1813: 93–107). The model of treatment practiced at The Retreat - classification, activities, rewards and punishments and the direct influence of the medical officer - was taken up as part of the non-restraint system, with the emphasis being placed on providing an appropriately designed environment to support the regime.

THE NON-RESTRAINT MOVEMENT

The clean domestic setting and individual treatment regime of The Retreat was in sharp contrast to the reality of the madhouses, hospitals, and asylums of the eighteenth and early to mid-nineteenth centuries. Until the advent of moral treatment and the belief in the curability of the insane, the primary focus of treatment had been control. This was primarily through mechanical restraints, whether the lunatic was being 'cared' for at home, by a member of the clergy, or in a madhouse or hospital for the insane. Pinel had been one of the first to realize that the newly recognized rationality of the insane was undermined by continuing abuse, and he was to become legendary for his freeing of the patients of the Bicêtre and Salpêtrière (Skultans 1979: 53). Reformers such as Robert Gardiner Hill believed they were continuing his work in arguing for a new treatment regime of non-restraint (Hill 1838: 13, 21).

For Hill, the use of instruments of restraint deprived the patient of all power and command over themselves (Hill 1838: 20). He argued that self-government would lead to self-control and, ultimately, to a cure. But what was restraint to be replaced by? For the reformers of the non-restraint movement the answer lay in providing an appropriate environment in which an insane person might be cured, or if not, then at least cared for humanely for the rest of their natural life.

In 1838 Robert Gardiner Hill described what he considered to be four essential requisites of the new system of management:

1. A suitable building must be provided, in an airy and open situation, with ground sufficient for several court-yards, gardens, and pleasure-grounds, commanding (if possible) a pleasing and extensive prospect.
2. There must be proper classification of the patients, more *especially by night* (original italics)
3. There must also be a sufficient number of strong, tall, and active attendants, whose remuneration must be such as to secure persons of good character, and steady principle, to undertake their arduous duties.
4. The House-Surgeon must exercise an unremitting control and inspection, in order that the plan may never, under any circumstance whatever, be deviated from in the slightest degree. (Hill 1838: 38–39).

The treatment regime was based on moral treatment with a view to inducing habits of self control (Hill 1838: 45). The classification of patients within the asylum allowed those recovering or convalescent to be kept in a quiet and calm state without the stress of being exposed to the noise and disturbance of those at the height of their illness. This supported their cure. The number of attendants was to be sufficient so that restraints were not required, as the patients were to be observed at all times and, if necessary, shut in their bedrooms to quieten them. Following on the preliminary work of Dr. Charlesworth, who had removed the worst restraints, Hill instigated the non-restraint system at Lincoln Asylum, and by 1836 was able to report that three months had passed without a single instance of restraint (Hill 1838: 100).

Robert Gardiner Hill's suggestions were expanded in W. A. F. Browne's series of lectures on *What Asylums Were, Are and Ought To*

Be, presented in 1836 at the Montrose Lunatic Asylum in Scotland. Browne argued that in the asylum:

> ... Every arrangement, beyond those for the regulation of the animal functions, from the situation, the architecture and furniture of the buildings intended for the insane, to the direct appeals made to the affections by means of kindness, discipline, and social intercourse, ought to be embraced by an effective system of moral treatment. (Browne 1837: 156).

Above all, the insane within the asylum should be treated as individuals, with treatment regimes responding to their condition and patterns of behavior. If restraints were to be removed, some system of controlling or managing the patients had to be in place to prevent disorder. The regime as envisaged by Browne was based on the employment of keepers with strong, healthy, and well-constituted minds; the classification of patients; and "by the exercise of sound selection of those who are to associate together" (Browne 1837: 152).

John Conolly in his *Treatment of the Insane Without Mechanical Restraints* (1856) expanded on Hill's ideas and described his application of the non-restraint system at the Middlesex County Asylum at Hanwell from 1839 onwards. Hanwell had initially accommodated 300 patients and was expanded to house over 1,000 patients within a few years of its opening. The ideal world of asylum life, as envisaged by Conolly, was based on personal knowledge and kind care of the individual, who in turn would have access to good food, proper clothing, occupations, and religious consolation (Conolly 1856: 57–60). By allowing some kind of activity, whether work or amusement, the mind was distracted from its cares, and the monotony of asylum life was broken. Above all, the patient was not to be forced into any activity before they were ready (Conolly 1856: 67, 71, 73). In place of restraints, a padded room was used for patients who were experiencing a manic episode or were disruptive, or distressed in some other way. Alternatively, the patient was allowed to retire to their room for quiet time or walk alone in the airing court (Conolly 1856: 42 & 44). Interestingly, time spent in improving the physical health of the patient through the provision of good quality food and through allowing patients out to exercise in the gardens or airing courts, often led to a marked improvement in some patients' mental state. Clean wards and rooms and regular times for meals and activities often promoted calmness and quiet in the wards (Conolly 1856: 55).

In summary the key elements of the non-restraint movement were:

- the removal of mechanical restraints;
- the classification of patients;
- their employment in some form of activity;

- exercise - preferably outside;
- a good diet;
- provision of appropriate clothing and bedding;
- clean wards and beds;
- religious consolation;
- amusements to break up the hours in the asylum;
- the appropriate treatment for each patient's condition;
- the treatment of patients with kindness.

Ideally, the asylum environment should support this management system and facilitate its operation. It was this ideal environment that was to become the focus of a number of writers directly involved with the care of the insane, including John Conolly who had published his *The Construction and Government of Lunatic Asylums and Hospitals for the Insane* in 1847.

Importantly, it was not just those involved with moral treatment and non-restraint who emphasized the importance of the removal of the insane person from their home to a specialized environment. A growing emphasis on the role of the doctor as a professional specialist in the treatment of the insane (Scull et. al. 1996: xiv) and the advocacy of the early removal of the insane person into the doctor's care in the setting of an asylum or private madhouse also focused attention on the lunatic asylum. As George Man Burrows indicated "Cases which in the early stages are comparatively manageable, obedient to medical discipline, and commonly curable became obstinate, tedious, and too often incurable if left at home" (Burrows 1828: 696). Burrows himself favored remedies that firstly treated the body followed by moral treatment.

As a consequence of these new ideas the modern asylum became the symbol of the possibilities for the cure of the insane, rather than simply a place of imprisonment. This was the ideal vision of the asylum and its role. The asylum world would be one of kindness and comfort, where patients worked with attendants and the medical superintendent to control their thoughts and emotions and to achieve a cure.

This focus was coupled with an increasing humanism within English society, which in turn saw a growing interest in social causes that expressed itself in tours of inspection by interested gentlemen of places such as madhouses (Porter 1981: 16). Revelations about the treatment of the insane led directly to reform of the laws covering their treatment and the provision of places for their care. Again the lunatic asylum was the focus as the primary means of caring for the insane, as the English Parliament sought to establish a country wide system of county lunatic asylums. These provided an opportunity for lunacy reformers to put their ideas about moral treatment and non-restraint into practice, as they had the opportunity to influence the design and operation of the new lunatic asylums.

THE RISE OF THE LUNATIC ASYLUM

In eighteenth century England the insane were generally kept in private licensed houses or under the care of an individual such as a minister of religion. Anyone could establish a madhouse. For families with insane family members these madhouses provided the main means of caring for the afflicted persons.[2] The only alternative was a charity hospital. The oldest and most famous of these charity hospitals was Bethlem which was to become the focus in the nineteenth century of accusations of cruelty and poor management in the treatment of the insane (Browne 1837: 116–118; Allderidge 1985; Jones 1993: 7–10, 48–50)[3]. With the growing perception of the insane as individuals capable of being cured, and no longer subject to their animal nature, attention began to focus on conditions within the madhouses and charity hospitals.[4] This found public expression in a number of Select Committees of the English Houses of Parliament, which were in turn prompted by a number of changes within society, including the rise of the Evangelical Movement (started by the Clapham Sect) which focused on social reform, including the abolition of the slave trade, and the rise of philanthropic groups with a wide range of interests (Jones 1993: 34; Harrison 1966: 356–7). Both groups sought to correct perceived failings or faults within society through their work, even if at the same time they sought to enforce their own moral values (Harrison 1966: 359). It was the work of these groups, whose members took a personal interest in the poor and insane which led them to visit the asylums and madhouses, and revealed to wider society the abuses occurring in these places.

The first of these Select Committees was the House of Commons Select Committee of 1807, appointed to enquire into the State of Criminal and Pauper Lunatics in England and Wales (Parry-Jones 1972: 14). While only briefly surveying conditions affecting the insane, the Select Committee Report was of fundamental importance because of its recommendation

---

[2] See Parry-Jones 1972 for a discussion of the mad-house system.

[3] For a more complete history of the hospital see Andrews et al. 1997. Allderidge has contested the accuracy of the claims relating to the level of abuse at Bethlem Hospital (1985: 17–27).

[4] The late eighteenth to mid-nineteenth century saw a growing recognition of the rational qualities of the insane and with this the possibility of a cure. Prior to this the perceived loss of the ability to reason had reduced the insane to the level of animals and with this had come the treatment of the insane with harshness and the use of restraints (Porter 1987: 40–41; Scull 1981: 108).

The Rise of the Lunatic Asylum

that each county of England should have its own asylum for pauper and criminal lunatics. These asylums would be under the control of a committee of governors nominated by local magistrates and financed through a county rate (a form of tax) (Jones 1993: 35). Believing the power of public opinion was on their side, they recommended that the building of county asylums not be made compulsory. These recommendations were embodied in the County Asylums Act of 1808 (48 Geo. III, c. 96). The new asylums were to be built in healthy situations with a good supply of water. Patients were to receive constant medical assistance, be accommodated in separate wards for men and women, and with separate wards for convalescents and incurables (Jones 1993: 36–37). It is unclear at this stage whether these provisions were in response to the changing ideas about the insane which advocated a specific environment for their care, or more in response to the appalling living conditions in which visitors to the madhouses found the patients. What did emerge most clearly was the role of the public institution in the care of the insane.

The Report of the Select Committee of 1827 included a guide to what the ideal asylum should be including its physical characteristics and management of the patients. The sexes were to be completely separated, dormitories should be properly ventilated, courtyards airy and dry, offering some kind of view. The management regime was to be based on moral treatment. Patients should be clean, bathed regularly, allowed outside to exercise, and while on the wards a range of amusements and employments should be offered to occupy them. The wards should be furnished with flowers and birds, while musical instruments and art materials should be available for the patient's enjoyment (Jones 1993: 63).

However, few lunatic asylums were actually built under the 1808 Act. In 1828 nine county asylums had been erected under the permissive Lunacy Acts: Nottingham (1811); Bedford (1812); Norfolk (1814); Lancaster (1816); Stafford (1818); West Riding, Yorkshire (1818); Bodmin, Cornwall (1820); Lincoln (1820) and Gloucester (1823). These were built to accommodate various numbers of patients. Bedford, for example, accommodated 52 patients, Norfolk allowed for 102, while Lancaster and West Riding respectively took 170 and 250. As the magistrates of each county could choose their own style and plan, architectural styles and costs varied considerably. Nottingham Asylum cost £21,000 or £262 per head (designed for 80 patients), Lancaster cost £60,000 or £354 per head (for 170), while Bodmin cost £12,000 or £147 per head (for 102) (Halliday quoted in Jones 1993: 60). The variation in the sizes of the asylums resulted from the county authorities estimates of the number of insane requiring treatment. This was usually based on existing numbers with no provision for increases over time. In the next 14 years, a further seven county asylums were built: Chester, Dorset, Kent, Middlesex, Suffolk, Surrey and Leicester (Jones 1993: 64).

Despite the appearance of these county asylums, in 1844 there was more than double the number of lunatics in workhouses than in county asylums. The abuse of lunatics continued as before and further reform was called for (Art. 5 1844: 427, 430–2). Consequently the Lunatic Act of 1845 (8 & 9 Vict., c. 100 & c. 126) made the building of county asylums for pauper lunatics compulsory in England. By 1857 there were 33 county asylums and four borough asylums in existence accommodating 14,309 lunatics with a further four planned (11th Report Comm. in Lunacy 1857: 14).

The county asylum initially offered the possibilities of a curative environment, but this vision became submerged under the increasing number of the insane requiring care in the county asylum system. The main problem facing the reformers was the apparent rise in the number of insane in England and Wales.[5] This rise effectively meant that as soon as an asylum was built it was filled to overcrowding. This led to a cycle of additions and expansions of existing asylums and the building of ever larger asylums. In 1860 the average number of patients in the 41 county asylums was 386.7; in 1870 even with 10 more asylums available, the average number in each had still risen to 548.6 (Scull 1979: 198). In the 1860s and 1870s this increase led to the modification of ideas about what was required in a lunatic asylum environment.

DISCUSSION

This, then, is the background against which the lunacy reformers developed the 'ideal' asylum models. The new treatment regimes of moral treatment and non-restraint required the insane person to be removed to an appropriate and curative environment, where through a structured plan of management, including various activities, exercise and the personal attention of the Medical Officer, they could be returned to sanity and their families. The accompanying recognition of the appalling treatment the insane were experiencing within existing

---

[5] This apparent increase in the number of the insane was actually a product of several different forces. These include: the faulty collection of the original figures about the number of the insane (Scull 1979: 225; Arlidge 1859: 3, 6, 10, 20); broadening definitions of what constituted insanity as held by society generally (see Arlidge 1859: 58, 91 & 94; Scull 1979: 240; Jones 1997: 60; Piddock 1996: 27–28); and the accumulation of the chronic insane in asylums.

Discussion

lunatic asylums, charity hospitals and madhouses, provided a powerful incentive to provide better care. The two forces came together in the creation of the county lunatic asylum system. Here, then, was the opportunity for those interested in non-restraint, moral therapy and in the simple care of the insane to actually specify what was required in a curative environment - an environment that would also support the effective management of the insane. The construction of the county asylums provided a further opportunity for adaptation of ideas about what the lunatic asylum should be, to reflect the realities of these asylums. What, then, were the features of the 'ideal' asylum? And how influential were the 'ideal' asylum models? These questions will be addressed over the next two chapters.

Constructing the 'Ideal' | 5

As was discussed in Chapter Three, to answer the questions posed in the research design it is necessary to develop a descriptive framework of what lunatic asylums should be that then can be tested against the reality of the built asylums, and the discrepancies between the two be used to understand life within the asylums. The descriptive framework acts as a launch pad to explore ideas about the asylum, and gives us a starting point in understanding asylums, which in turn can go beyond a simple list of rooms and spaces provided. As was seen in Chapter Four, lunatic asylums were not simply buildings rather they were to provide a curative environment that would return the insane person to sanity and society. This chapter will explore the ideas about what asylums should be as written about by those interested in seeing the new regimes of moral treatment and non-restraint applied. It is important to realise that these ideas did not just appear but developed with the passage of time in response to the fleshing out of the new treatment regimes, and in response the provisions made for the insane in madhouses and county asylums. Consequently in this chapter the 'ideal' asylums discussed are presented chronologically with some of the earlier works discussed first before the discussion of John Conolly's 'ideal' asylum, which as l mentioned in Chapter Three is the most detailed and useful for understanding lunatic asylums and forms the core descriptive framework in the case studies. The chronology is based on the publication date of various books and pamphlets rather than on the date of the erection of an asylum which may be discussed in the particular text. For example, while The Retreat was built earlier than some of the asylums discussed below, the book on its management and design was not published until 1813 and this then can be seen as the point when the ideas about the use of the built environment at The Retreat in York became more widely available to those constructing lunatic asylums.

THE 'IDEAL' LUNATIC ASYLUM: EARLY EXPERIMENTS 1807–1809

The earliest descriptions of lunatic asylums reflecting the requirements of the new modes of treatment were provided initially by architects rather than those directly involved in the care of the insane. In 1807 the architect William Stark published his paper *Remarks on the Construction of Public Hospitals for the Cure of Mental Derangement*, which was originally read before the Committee appointed by the City of Glasgow to receive plans for a new public asylum. As with many works dealing with the design of lunatic asylums, this paper presented not only the design features but also a discussion of the underlining ideas about the treatment of the insane. Often the two are inseparable. William Stark, who had himself, visited existing asylums and madhouses to study their failings based his design for the Glasgow Asylum on the principles of minimal restraint and the moral treatment of the insane as practised at The Retreat (Stark 1807: 5–8). Consequently, the focus of Stark's design was the constant observation of patients by attendants, which had replaced physical restraint, and classification.

Stark's design for the Glasgow Asylum, which was incidentally never built, was based on the panopticon principle first advocated by Jeremy Bentham, a leading radical philosopher and social reformer. The panopticon was intended to be used for the new workhouses and prisons; its design allowed the constant inspection of the patients and their classification into various classes (Knott 1986: 47; Casella 2001: 51; De Cunzo 1995: 45). Stark's plan for the proposed asylum had four wings or arms and a central hub creating a radial asylum. These wings were composed of a number of single rooms with circular stairways halfway along their length. Stark's paper indicates that the wings were three storeys in height, with the ground floor wings extending out further than the upper storeys. The ground floor had two wards, while the first and second floors had one ward to a floor, allowing eight wards for women and eight for men. The male and female sides, in effect, were composed of two 'spokes' each. The centre was an octagon and had four day rooms accessible via the ward galleries. The central space was occupied by a circular staircase. Situated between the two sets of wings on each side was the keeper's room. This allowed the keeper to directly access the wards and the day rooms directly opposite. This theme of observation continued in the placement of the keeper's room overlooking the space between spokes, which was divided up into two airing courts. A central corridor inside the day rooms allowed the superintendent easy access to any part of the asylum. Stark indicates there was to be an attic over the central space, which may have been intended as rooms for the superintendent

(Stark 1807: 25). While initially designed for 60 patients, Stark believed that the asylum should be expanded to accommodate a minimum of 100 patients (Stark 1807: 27–28).

Moral management and the early form of non-restraint both required many of the same features in a lunatic asylum. How were these realised in Stark's 'ideal' asylum? Classification was given a high priority within the design, with both male and female patients divided into higher and lower ranks, with each having their own spoke. Those of liberal education were being mixed with those of 'brutal manners' in other asylums, to the distress of the former. Consequently Stark separated them. The remote wards on the ground floor were for the frantic, furious and highly disorderly patients with 'habits and propensities ... offensive to the others' (Stark 1807: 6, 10, 26). The ground floor ward nearest the centre was for the incurable. The first floor ward was for the convalescent and the second floor for those in an 'ordinary' state. Movement through differently furnished wards was to be a punishment or reward for appropriate/inappropriate behaviour. The design allowed limited exercise yards for the patient's use but the plan appears to have made no provision for work or other activities. In the asylum the patients' movement was limited to the sleeping room, the day rooms where meals were taken, and the airing court.

Stark's plan for the Glasgow Asylum was an *architect's* interpretation of what an asylum should be if moral management and non-restraint were practised. Robert Reid's plan and notes for the planned Edinburgh Lunatic Asylum published two years later in *Observations on the Structure of Hospitals for the Treatment of Lunatics, and on the General Principles on which the Cure of Insanity may be most successfully conducted* (1809), offers a different arrangement of the rooms and spaces, though similarly from an architect's view point. Reid in his design was particularly concerned with providing a secure, healthy and comfortable environment. The asylum was to have a thorough and complete system of ventilation and sanitation (*Observations* 1809: 9–10; see also Art. V. 1844: 432).

The illustrations included in *Observations* indicate that the asylum was to be composed of a series of buildings, which could be added to as needed. Each series was composed of three buildings joined in the Palladian manner by single storey arcades. Each building series was intended to house 40 patients. Reid indicates that the Edinburgh Asylum was to be composed of four large houses which, with the smaller buildings, would form four sides of a square. The interior courtyard would be divided into four courtyards by the connecting passages (*Observations* 1809: 1–2, 4, 10).

The central building of each sequence contained three storeys, while the two flanking buildings had two storeys each. Reid indicated that each building would be complete in itself, having its own kitchen and servants' rooms. This would allow for internal differences, reflecting the different ranks of the patients and the different fees they would pay. These buildings would be shared by both sexes who would be kept separate. On the plans the right side of the central building was female, and the left, male. Logically each of the two smaller buildings would be single sex, reflecting the division of the main building. These small buildings were reserved for patients of an even higher rank (sic) than those housed in the main building (*Observations* 1809: 2, 3, 4, 10–11). Reid's plan included baths and water closets, but made no provision for work or leisure activities. As with Stark's plan living and exercise spaces were limited, with emphasis being placed on classification and observation.

Stark and Reid, while familiar with moral treatment and the new concerns for providing improved accommodation, were not directly responsible for their care. Their interpretations of what was required in a lunatic asylum were from a lay person's perspective. For Stark and Reid the 'ideal' asylum supported:

- Observation at all times.
- Classification.
- Social ranking.
- Sanitary conditions.

Within a few years books began to appear written by those who were directly involved in the day to day care of the insane. Samuel Tuke's *Description of The Retreat* published in 1813 was the first of a number of works that dealt with the role of the physical arrangement of the asylum as part of the cure of the insane. Tuke's work was followed in 1837 by W. A. F. Browne's *What Asylums Were, Are and Ought to be,* and Robert Gardiner Hill's *Total Abolition of Personal Restraint in the Treatment of the Insane* (1838).

THE MORAL ENVIRONMENT: TUKE, HILL AND BROWNE 1813–1838

The Retreat was the first asylum to be built with the ideas of the curative or the moral environment in mind. Opened in 1796 it sought to provide Quaker lunatics with a non-threatening environment that would remind them of home. As the Retreat's architect noted: "if the outside appears heavy and prison-like it has considerable effect upon the imagination" (Digby 1985: 37). Consequently The Retreat was designed to appear as a country home.

As the illustration included in the book *Description of The Retreat* by Samuel Tuke (1813), indicates The Retreat was built in a plain Georgian style, with the only decoration a small portico over the front door. The asylum was to be composed of a three storey square building with flanking wings of two storeys on each side. Each wing had a further smaller building attached to it. The illustration is difficult to date, but would appear to pre-date 1810 as do the plans as by 1810 another separate building had been added (Tuke 1813: 65–66). The Retreat was located half a mile from the city of York on an elevated site of 11 acres surrounded by picturesque scenery (Tuke 1813: 41 & 93). The attempt to create a home-like environment was enhanced by the lack of bars on the windows. Rather windows were composed of small panes of glass set in cast iron sashes. But like Glasgow the windows in the bedrooms were small (3ft. by 3½ ft.) and set six to seven feet high in an attempt to prevent injury to the patients (Tuke 1813: 100 & 105). Thus there was an inconsistency created, The Retreat which was intended to be a surrogate home had no windows that allowed a view of the outside world. The airing court walls followed the same pattern. They were eight feet high, yet Tuke believed that the slope of the ground lessened their height visually (Tuke 1813: 95). The Retreat had a public face where the patient entered, which presented a hedge as the only barrier between the patient and the outside world, and a private face where the patients' day room windows looked only onto walled airing courts behind the asylum.

Tuke's book did not provide details of what was required in a curative asylum per se. Rather by giving a description of the buildings themselves and the mode of treatment within it, it was hoped to demonstrate what was required in a curative asylum. As Tuke indicated The Retreat was not perfect in its design (Tuke 1813: 109).

The rooms and spaces of The Retreat were used to classify the patients, based on their state of mind and behaviour. For example those men who were more violent and 'least capable of rational enjoyment' occupied the day room in the extreme east wing; as a reward, those who were regarded as 'superior' in their behaviour were allowed to use the day room closest to the central section. In keeping with moral treatment a "room [off the day room] affords an opportunity of temporary confinement by way of punishment, for any very offensive acts" (Tuke 1813: 98). The ultimate 'reward' for the male patients was to take their meals with the superintendent and the females in the central dining room. The same arrangement was followed for women patients who used the three day rooms on the first floor, with the refractory patients using the extreme west wing. Five to six patients of the 'superior' class occupied the attic rooms and used the dining room as a day room. The two downstairs rooms in this wing were used to isolate patients during the day as needed (Tuke 1813: 98–102). The Retreat distributed patients throughout the asylum on the basis of mental condition and social rank, although its size limited the physical separation of the various groups. While being 'home-like' The Retreat presented a highly organized environment with movement towards the centre of the house physically indicating control over the self and a return to sanity.

The Retreat, by example, embodied some of the attributes of what was considered important in a curative environment:

- It was located in a rural setting.
- It provided enough space to classify the patients and to use access or the denial of access to particular rooms as a privilege or a punishment.
- It provided day rooms where the patients might engage in activities.
- It provided gardens where patients might be employed and exercise areas complete with animals to distract the mind.
- Most importantly its size allowed the patients to be treated as individuals with their own treatment plans.

These themes of classification and the movement of the patient through the asylum space as a reward for acting appropriately could also be applied within a larger scale asylum.

Opened in 1820 in response to the call for public county asylums under the permissive lunacy acts, Lincoln Asylum was to be one of the first asylums to fully apply non-restraint. Here, again, access to better wards was a reward for appropriate behaviour with a complex arrangement distributing patients over a series of wards, galleries and sitting rooms. Classification was again based on social rank and three classes of mental condition: convalescent and orderly; moderate; and disorderly. The wards included a range of small dormitories, single rooms and infirmary rooms (Hill 1838: 39–1). The move to a single room with its attendant privacy was a reward for good behaviour, one of the fundamental indications that a patient was seeking to control their irrational thoughts. The arrangement of sleeping accommodation allowed the attendants to focus their attention on problem cases at night, replacing the need to restrain suicidal or destructive patients.

For Robert Gardiner Hill, author of *Total Abolition of Personal Restraint in the Treatment of the Insane* (1838), which was based on his experiences at Lincoln Asylum, an essential part of non-restraint was the provision of a suitable building with several courtyards, gardens and pleasure-grounds allowing the patients to exercise. In this building there would be a proper number of apartments, dormitories, and galleries to allow the proper classification of patients, particularly at night, and to allow appropriate treatment for each class (Hill 1838: 38). However Hill provides no specific details about any of these rooms.

If Samuel Tuke and Robert Gardiner Hill indicated by example, W. A. F. Browne in his *What Asylums Were, Are and Ought to be* (1837) was to be far more explicit in identifying what was wrong with the environments and care provided by many existing asylums. For Browne, an advocate of non-restraint, the English asylums of the 1830s, while an improvement upon earlier asylums, were lacking in the requisites of moral treatment. In particular, there was no classification, no occupations or amusements for the patients, no exercise areas, and no control of the internal climate (Browne 1837: 122, 140, 144, & 146). Believing there was no systematic plan for managing the asylum in its totality; Browne's book went some way to outlining this plan. His series of five lectures briefly touched on the built environment of the asylum as part of a holistic approach that saw the asylum, its attendants and the role of the superintendent as all part of the cure (Browne 1837: 156). These arrangements began with the most basic starting point for an asylum - the site.

A site should be generally healthy, should possess a dry cultivatable soil, an ample supply of water, and: "should be so far into the country as to have an unpolluted atmosphere, a retired and peaceful neighbourhood". However it should not so isolated that the benefits of a town, which provided "comforts and privileges and intercourse", could not be experienced (Browne 1837: 181). The placement of asylums in semi-rural or rural settings was important, as this provided the prospect of a view, allowed for future expansion, and the inclusion of airing courts and gardens. The gardens were intended to provide vegetables for the asylum and employment for the patients.

Browne believed that "the locality in which the building is erected may be made to contribute to the cure of insanity, and to the enjoyment of those under treatment" (Browne 1837: 182). If the asylum was placed on a slope or summit the view would be limitless and have profound psychological advantages, for it would remind the patient of the world outside and what they must do to return to that world. The changing seasons provided further intellectual stimulation. In this view the landscape is the bond that links the patient with the external world while they reside within the walls of the asylum. An interesting view acted as an encouragement to patients to exercise, while an irregular surface was necessary for exertion and exhilaration (Browne 1837: 182–183).

In terms of the internal arrangements of the asylum, Browne placed greatest emphasis on classification, ventilation and heating. The best form of asylum, in his view, was composed of a series of separate houses. Ideally a large part of the asylum would have only one storey, to prevent the dangers of suicides and injuries arising from ascending and descending stairs, and to remove the gloomy iron screens and cages associated with them. For those who could not afford a servant to attend them, Browne favoured dormitories over single rooms, where beds were widely spaced and an attendant slept with the patients, for:

> ... it yields the pleasure of society and protection, as it prolongs the influence of moral training into the silent watches of the night. (Browne 1837: 186).

Browne was particularly concerned that the interior climate of the asylum should be healthy, as disease and physical illnesses affected the possible recovery of the patients, and problems of ventilation led to offensive smells and stale air. Small, ill-ventilated cells collected air that affected the breathing of the patient, and disturbed their sleep which should be 'quiet and refreshing'. Consequently sleeping apartments should be large and lofty and well aired. To aid ventilation sleeping rooms should open onto a long and spacious gallery, which could be used as a common hall, or a work area. Classification allowed the windows to be placed a few feet above the ground allowing a view out for convalescent patients, who should also have free access to the airing courts. The houses should be provided with baths and showers for keeping the patients clean and comfortable, and on occasion to act as therapy. Self-cleansing water closets were also essential (Browne 1837: 183–186).

Browne's 'ideal' lunatic asylum features can then be defined as:

- A healthy site with a dry cultivatable soil, and an ample supply of natural water.
- A country site, elevated or on a slope, near enough to a town for supplies and activities.
- The asylum be composed of a series of one storey houses.
- Accommodation should be in the form of dormitories which aided ventilation and observation.
- Rooms should open onto a gallery.
- Galleries should be wide enough to be used as a common hall and work area;
- Windows should be placed low in the walls to allow a view out.
- There should be free access to airing courts for exercise.
- There should be baths, showers and water cleansing privies.

The 'ideal' asylum thus encompassed a range of features considered necessary for the cure of the patient as defined by moral treatment.

Browne further emphasised sanitation, cleanliness, ventilation and heating in response to the appalling living conditions of older asylums. The 'ideal' asylum was one that provided a healthy and comfortable environment while fulfilling the requirements of a curative environment. Browne's recommendations form only a small part of his book. The works of Maximilian Jacobi and John Conolly were to provide a much more detailed view of the lunatic asylum and what it should be.

THE 'IDEAL' ASYLUM DETAILED: JACOBI AND CONOLLY 1841–47

Jacobi and Conolly continued the trend of presenting the asylum environment as part of a holistic system of patient management. Both wrote from their own experiences of asylum management. While Maximilian Jacobi was writing from his experience in Europe where he was at the Seigburg Asylum in Prussia, his book *On the Construction and Management of Hospitals for the Insane* was published in England in 1841 and became part of the English canon of works dealing with the arrangement of lunatic asylums.

Jacobi does not advocate moral therapy as such, but his descriptions of the treatment and classification of the patients does in many ways parallel some of the views of the moral therapists. Above all Jacobi believed that the lunatic asylum should be a curative institution and this was, in the middle decades of the nineteenth century, a fundamental aspect of the 'ideal' asylum.

In Jacobi's view the private home was an inappropriate environment for the care of the insane. They required careful treatment in an environment that offered security, attendance, oversight, restraint (applied in the most humane manner), remedies of all sorts, and due medical assistance. This could only be achieved in an asylum (for his arguments see Jacobi 1841: 1–13). The asylum population should never exceed 200 and all treatment and higher government should rest with the director alone. To achieve a cure all forms of medical treatment should be used, including baths, electricity, diet, wholesome air, suitable temperatures, and means of bodily exercise and employment, the manipulation of the feelings of the insane, and the strengthening of the will. To achieve these ends patients were to be divided into strict classifications which could change hourly (Jacobi 1841: 16, 23 & 61). This division was based on the degree to which their disease influenced their moral and social behaviour, and:

> ... according to the degree, dependent upon the measure of this influence, of their ability or inability to conduct themselves in a quiet, cleanly, decent

and orderly manner, to observe prescribed rules, and to employ themselves usefully, &c. (Jacobi 1841: 50).

In these rules Jacobi was following the ideas laid out by Tuke and the other advocates of moral therapy. Jacobi envisaged five divisions of patients, reflecting behavioural and physical classifications (Jacobi 1841: 55, 57). These divisions were reflected in both the arrangement of the asylum and its internal fittings, which Jacobi discusses at length based on his own experiences at the Seigburg Asylum.

Treatises such as Jacobi's went into precise detail about the physical arrangements of the asylums. They detailed arrangements for water-closets, ventilation systems and drainage. Jacobi himself provides details about the measurements and construction of windows, doors, the shape of walls below windows, lighting, the furnishing of the laundry and kitchen, bath construction, and the building materials that should be used for walls, ceilings, floors etc., for each part of the asylum. These works provided, in effect, a building guide by a person having a direct experience of actually living and working within the institution. For the purposes of this study, however, the focus will only be on those features that are archaeologically testable.

Jacobi agreed with Tuke and Browne's views of a suitable site and that a building should be cheerful in its aspect and unlike a prison, as well as having a good water supply (Jacobi 1841: 26, 27, 28). Unlike Browne, Jacobi considered the physical layout of the asylum buildings and how this might support the purposes of the asylum and the daily management of the patients. Jacobi believed that arranging the asylum into quadrangles was by far the most adaptable form. The H, linear, and panopticon layouts were all problematic if large numbers of patients were to be accommodated (Jacobi 1841: 33–48).

Within Jacobi's 'ideal' asylum the internal arrangements conformed to the needs of the particular divisions, these were based on the patient's behaviour, their ability to care for themselves and their social rank. The asylum would resemble a home with coloured walls, pictures, and caged birds; while musical instruments, games and books would be readily available. Gardens would have benches, fountains, flower beds and fruit trees. Other provisions included a bake house, dairy, carpenter's and tailor's shop, a separate administrative section, a fully equipped bathroom with a range of baths, and a playground complete with a nine pin stand, a tilting yard, swings, and a cross bow range (Jacobi 1841: 64–73, 83, 91–93, 99–101, 108, 109–110, 119–120 & 129). In effect, the asylum was a complete world providing the patient with security, medical care, amusements and work appropriate to their level of wellness or insanity as well as their social class.

Treatises like Jacobi's provided a detailed guide to the curative environment as it was to be expressed as a physical reality. Such studies argued that the human mind was fundamentally aware of its surroundings even in illness.

From Jacobi's book it is possible to define the following key points for an 'ideal' asylum in terms of its built environment:

- Houses should be arranged around courtyards.
- It should allow classification, in particular the separation of the sexes, and the noisy and violent patients from the convalescent.
- It should be placed in the country and close to a town.
- There should be a good water supply.
- The building should be arranged so as to prevent contact between the sexes, and the divisions of the insane, to the point that no group could see another via windows.
- There should be appropriate rooms for each group, and, if necessary, rooms should reflect the social class of the patients to some extent.
- The physical arrangement of the building should prevent the noisy from disturbing the others but not prevent their effective supervision by the superintendent.
- The building should be not more than two storeys or go to an excessive length.
- Patient numbers should be limited to 200.
- The convalescent should have well lit rooms, furnished appropriately.
- There should be work areas and pleasant exercise areas and gardens for the patients.
- There should be a chapel.
- The building should be sufficiently lit and ventilated.

A comparison with Browne's features shows the same basic features of classification, ventilation, and location. However Jacobi went further, placing a greater emphasis on the physical layout of the building and on the interior furnishings, which, while not detailed here, sought to make the asylum home-like for those on the road to recovery. Above all Jacobi followed Browne in arguing for an asylum of a manageable size that supported supervision. Browne had advocated houses and Jacobi recommended small buildings based around courtyards. Jacobi further recommended the provision of specialised work areas.

John Conolly published his work, *The Construction and Government of Lunatic Asylums and Hospitals for the Insane* in 1847. In this book Conolly presented a system of patient management that was based on an appropriate environment for the care of the insane. Conolly was one of the leading advocates of the non-restraint system and had brought the system to the Middlesex Asylum at Hanwell. Following his experience at Hanwell, Conolly outlined his ideas about the best environment for the treatment and care of patients in a pauper or county asylum and for their supervision by attendants. Conolly's book was published two years after the English Lunatics Act of 1845 had made the building of county asylums compulsory. It appeared at a time when ideas about the appropriate site and built environment could have the most sway as county magistrates sought designs for county asylums. As Conolly himself indicates, there were few reference works available for the English reader to consult (Conolly 1847: 6). He felt that while Jacobi's work had useful suggestions, the book written 13 years before was "all comfortable to the old system of restraint and force, although tempered by the author's evident kindness of heart and good understanding" (Conolly 1847: 7).

Conolly followed the reasoning of Jacobi and Browne, recommending a healthy country site with views and room for gardens, with ready access to a high road, railway or canal, and a town for the supply of stores and to allow friends to visit the patients (Conolly 1847: 8, 9). However unlike Browne and Jacobi who favoured separate buildings, Conolly favoured the linear form or modified H where wings only extended to the rear of the asylum, and was limited to two storeys. Any more wings brought with it more problems, particularly those associated with disease:

> ... By the accumulation of so many persons, day and night, in a lofty building, many of whom can seldom leave the wards, and no one of whom is in perfect health, the asylum becomes subject to every atmospheric and terrestrial influence unfavourable to life. (Conolly 1847: 11).

Ideally, there should be no bedrooms in cellars and attics, and all patients should be able to freely exercise outside. Conolly favoured accommodation for a maximum of 360 to 400 patients, higher than that proposed by those seeking to make the asylum a curative place with some level of individual care. It is likely that Conolly was responding to the experiences arising from the construction of public asylums under the previous permissive English County Asylums Acts. For he roundly condemned the lack of forethought in the construction of asylums only for the known number of insane, which did not allow for the accumulation of chronic and new cases, and where avarice played a part in how much funding was provided. This had led to poorly thought out additions. The Middlesex County Asylum at Hanwell for example, was facing ongoing problems as it was expanded from an asylum for 300 patients in 1831 to one housing 1000 in 1847 as more additions were made to meet the every increasing number of insane requiring care (Conolly 1847: 10–12).

In terms of the arrangement of the various parts of the asylum, Conolly recommended placing the chief physician's residence, offices, a chapel, large recreation room, and school rooms in the centre of the asylum, with the kitchen, laundry, workshops, and various offices located behind. The galleries were to extend out from the central administrative block, with two galleries on each storey. This allowed the easy division into male and female sides. The second gallery would be slightly offset from the first wing. A third gallery could then be extended at right angles from the junction point. Through this arrangement all wards had an equal share of light and, with the rooms situated on only one side of the gallery, cross ventilation would occur (Conolly 1847: 12–13). Similarly the airing courts were not to be overshadowed by the buildings. A north-south orientation was favoured to allow for the best lighting with the galleries facing south and the bedrooms facing north. Similarly the galleries of the east-west wings faced either the rising or setting sun, with the bedrooms on the darker side.

Reflecting the nature of the large county asylums, Conolly did not support the extensive classification of patients. At Hanwell the most tranquil patients, some convalescents and some newly admitted cases occupied the wards nearest the centre. Then came the infirmaries, followed by a ward housing the 'epileptic, imbecile, loquacious, and troublesome'. A further ward housed the clean and industrious patients, and at the furthest point was the ward for the 'noisy, the refractory, and the dirty'. Conolly recommended these divisions be followed in all large asylums. Each ward should accommodate 30 patients and have two attendants (Conolly 1847: 16 & 18).

Many of Conolly's recommendations for the construction and layout were directly reflective of his experiences in a large scale asylum. He argued for a preponderance of single rooms over dormitories, as patients appreciated the quiet and solitude, and too large dormitories meant one patient could disturb the sleep of others in the room; that attendants should have separate rooms and dining rooms to allow them some respite from the constant demands of patient care; and he favoured open day spaces as these allowed the easier observation of all patients by the fewest attendants (Conolly 1847: 16–17, 21 & 24–5, 95, 100). These suggestions were then all based on his direct observation of the human experience of the lunatic asylum. This also led Conolly to recommend the provision of reception rooms for newly arriving patients and external corridors so that staff and patients could move around the asylum without disturbing the wards (Conolly 1847: 14, 38–40).

Following the emphasis of earlier writers, Conolly argued for baths, lavatories and water closets on every ward, and for large windows that allowed a view, along with fresh air. Importantly, there should be a large apartment for musical activities and dances (Conolly 1847: 40–42, 55). Non-restraint and moral management recommended activities and exercise for the patients, and for Conolly this meant the provision of gardens, a bowling green, a cricket ground, and an area for ball games. Shallow ponds attracting ducks and other birds could provide further diversions, along with other tame animals, while walls should be low at around 7 ft. compared to the 10 to 15 ft. of older asylums. Airing courts were to be landscaped and provided with seats and summerhouses. To complement the outside recreation, the tranquil wards should have a range of amusements including books, journals, illustrated papers, picture albums, soft balls, bagatelle, draught boards, dominoes, cards, and puzzles (Conolly 1847: 52–4). Workshops should be large and airy, and those at Hanwell included a carpenter's shop, upholstery room, tailor's shop, shoemaker's shop, tinman's shop and a printing office (Conolly 1847: 81). Women were generally employed in the kitchens, laundries and wards and were not provided with separate work areas beyond needle rooms. Under the asylum system the need to create a self sufficient institution served the need to employ the patients as part of the moral regime. In effect there were no work areas that reflected the range of activities pursued by the patients outside of the asylum.

There were in essence four areas to be considered in the design of a lunatic asylum: the wards; the central administration and domestic offices; work areas; and airing courts and gardens. The county lunatic asylum generally required a number of particular rooms for its day-to-day functioning (Table 1). However, the arrangement of the wards with their sleeping accommodation, attendant's rooms, day rooms, and baths/lavatories was the main concerns for Conolly and others.

Table 1. Required Rooms and Spaces of the Asylum

Living Space	Administrative Space	Domestic Space
Sleeping Cells	Staff offices	Kitchen
Dormitories	Medical Superintendent's Rooms	Bakehouse
Day Rooms	Attendent's Rooms	Brewhouse
Baths, Water closets	Committee Room	Dairy
Lavatories	Dispensary	Vegetable Gardens
Airing Courts and Gardens		

The 'Ideal' Asylum Detailed: Jacobi and Conolly 1841–47

For Conolly the 'ideal' arrangement of these spaces was found at Derby Lunatic Asylum, the plan of which he included in his book. It was "in almost every material point accordant with the principles maintained" (Conolly 1847: 181). Reflecting the nature of the patients and the need for constant observation, the refractory wards had bays for day rooms as opposed to closed rooms. The wards for the aged and infirm and moderately tranquil, who required less strict observance, had separate dining rooms at each end. The Derby asylum had a chapel and music/school rooms over the kitchen and offices, so as to be centrally located and easily accessible. It also had discrete work areas at the rear of the asylum, and provided airing courts with shelters and pavilions. Thus, although for John Conolly the 'ideal' asylum had already been constructed, what was important was that these features be clearly defined and recognised, and even improved upon. The features of an 'ideal' asylum in Conolly's view were:

- An appropriate site with some form of scenery.
- An arrangement of the buildings that allowed light in and cross ventilation, with no building overshadowing another or the airing courts.
- A linear layout.
- It terms of size, it should accommodate no more than 360 to 400 patients.
- A building that offered a range of wards for classification, with each ward having its own attendant's rooms, and open areas as opposed to day rooms for patients.
- Each ward should have access to a bathroom, lavatory and water closets without the patients being required to go outside.
- Each ward should have a wide gallery furnished as a day room with windows low enough to allow a view outside and with as discrete security as possible.
- There should be a large recreation room, school rooms, work rooms and workshops, and a chapel for the use of patients.
- The offices should be centrally located and there should be a means of accessing the various wards without passing through each.
- Attendants should have their own dining hall.
- Accommodation should primarily be in the form of single rooms with a few dormitories.
- Above all, the asylum should be light, cheerful and liberal in the space it offered.

Conolly's 'ideal' asylum model builds on the features of Browne's. The principal difference was that Browne envisaged the gallery as the main living space functioning as a combined day room, recreation area and work area. In Conolly's view there should be separate rooms for these activities, i.e. work rooms and workshops, a large recreation room, day alcoves along with furnished galleries, and additional spaces such as school rooms and a chapel. Conolly also emphasised the provision of centralised offices and staff areas in the form of attendant's rooms and dining halls. Where Browne had spoken in general terms, Conolly and Jacobi had supplied blueprints for the exact placement of the various spaces and rooms. They had indicated how the spaces would work in relationship to each other.

Jacobi and Conolly's 'ideal' asylums shared a number of features in common, but were significantly different in how they arranged the space used by the patients; for example Jacobi had advocated dormitory accommodation for everyone except refractory patients, whereas Conolly favoured single rooms. In Jacobi's asylum the world of the patient was more limited, often restricted to one room for living and sleeping unless one was socially and financially better off. In Conolly's asylum each group of patients was accommodated in the same type of ward with galleries wide enough for exercise. All patients had access to workshops, a central recreation room, school and music rooms to provide some variety to the day. Equally important for Conolly were the airing courts and exterior spaces available to the patients for exercise and fresh air. In Jacobi's asylum the staff slept and lived in the same rooms as the patients; in Conolly's asylum they had their own spaces. At a fundamental level there was the question of the size of the asylum: Jacobi's asylum was half the size recommended by Conolly, who was working in the context of the English county lunatic asylum system. Conolly's 'ideal' asylum was above all practical, with particular emphasis placed on what could be called quality of life which considered both the physical and mental health of the patients.

FURTHER IDEAS ABOUT THE 'IDEAL' ASYLUM: SANKEY AND ARLIDGE

Following Conolly's initial work other reformers came to focus on the requirements of the 'ideal' asylum. The period 1850 to 1870 saw a range of works appearing that built on Conolly's basic features and sought to modify and improve the functioning of the asylum space. This in turn affected patient management.

In 1856 W. Sankey, physician to the Female Department of the Middlesex Asylum at Hanwell, offered a different approach in his article "Do the Public Asylums of England, as presently constructed, afford the greatest facilities for the care and treatment of the Insane?" published in *The Asylum Journal of Mental Science*. He advocated the movement of patients and staff to various parts of the asylum space at different times of the day and for different activities. This was in contrast to the asylums of Jacobi and Conolly where the patients spent the majority of their time on the ward, apart from when they were employed or exercising.

Sankey followed Conolly in his views on the treatment of insanity which did not need: "a well-furnished dispensary", instead a cure rested with "careful nursing, wholesome diet, regular employments, diversified amusements, cheerful dwelling [sic], personal cleanliness" (Sankey 1856: 466–7). Rather Sankey's preferred treatment depended greatly:

> ... upon the regulation of the ordinary occupations and pursuits of the patient, and the facilities for these, upon the architectural arrangement of the building, that the form of the edifice, and the disposition of its offices becomes of paramount importance to the medical attendant (Sankey 1856: 467).

As indicated earlier, the rooms and spaces of the built asylum had to support the curative regime, which was primarily about controlling the activities of the patients. The building had to be designed in such a way that the attendant could always observe and monitor the activities of the patients. In a way physical restraint had been replaced by a form of psychological restraint exercised by the attendant and the superintendent. Thus while Conolly had trees and shrubs in his garden, they were not to obstruct the view of the attendant (Conolly 1847: 52). Day rooms, for example, could be arranged so that the attendant had a full view of all his patients at a glance "without the necessity of his following them from place to place, or dogging them like a spy" (Sankey 1856: 470). Sankey believed that, if the rooms of the asylum were properly arranged, fewer attendants would be required, reducing the running costs of the asylum (Sankey 1856: 467).

Sankey noted that in existing asylums the ward consisted of a day room, sleeping rooms containing one, three, or five to eight beds, and a gallery or wide passage. Each attendant had their own ward of 30 to 35 patients. Patients took their meals in the ward as well, making it "a little system of itself; a distinct and separate division" (Sankey 1856: 472). These divisions grouped together formed the asylum. As each ward was a separate division this led to duplication of amusements in the wards or less variety in each, and two attendants were required in every ward at all times. Sankey believed that there was a better way to arrange space than this. In Sankey's 'ideal' asylum all the day rooms would be concentrated together on the ground floor, and with the rooms close together only one reading or music room, and a billiards room would be needed (Sankey 1856: 473).

Taking this a step further, Sankey felt that the classifications used during the day and at night did not necessarily need to be the same. A patient could belong to two classes, one for the day, reflecting work assignments, and a night classification based on the need for care. Sankey believed that dormitories were more practical for supervision, as under the present system of single rooms only one or two patients could be observed at a time, running the risk of patients having fits unnoticed by the night attendant. By the provision of dormitories all could be observed, although four to five rooms per hundred patients were still required for the noisy cases who would disturb the whole dormitory (Sankey 1856: 474–5). In this Sankey was favouring practical management over the patient's comfort.

Sankey believed that the patients' lives should be regulated to the extent that each activity had its own time and place. Thus, during the hours of work, no patient should be enjoying amusements. When work finished it should end throughout the asylum, and only amusements should occupy the patient, and "the parts of the building devoted to each should be entirely vacated and closed" (Sankey 1856: 477). By keeping all the patients together it was easier for the attendants to observe them and allow parts of the asylum to be ventilated freely. Sankey's 'ideal' asylum for 1,000 patients had:

- A central building dividing the asylum into male and female sides.
- A chapel, entertainment room, kitchen etc., and the residence for the chief or superintending officer in the centre building.
- Rooms for the male and female divisions' officers in the divisions themselves rather than in the central building.
- Wards divided into two classes, those for day time use and those for night time use.
- Separate infirmary wards on each side of the asylum.
- Day and night areas which would be completely distinct and separate to the point of having separate sets of staff.
- Day time areas, preferably located on the ground floor, and including the indoor areas of day rooms, workshops, dining rooms, halls for amusement, and the exterior areas of the garden, the airing courts, and the skittle ground.
- Areas that freely communicated with each other.
- Sleeping rooms only on the first floor of the building. These would be divided down the centre by arches and dwarf partitions, effectively creating four walls against which beds could be placed (Sankey 1856: 476–477).

The problems of ventilation that concerned Conolly would be partially solved by the fact that the dormitories were only occupied at night, not for 24 hours. If the dormitories were arranged in a cruciform with arms of various lengths, the nurses' station could be placed in the centre. The longer arms would house the quiet patients, with the quietest at the furthest point from the nurses' station. The shorter arms would house the epileptics, the refractory and those requiring attendance (Sankey 1856: 478).

Sankey's arguments for a different room arrangement and classification were taken up by John Arlidge in his *On the State of Lunacy and the Provision for the Insane with Observations on the Construction and Organisation of Asylums* (1859). Judging by Arlidge's comment that there was little attention given to the special subject of asylum architecture in England beyond John Conolly's book, Tuke's introduction to Jacobi and a few pages in Browne, however he appears to be unaware of Sankey's article even though they make very similar suggestions (Arlidge 1859: 200). Arlidge, like Browne, Conolly and Sankey was familiar with the world of asylums, having been the medical superintendent of St. Luke's Hospital in London (Digby 1985: 38).

The basic fault with asylums, Arlidge believed, lay in the fact that they were designed by architects, who, having no personal experience of the requirements of the insane, were purely copyists "of the generally-approved principle of construction, which they have only ventured to depart from in non-essential details, and in matters of style and ornamentation" (Arlidge 1859: 200). This led the majority of built asylums to be slight variations on the one model: that of a corridor, with sleeping rooms along one side, and one or more day-rooms at one end or in a recess, in lieu of a separate room. This constituted an apartment 'fitted for constant occupation day and night' and was called a ward. These wards were arranged over two, three, or four storeys to form an asylum (Arlidge 1859: 199–200). Variations in asylum designs occurred in the way in which wards were juxtaposed and disposed in reference to the block and ground plans, or in the introduction of accessory rooms. Arlidge believed this arrangement originated in the design of monasteries that had been appropriated for the use of the insane who had been shut away under the old system of treatment. Asylums as they were now resembled barracks, workhouses and factories, removed as far as possible from the familiar world of the patient's home (Arlidge 1859: 143, 200).

For Arlidge the world of the asylum above all should be as close as possible to the ordinary home-life of the patient and in effect a home. In the ordinary home there were discrete spaces for the various parts of daily life: a bedroom, sitting room, and a kitchen or dining room for meals. On entering the ward of the asylum the new patient found themselves in a corridor peopled with a number of eccentric people pacing up and down, or huddled in groups (Arlidge 1859: 201). This ward formed the patient's world apart from when they were taken to the workroom to work or outside to exercise:

> ... within it he will have to take his meals, to find his private occupation or amusement, or join in intercourse with his fellow-patients, to take indoor exercise, and seek repose in sleep; he will breathe the same air, occupy the same space, and be surrounded by the same objects, night and day. (Arlidge 1859: 201–202).

This ward system was "an inversion of those social and domestic arrangements under which English people habitually live" (Arlidge 1859: 201). The gallery or ward system had other disadvantages. The gallery gave refractory patients room to run, jump, and dance about, inciting others to join in. Attendants could not properly monitor patient activities, and were frequently absent from the ward collecting meals, and performing other tasks. Stairs presented a constant danger for patients and attendants going to the airing courts, workshops and offices (Arlidge 1859: 207, 210–11). Under the system Arlidge was proposing the stairs would only be used twice a day. Arlidge, like Sankey, argued for a ground floor devoted to day rooms and for the upper floors to be used as sleeping rooms. The ground floor should be composed of a number of sitting rooms, which through the use of folding doors could be made into a larger room for entertainments. These sitting rooms would be furnished and fitted for different activities such as light work, indoor amusements, reading, or for meals (Arlidge 1859: 204–5), bringing them far closer to being home-like. A number of sitting-rooms further allowed the patients to be classified according to their capacity to work or to take part in amusements. Following in Sankey's footsteps, Arlidge suggested that day time classifications could vary from night classifications (Arlidge 1859: 205 & 208).

An article written in 1858 provides an illustration of the design of the asylum as Arlidge envisaged it. The article "On the Construction of Public Lunatic Asylums" in *The Asylum Journal of Mental Science* contains essentially the same material which Arlidge included in his 1859 book, with the exception of the plan and his description of it. This is an interesting omission and may reflect a change of mind about the precise form of the asylum rather than the ideas he was expressing. The plan proposed is for an asylum:

> ... unbroken or continuous, under one roof, and presented a long front (sic) with a wing extending backwards from each end, at right angles, and a central block of buildings, for general offices, also extending backwards from the officers' residences, which were placed in the middle of the front line of the building (Arlidge 1858: 193).

Arlidge's asylum for 220 patients offered accommodation for the following classes: "1, the convalescent, with the quiet, clean and industrious patients; 2, the epileptic; 3, the demented feeble with the paralytic; 4, the sick, in an Infirmary; 5, the refractory." (Arlidge 1858: 194). On each side of the central block were three large rooms fitted out as a day room, dining room, and multi-purpose room that would be a library/reading-room/school room/billiard/reception room for visitors. While apparently more home-like in its assignment of different activities to different rooms, the functional description of the third room reflected middle class rather than working class values. The paupers in the county asylum were unlikely to have music, library, or billiards rooms in their houses. Rather, these designations represented suitable activities for the patients which would in turn reinforce particular moral values. The dining room was to be separated from the sitting room to allow the latter's use to be a privilege and reward for better behaviour and orderly conduct. Consequently the sitting room was to be better furnished with ornamental fittings. In close proximity would be a bathroom, lavatory, scullery, water closet and store-cupboard to meet the daily needs of the patients. At the end of the day rooms were areas for the sick and bed-ridden cases, epileptic, chronically dirty (incontinent) and refractory patients. To prevent noise and disruption to the patients these rooms were separate from the day rooms. The first floor would be devoted to dormitories and single rooms, 'ideally as few patients as possible would sleep downstairs. Sleeping on the ground floor was to be a punishment (Arlidge 1858: 194–196). Presumably the rooms were better furnished upstairs.

In 1858 when Arlidge drew up the design for his asylum he envisaged it as one large building. By 1859 he had changed his mind, perhaps in response to the rising size of asylums, and favoured the block system of a series of separate buildings, each furnished to suit the needs of the patients (Arlidge 1859: 143).

Sankey's and Arlidge's 'ideal' asylums saw almost totally different arrangements of the day and night time spaces of the asylum compared to Conolly's model. From Sankey and Arlidge's perspectives the use of the ground floor for day rooms allowed the more effective supervision of the patients and allowed easier access to work and recreation areas. The patients were not required to travel up and down stairs several times a day. A number of day rooms and dormitories were freed for differing day and night classifications. The use of day rooms downstairs allowed the upper floor space to be freed up and offered different possibilities for ward arrangements. It seems likely that the reduction in the duplication of rooms and service areas, such as baths and water-closets with their associated costs, would have been a powerful economic argument for building asylums along such lines.

VARIATIONS ON A THEME: PAVILION AND COTTAGE ASYLUMS 1860–1865

By the 1860s 33 county and four borough asylums had been built in Britain, and a further four were planned (11th Report Comm. in Lunacy 1857: 14). In response to the new problems arising from the construction and operation of these county asylums (constant additions and an increasing resident population), papers appeared that offered alternative asylum designs, and responding to the actual composition of the asylum population.[1] Writers of the 1860s focused on how to provide for the growing number of the insane in an asylum that was workable in terms of building size, ventilation, heating and patient management. An alternative to the linear asylum under one roof was the block or pavilion system. The pavilion system had first been developed as a response to the appalling conditions within hospitals, which had become centres for disease transmission between patients.[2] Florence Nightingale in her *Notes on Hospitals* recommended that for a hospital of 120 beds or more, buildings could be placed side by side, while smaller hospitals could have blocks arranged in echelon. Each block would be self contained with nurse's rooms, lavatories (rooms with taps, sinks, and mirrors), baths, and water closets (Robertson 1867: 468). The same system could be applied to asylums where there would be a number of discrete buildings linked in some way, usually by a communication corridor that allowed comfortable access in all weather.

Two block plans were published in the 1860s, one by the anonymous author of "Description of a Proposed New Lunatic Asylum for 650 Patients on the Separate Block System, for the County of Surrey" in the *Journal of Mental Science* of 1862, and the other by Dr C. Lockhardt Robertson in 1867 in his "Pavilion Asylums" article in *The Journal of Mental Science*. These articles show two possible systems of arrangement for the blocks. The proposed Surrey County Asylum consists of two ranges of buildings, one behind the other linked by an administrative block, while Robertson's favoured the placement of buildings either side of a central corridor, again with a central administrative block. The primary difference between the two lay in the size. Robertson's plan was for 250 beds, although he noted that it was capable of expansion to 400 and 550 beds, while the Surrey plan began with 650 beds (Robertson

---

[1] For a discussion of the nature of asylum populations see Andrew Scull (1979) *Museums of Madness. The Social Organization of Insanity in Nineteenth-Century England*.
[2] See Anthony King (1966) "Hospital Planning: Revised Thoughts On The Origin of the Pavilion Principle in England." *Medical History* 10: 360–3.

1867: 471; *Description* 1862: 600). The latter reflected the high level of chronic cases that were beginning to emerge among the asylum population. These people would generally live in the asylum until they died.

For the author of the Surrey article the importance of the design lay in the breaking down of the 'thick atmosphere of insanity' that arose from accumulating large numbers of insane persons in a limited space. The block system afforded natural ventilation, and diminished the risk of fire. Within the asylum the administrative officers were to have their residences spread across the blocks to allow effective supervision, countering one of the possible arguments against a move to such a system. The asylum was to consist of six separate blocks, three each for men and women arranged either side of the central block. The chapel was set in front of the central block and was free-standing. The second and fifth buildings were set back 60 yards from the others, but as the author noted the visual effect was of one continuous frontage. To avoid wasting space, galleries were not used, rather the ground floors were to be fitted out as spacious day rooms, with some infirmary accommodation. The upper floors would be given over to sleeping wards, primarily of dormitories but with a few single rooms. The quiet tranquil patients would occupy the front buildings, giving them ready access to the dining room in the centre block and to the laundry, kitchen and workshops. The noisy and dangerous patients would be accommodated in the rear blocks (*Description* 1862: 600, 603 & 605–607).

Lockhardt Robertson was of the view that all English county asylums erected in the previous 20 years were copies, with slight modifications, of the original monastic hospital of St. Mary of Bethlem, which in turn provided the model for the third Bethlem Hospital built in 1815 (Robertson 1867: 469). In this he echoed Arlidge's view. Under this system each ward was a distinct asylum with its own sleeping cells and dormitories, day room, attendant's room, baths, scullery, water-closet and work room. Derby (Conolly's 'ideal' asylum) and Essex asylums represented the best of this arrangement, while Bethlem and St. Luke's Hospitals represented the worst (Robertson 1867: 469). While asylum architects and planners had adhered to the gallery system, Robertson noted that where additions had been made to existing asylums, there was a departure from the gallery system. Instead, at the behest of the medical superintendents, the additions were freed from the gallery system, often with separate day and night rooms, as advocated by Sankey and Arlidge (Robertson 1867: 470).

Robertson believed it was possible to adapt the hospital pavilion system to lunatic asylums, allowing for single rooms, security against escape and employment of the patients. The asylum was to be divided into a series of blocks arranged on either side of a central corridor.

The administrative block and kitchen block straddled the corridor in the centre, with infirmary blocks flanking each side of it. Beyond the infirmaries were the blocks for chronic and acute males and females. Across from the acute blocks, on the other side of the corridor, were the laundry and washhouse, and the workshops respectively, while free-standing bath-houses were sited opposite the chronic wards (Robertson 1867: 473).

The ward pavilions were slightly different in arrangement and included a mix of single rooms, dormitories and day rooms reflecting the requirements for nursing and supervision. The pavilion for chronic patients, for example, had day rooms opening freely onto the airing court, while the refractory block had more single rooms than the chronic block, reflecting the possible level of night time disturbance. There was a growing trend of placing chronic quiet cases in dormitories as a cheaper accommodation solution than single rooms. But, as Conolly had indicated twenty years earlier this was to deprive patients of all quiet and privacy. In Robertson's asylum the proportion of single rooms was one bed in each single room to every four dormitory beds (Robertson 1867: 472–473). The key features of the pavilion asylum as envisaged by Robertson were then:

- A series of blocks dedicated to a particular class of patient.
- The provision of single rooms and dormitories in a percentage reflecting the classification (acute and chronic).
- Ground floor day rooms and sleeping rooms on the first and second floors.
- The provision of central male and female dining rooms.
- The provision of workshops and the laundry on the male and female sides of the asylum respectively.
- Division of the floors into day and night roles.
- The provision of a separate recreation hall, attendant's rooms and chapel.

The placement of the laundry and workshops reflected perceived gender roles for men and women, associating domestic tasks firmly with women. Robertson further retained the day and night division that had been central to Sankey's asylum, but not a diversification of day rooms as recommend by Arlidge.

In the asylums of the 1860s the extensive classification advocated by Jacobi had almost disappeared. These asylums reflect a much simpler classification, into acute and chronic. Both the proposed Surrey asylum and Robertson's plan offered this most basic of classification. This shift in the classification of patients may have been the product of the rapidly increasing number of chronic patients in the county asylums.

The idea of a curative asylum that had offered such hope at the turn of the century was to disappear by the mid to late nineteenth century. The sheer number of lunatics being sent to the asylums and their poor condition on arrival overwhelmed the possibility of a cure for the majority, for curative regimes placed emphasis on the treatment of insanity on its first appearance. Many individuals were sent from the workhouses to the asylum only when near death. The problem was inadvertently worsened by the better diet and sanitation found in these new county asylums which led to the extension of the lives of many lunatics who subsequently were seen as incurable or suffering age- related dementia (Conolly 1859: 411). The cure rate of 15.4% in 1844 had dropped to 7.7% in 1870 despite increasing numbers of the insane being housed in asylums (Scull 1979: 190 & 192).

In response to the changing nature of lunatic asylum populations, writers on lunacy began to give serious consideration to the options for housing the chronic patients who would spend the rest of their lives within institutional walls. As early as the 1840s there had been suggestions for housing the chronically insane in low cost purpose-built asylums. But for reformers such as John Conolly these asylums were objectionable as they suggested a patient was beyond cure. Conolly believed patients might recover after many years, and they would be aware of their removal to a chronic asylum with its plainer environment. Chronic patients, he believed, required more stimulation and variety in their surroundings and in the employments and amusements on offer to them (Conolly 1847: 4–5).

E. Toller offered a variation on the separate block system to deal with chronic patients. He proposed a design based around a series of cottages. Toller's design arose from his own experiences as the medical superintendent of Gloucester County Asylum, where there was no room for conventional additions (Toller 1865: 342). Toller believed cottages offered a form of accommodation suitable for both chronic and harmless cases. One argument for the separation of chronic and acute cases was that it allowed treatment and attention to be focused on the acute cases who had the greater possibility of being cured, and the cottage system would facilitate this. Those requiring treatment would be placed in cottages closest to the administrative offices where the Medical Superintendent worked and in some cases lived.

In response to the criticism that chronic patients would receive a lower standard of care, Toller argued that under the cottage system, greater attention would be given to each patient by the attendant, as each cottage would house only 15 patients. By separating the larger groups of patients into smaller groups within the Gloucester Asylum, Toller had found they were better behaved and more industrious.

Patients who would not formerly work undertook work when moved into cottages. This made the use of cottages equally worthwhile, as employment - a part of moral treatment - was seen to improve the mental and physical health of patients, an effect Toller directly observed himself (Toller 1865: 343–344).

Toller's design for a cottage asylum was intended for 525 patients, the maximum number he believed a superintendent could supervise. The asylum consisted of 29 cottages housing 15 patients each and two infirmaries for 45 patients each. There were 14 cottages on the male side and 12 on the female side. The administrative offices were housed in five detached buildings in the centre with the male and female cottages on either side forming two parallel lines. The central building housed the committee room, superintendent's office, the assistant superintendent's rooms, and visiting and reception rooms on the ground floor. On the first floor was an entertainment room (80ft. by 40ft.). Flanking this building were the male and female infirmaries and stores buildings. Behind these buildings was the chapel and beyond this the laundry (with a bathhouse on the first floor) which was flanked by three cottages for the female patients who worked in the laundry. The bake house, brewery and farm buildings were set on the boundary of the male side, while on the female side was the cemetery. The superintendent's residence was separate and to the front of the asylum. There was no central kitchen as each cottage would have its own, along with a living room, single rooms and dormitories.

In terms of classification, on the male side there were seven cottages for the different trades with the appropriate workshops attached (i.e. carpenter, bricklayer, painter, shoemaker, tailor and upholsterer), three for agricultural workers, three for epileptics, and one for a school. Patients without a trade would be placed where they might learn one. For the women, three cottages were for epileptics, three for laundry workers, and the rest for domestic activities (Toller 1865: 345). Each cottage would become a home with its own games and books, and the retirement time could be varied to suit the patients (Toller 1865: 345). The rest of the 100 acres of the estate could be devoted to gardens and agriculture.

Toller's asylum, more than any other asylum design, most resembled the homes of the patients and was least like an institution. The design did not allow for the vagaries of the weather, however, and it seems likely that those patients who were not entirely healthy probably would not be taken to the chapel and recreation rooms. Thus while the cottages were home-like, they were in fact equally limiting in the world they offered the patient - a world where movement may be restricted to a living room and the attached workshop. Another danger of such arrangements was that patients might be constantly employed and not taken out to exercise as there were no safe enclosed airing courts. The ratio of one attendant to 15 patients would present problems of supervision unless courts were attached to the cottages themselves. In 1859 Arlidge had warned of the dangers of industrial classification whereby in some asylums the day rooms and sleeping accommodation were situated over the work area, such as the laundry:

> ... Instead of being thus scarcely allowed to escape the sphere and atmosphere of their toil, they should have their condition varied as far as possible, be brought into new scenes, mixed with others who have been otherwise engaged, and made to feel themselves patients in an asylum, not washerwomen. (Arlidge 1859: 143).

Rather than breaking away from the lifestyle that may have induced their insanity, the problems of a patient's life were reinforced by their work in the asylum. Arlidge favoured the use of medical classification within the main asylum, with cottages for the chronic perhaps being further subdivided (Arlidge 1859: 145).[3]

CONCLUSION

This survey of the literature shows that there was no one design for the 'ideal' asylum. Rather the 'ideal' reflected a range of ideas about the building arrangements required. At the turn of the nineteenth century ideas about the 'ideal' asylum were very much focussed on providing an appropriate environment that allowed for the classification, observation and humane care of the insane. This came in response to the appalling conditions under which the insane had been kept in the eighteenth and early nineteenth centuries, and formed a part of the new curative regime. The asylum would provide an environment in which the insane would be cured. By the 1860s under the County Asylums Act a number of county asylums had been built and writers on lunacy began to focus on what was needed in practical terms based on the experience of these asylums.

---

[3] While this chapter finishes at 1870, the interest in asylum designs was to continue. See from example T. S. Clouston's 'An Asylum, or Hospital-Home, for Two Hundred Patients: constructed on the principle of adaptation of various parts of the needs and mental states of inhabitants; with Plans, &c.'(1879) and Richard Greene's 'A Public Asylum, Designed for 414 Beds, capable of Extension to 600'(1880), as well as the later three volume work, *Hospitals and Asylums of the World* by Henry Burdett (1891) and George T. Hine's 1901 article 'Asylums and Asylum Planning.'

The 'ideal' asylum core principles as described by John Conolly were to continue down through the decades and can be found in some form in all the works of subsequent writers discussed. Later changes to Conolly's model included the shift from single accommodation to dormitories, the use of central dining halls, and a greater variation to the physical arrangements of the wards into blocks and cottages, not just the linear form. The use of classified space had moved from clearly delineated groups to the broader acute and chronic groupings, with patients also being classified as workers and given their own buildings. The subtle shift from the curative asylum to one with long term resident populations was reflected in these changing classifications. The separate cottages for workers, which offered less observation by the medical officers, speak of a long term resident population who could be employed to the economic advantage of the asylum.

The shift to the pavilion or block system was a response to the changing ideas about the role of the asylum in curing the patient, and the problem of the congregation of patients together. In effect the 'ideal' asylum had two parts: the first related to the regime of patient management and required the provision of certain types of space for the use of the patients and staff; the second related to prevailing ideas about healthy buildings and the provision of light, ventilation, sanitation and heating, which formed a significant part of most of the published works discussed above.

Each author's version of the requirements of the 'ideal' asylum included a range of features that are testable to varying degrees by the archaeologist. These include the physical layout of the buildings and their relationships to each other; the provision of appropriate rooms and spaces; the relationships between these rooms and spaces; and the location and settings of the lunatic asylum itself. As John Conolly provided the most detailed and testable of the models and as his features were included in most later models, it was decided to use his model as the core of the descriptive framework against which the built lunatic asylums of Britain and Australia could be compared. Consequently, in the following chapters the focus of the analysis is on Conolly's model, with some consideration of the other 'ideal's' to determine the influence of such works on the asylums constructed, and to understand the gap between the 'ideal' and reality, and what this can tell us about life within the lunatic asylums.

The British Lunatic Asylum: Ideals and Realities | 6

In 1859 John Arlidge argued that most, if not all; lunatic asylums were based on the design of Bethlem Hospital, itself based on the design of monasteries which had provided the early accommodation for the insane (Arlidge 1859: 200). Was this true? Were those given the task of designing and constructing lunatic asylums merely copying an established template? Or were they responsive to the current ideas about what was required in an 'ideal' asylum environment? This chapter examines a collection of British lunatic asylum plans to try and clarify to what extent the models of the 'ideal' asylum were realized in nineteenth century lunatic asylums. This is done by analyzing the buildings, their layouts, and the use of rooms as indicated on the plans or in accompanying legend, and comparing the results to the features detailed in the 'ideal' asylum models, such of those of Conolly, Jacobi, Sankey and Robertson as discussed in the last chapter. If the 'ideal' was not realized do they instead show an internal consistency that might be based on a replication of the Bethlem design?

A sample of asylum plans was collected by the author and included those of Bethlem and 19 lunatic asylums from across Great Britain including England, Wales and Ireland. For ease of discussion all of them have been classed together under the heading of 'British'. Many of the plans appeared in nineteenth century magazines and reports, and consequently they could not be reproduced here because of image quality problems. Consequently in Appendix 1 the locations of the plans discussed can be found.

The construction dates for these asylums range from 1814 to 1873 and cover the period during which the authors discussed in the previous chapter were writing. The date range used allows for a slight time lag, as such large scale building projects would have taken over a year to complete, and it is unlikely that building designs would be instantly responsive to new ideas. It is anticipated that these built asylums would change over time in response to the writings about what an asylum should be and the realities of actually using these buildings to care for the insane; in much the same way that the writings on what the 'ideal' asylum should be responded to the realities of accommodating large numbers of the insane in asylums, which in turn saw the proposal of cottage and pavilion asylums.

By looking at the asylums which were constructed, even using a small sample such as this one, it is possible to achieve a better understanding of the relationship between text and the reality of the built environment; and to understand the development of asylum design.

VARIETY AND EXPERIMENTATION: CHARITY HOSPITALS AND EARLY LUNATIC ASYLUMS 1800–1844

There are five lunatic asylums from this early period in the sample, and these asylums are also the ones for which the least detailed information is available. They are included as it is important to understand what came before the county asylums. These asylums did not just appear but were part of a development process that saw the rise of the large scale lunatic asylums where hundreds of patients were accommodated in one asylum. As the first detailed outline of the 'ideal' asylum did not appear until 1837 with Browne's work *What Asylums Were, Are and Ought to be*, these early asylums will be considered against the basic requirements of moral management and non-restraint, which included: classification, observation, freedom for the patients to undertake activities and exercise, kind and individualized treatment, and no restraints. Both these movements placed an emphasis on the provision of an appropriate environment for the care and cure of the insane person and formed the basis of the early descriptions of the 'ideal' asylum.

Classification

All of the asylums in this date range supported classification of the patients based on their mental condition by offering a range of wards. The new Bethlem Hospital opened at Southwark in 1812, offered wards over three full storeys and an attic floor. The men and women were accommodated in mirror wings on either side of a central administrative section. Accommodation was primarily in single cells with a small spur ward on either side providing three cells for the noisy patients.

James Bevan's design for the London Asylum of 1815 followed Stark's idea of the radial asylum discussed in the previous chapter, and offered seven arms of three storeys each, with all but one arm devoted to patient accommodation. The seventh arm housed the staff rooms, offices, laundry, and service rooms. The space between the arms was given over to airing courts, allowing three classified airing courts for men and three for women reflecting their classification in the arms of the asylum.

Watson and Pritchards's plan for the West Riding Asylum at Wakefield offered a similar design with two central spaces or hubs linked by a ward and wards extending out north/south and east/west from each hub. It is likely that the rooms in the hubs may have been offices, day rooms for the patients or something similar. Each side of the asylum had five airing courts with smaller cells and yards to the north of the main building possibly for refractory or noisy patients. Unfortunately the illustration is not clear enough to determine the legend on the rooms.

An adaptation of the radial design was used at the Devon County Asylum. Designed by Charles Fowler, it opened in 1842 with 420 beds. Here the wards were housed in the spokes radiating from the horse-shoe shaped main building. The spaces between the spokes were given over to airing courts and the ends of the spokes connected by single storey buildings with service rooms.

Not all early asylums followed this radial plan. The Middlesex County Asylum at Hanwell built, between 1829 and 1831, offered a return to the linear design of Bethlem. The original building consisted of a central octagonal pavilion with wards placed in an open U-shape around it. Each ward, in turn, ended in a pavilion. The asylum offered 300 beds over two storeys and was eventually expanded by the addition of further wings to accommodate 1,600 patients by the 1850s (Conolly 1847: 11; Arlidge 1859: 125).

While offering different designs, all the asylums offered a range of wards that were separate enough to offer a basic range of classification as required under the new treatment regimes, whether in the simple linear wards of Bethlem or the more complex radial designs. This would suggest that ideas about classification were moving from theoretical ideas to practical building designs.

Observation

The key to non-restraint had been the removal of restraints which were to be replaced by visual observation of the patients by the attendants and the medical superintendent. The radial design had first been recommended for prisoners, as its design supported the constant observation of the prisoners, by the staff in the central hub, and noise could be carried up and down the enclosed wings. This same design made it ideal for an asylum, and observation was further supported by the placement of day rooms close together in the hubs of both the London and West Riding Asylums, allowing easier observation by a few attendants. In contrast, the large wards of Bethlem presented more extreme difficulties for observation as the overall length of the building was 580ft. (Andrews et. al. 1997: 406–7).

Employment

Only one asylum, the West Riding Asylum, had work rooms marked on the plan. Reflecting a lack of awareness of the importance of diverse living spaces in the other asylums.

Amusements/activities

All the asylums provided day rooms for patient use, and the London Asylum provided a chapel for patients.

Exercise

All the asylums offered airing courts, from the basic level of three yards at Bethlem to the multiple airing courts of London Asylum.

Table 2. Ideal Asylum Features of W. A. F. Browne, 1837

A healthy site with a dry cultivatable soil, and an ample supply of natural water
A country site, elevated or on a slope, near enough to a town for supplies and activities
The asylum should be a series of one storey houses
Accommodation should be in the form of dormitories which aided ventilation and observation
Rooms should open on to a gallery
There should be galleries wide enough to be used as a common hall and work area
Heating through the asylum should encompass all areas
Windows should be placed low on the walls to allow a view out
There should be free access to airing courts for exercise
There should be baths, showers and water cleansing privies

THE 'IDEAL' ASYLUM OF BROWNE – 1837

In 1837, six years after Hanwell's opening, W. A. F. Browne published his book on what asylums were and should be. A comparison of his small list of recommended features (Table 3) with the asylums discussed above reveals only occasional matches. Certainly, none of the asylums were restricted to one storey, and all had single rooms instead of dormitories. Unfortunately, the question of galleries is more difficult to answer without a scale. The main function of Browne's gallery was as additional living space. Certainly, none of the asylums appear to have galleries wide enough to be used as a common hall and work area, although Bethlem and West Riding had galleries. They did however have the exercise yards to which one would expect reasonable access, and they also appear to have had baths. Water closets were provided. However some features such as heating and window position are not detectable on the plans. Clearly then, Browne's list of features reflects what was *not* occurring in the design of lunatic asylums during this period and what he felt was required instead.

Derby County Asylum – 1844

The Derby County Asylum, opened in 1844, continued the linear ward system of Bethlem and Hanwell. The primary modifications were firstly the extension of the wards at right angles to the main building line that gave a squared U shape to the central section (Figure 6.1), and the use of wings extending east-west from the central section at the point where the main line of the building meets the wards running north-south, and secondly the increase in the provision of administrative and service areas now placed in a centralized block. The extension of the wards into this three part layout most likely allowed the accommodation of the patients in spaces other than the attics and basement, as was the case at Bethlem Hospital. It is likely these latter spaces provided less than 'ideal' conditions.

If John Connolly considered Derby the embodiment of his 'ideal' asylum (Conolly 1847: 181), how then did it differ from the other earlier asylums? The features of the Derby Asylum included: 1) open day rooms and bays that allowed the attendant to observe activity in both these spaces and the gallery; 2) an external corridor that allowed passage around the asylum without a person passing through all wards; 3) it offered a smaller number of wards, allowing a simple classification of patients; 4) it possessed a number of beds reflecting the number of patients which the medical superintendent was capable of supervising directly; 5) it

Table 3. Conolly's Ideal Features Found in the British Lunatic Asylums

Lunatic Asylum	Date	A	B	C	D	Ea	Eb	Ec	F	G	Ha	Hb	Hc	Hd	Ia	Ib	J	K	L
Cheshire	1827–8	X		X		X	X		X	X		X				X		X		
Derby	1844	X	X	X	X	X	X	X	X	X				X	X	X	X	X	X	
Abergavenny	1852	X	X	X	X	X	X		X							X	X		X	
Eglinton	1852		X	X		X	X		X	X				X	X	X		X		
Lincolnshire	1852	X	X	X	X	X	X		X	X				X	X	X	X	X		
Buckinghamshire	1853	X	X	X	X	X	X		X	X	X	X	X	X	X	X	X		X	
Essex	1853	X	X	X		X	X		X	X	X	X	X	X	X	X				
Cambridgeshire	1858	X	X	X		X	X	X	X		X		X	X	X					
Cumberland	1858	X	X	X	X	X	X	X	X	X	X		X	X	X		X			
Sussex	1859	X	X	X	X	X	X	X	X		X		X	X	X		X			
Bedford	1860	X	X	X		X	X		X				X	X	X	X				
Bristol	1861	X	X	X		X	X	X		X	X		X	X	X		X			
Carmarthan	1862		X	X		X	X		X	X	X		X	X	X					
Surrey	1862		X	X		X	X		X	X			X		X					
Hereford	1871	X	X	X	X	X	X		X		X		X	X	X	X				
Whittingham	1873		X			X	X		X		X		X	X	X		X			

KEY

A - An appropriate site with some form of scenery
B - An arrangement of the buildings that allowed light in and cross ventilation, with no building overshadowing another or the airing courts
C - A linear form to the layout
D - It should accommodate no more than 360 to 400 inmates
Ea - A building that offered a range of wards for classification
Eb - Each ward should have its own attendant's rooms
Ec - There should be open areas as opposed to day rooms for patients
F - Each ward should have access to a bathroom, lavatory and water closets
G - Each ward should have a wide gallery furnished as a day room with windows low enough to allow a view outside
Ha - There should be a large recreation room
Hb - School rooms
Hc - Work rooms and workshops
Hd - A chapel for the use of patients
Ia - The offices should be centrally located
Ib - There should be a means of accessing the various wards without passing through each
J - Attendant's should have their own dining hall
K - Accommodation should primarily be in the form of single rooms with a few Dormitories
L - Above all the asylum should be light, cheerful and liberal in the space it offered

Figure 6.1. Simplified drawing of the wing arrangement at Derby County Asylum. (Drawn by author)

had a layout which did not block light or the flow of air from the wards; 6) it had workshops, women's workrooms, school and music rooms which allowed the employment of the patients and provided activity spaces for them; 7) there were centralized baths and water closets readily accessible from the various wards; 8) there was a range of exercise areas; 9) it had wide galleries, separate attendant's rooms and a dining hall for staff; and finally 10) accommodation was primarily in the form of single rooms (Conolly 1847: 21 & 24–5).

In effect, Conolly's 'ideal' asylum was achieved through a relatively simple design that used an existing asylum design, based on a linear arrangement. Derby was opened a year before the County Asylums Act was passed, which made the erection of county asylums for the pauper insane compulsory, and Conolly's book specifically addressed the design of asylums for paupers, with some comments made with regard to its modification for the middle classes (Conolly 1847: 43–44). It is important then to realize that Conolly's features were those required in an asylum for the lowest class within English society. Were later asylums to follow Derby's lead?

UNIFORMITY: THE COUNTY ASYLUMS – 1845 TO 1869

Thirteen of the sample plans collected fall into the period of 1845 to 1869 and reflect a period of major asylum construction. For ease of comparison to Conolly's 'ideal' asylum features, which are detailed in Table 3 and to the Derby Asylum, the asylums are treated as a group in this section. Conolly's requirements have also been broken down into components that can be directly compared with the plans in the sample, thus the grouping of school rooms; recreation room, workrooms and workshops, and chapel have been separated for the purpose of Table 3 which compares the asylums to Conolly's requirements. Cheshire Asylum is included in this period as the date for the plan is uncertain.

The plan was found in Frederick Manning's *Report on Lunatic Asylums* of 1868 and probably reflects a range of additions to the original.

A – An appropriate site with some form of scenery

From available information accompanying the plans, nine of the 13 asylums have this feature: Abergavenny and Lincolnshire both opened in 1852; Buckinghamshire and Essex opened in 1853; Cambridgeshire and Cumberland both opened in 1858; Sussex (1859); Bedford (1861); and Bristol (1861).

The Abergavenny Asylum, for example, was situated on a large tract of land which was being ornamentally laid out and cultivated (*The Builder* 1852: 299). Buckinghamshire, one of the smaller asylums, was situated on 20 acres, four miles from the town of Aylesbury; Essex County Asylum was built on 86 acres, 18 miles from London; and Sussex on 120 acres, 12 miles from Brighton (Crammer 1990: 31-2; *The Builder* 1857: 273; Robertson 1860: 248). Thus they all had room for airing courts, some level of privacy, and closeness to a source of supplies for the asylum's use.

Unfortunately, the question of scenery cannot be answered from plans, and even illustrations can be misleading, as the accompanying description in *The Builder* (1852: 299) notes that the artist had taken liberties with the scene in front of the Abergavenny Asylum.

B – An arrangement of the buildings that allowed light in and cross ventilation, with no building overshadowing another or the airing courts

All the asylums in this period achieved this feature through an adoption of a linear ward arrangement, often in the shape of an open 'W' with the bottom and side arms of the W accommodating wards and the central arm housing administrative and domestic rooms (figure 6.2). This period of asylum building saw an increasing uniformity in the design of the asylums. There was a central domestic/administrative area flanked on both sides by the male and female wards. This open design allowed the buildings to partially enclose a range of airing court spaces that could vary from two to three per side. Three generally supported the basic level of classification recommended by Conolly and allowed the separation of the refractory from the tranquil and convalescent. The presence and absence of scales on various plans makes direct comparisons difficult with regard to the size of airing courts; for example Derby appears to have more space in the interior airing courts

Uniformity: The County Asylums – 1845 to 1869

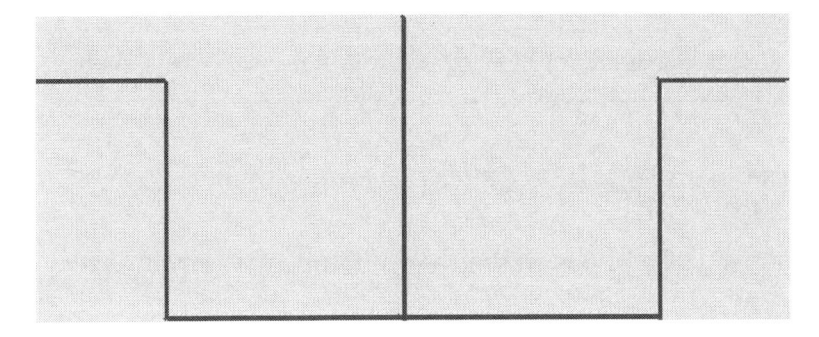

Figure 6.2. Simplified drawing of the Buckinghamshire County Asylum (Drawn by author)

than Abergavenny, but this may have been relative and distorted by the differing shapes.

The open layout of linear wards generally allowed for cross ventilation. Ventilation was increased, however, through the placement of sleeping and other rooms on only one side of the ward. Without a guide to window size and design, it is unclear how effective this might have been as design restraints, perhaps influenced by financial concerns saw day rooms and sanitary provisions being placed opposite sleeping rooms as at the Essex County Asylum and the Buckinghamshire Lunatic Asylum.

Not everyone accepted Conolly's ideas about cross ventilation. Cambridgeshire Asylum, which was built to the plans of an 'experienced superintendent and amateur architect, Mr. Hill' (Robertson 1860: 248), had dormitories opposite the single rooms on both the ground and first floors.

C – A linear layout

All of the asylums of this period saw an adoption of the linear form to the buildings. The primary variation lay in the placement of service areas. In some asylums they continued the corridor form as at Abergavenny, in others they formed blocks adjacent to the wards as at Cambridgeshire.

D – It should accommodate no more than 360 to 400 patients

In this respect the asylums in the sample varied, some such as Buckinghamshire and Lincolnshire were smaller in this case 200 and 250 beds respectively. Others such as Eglinton and Essex were larger at 500 and

450 beds respectively. A range of factors may have contributed to this variation, the primary ones being the known number of insane requiring accommodation in the county, and probably the cost.

Ea – A building that offered a range of wards for classification

All of the asylums in the sample fulfilled this requirement only varying in the number of storeys they had, although all most likely had at least two. Eglinton Asylum had three storeys (*The Builder* 1852: 754) as did Cambridgeshire; Lincolnshire had two floors (Palmer 1859: 73). Both the design and the number of floors decided just how many wards were provided, but there were generally two to three wards on the ground floor. These wards differed in their design and could form short infirmary wards of a few rooms, or much larger main wards as at Bristol, Cumberland and Westmoreland Asylums.

Eb – Each ward should have its own attendant's rooms

Table 3 shows that all the asylums in the sample had this feature which Conolly considered necessary for the well-being of the attendants who spent most of their days and nights with the patients.

Ec – There should be open areas as opposed to day rooms for patients

Conolly had made this recommendation with the ease of observation in mind, so that the patients would always be visible to the two attendants in each ward. However this feature was not generally adopted by the asylums. Cambridgeshire Asylum provided only large day rooms and no other day space, which meant the patients were always in view. A similar arrangement was followed at Sussex. However, plans can be misleading in some respects, as the Cumberland and Westmoreland Asylum had day rooms with glazed walls that prevented a sense of confinement and opened the room to observation (16th Report Commissioners in Lunacy 1862: 209).

F – Each ward should have access to a bathroom, lavatory and water closets

All of the asylums had these features. They did, however, vary in terms of whether each ward had its own bathroom and water closets. Buckinghamshire and the Bedford, Hertford and Huntingdon

(Three Counties) Lunatic Asylums, like Derby, placed these at the intersections of the wards meaning that they were shared by two or three wards. Other asylums such as Essex and Cheshire had provisions on each ward.

G – Each ward should have a wide gallery furnished as a day room with windows low enough to allow a view

Only the asylums from the early 1850s had gallery spaces as recommended by Conolly for use as additional day space. The later asylums converted the gallery space to dormitory space as at Cambridgeshire, or used differing arrangements of the day and sleeping rooms as at Sussex. The question of windows is not possible to answer from plans, nor can window size be accurately determined from the available illustrations.

Ha – There should be a large recreation room

Half of the asylums had large recreation rooms, and the asylums are spread over the date range. They tended to be centrally located and accessible to both men and women.

Hb – School rooms

Only three asylums had school rooms: Buckinghamshire, Essex and Cambridgeshire. The use of dedicated spaces allowed for a variation in the day to day routine of patients. Day rooms could be used for this purpose but did not allow variation in the daily routine.

Hc – Workrooms and workshops

All the asylums of this period had workshops and laundries where men and women respectively were generally employed. The provision of work rooms for women was variable, Abergavenny had several rooms for example, and others none.

Hd – A chapel

Of the sample, 10 asylums from this period had chapels and the remaining two might have had external chapels not indicated on the plans. This reflected the recognition of the role religion played in retraining the mind of the inmates.

Ia – Centrally located offices

The use of a linear design generally saw the centralization of offices through the natural division into male and female sides. The placement of the Superintendent's and Matron's rooms in the central area allowed them to be readily accessible day and night. Interestingly, the Three Counties Asylum provided the only variation to the placement of the offices with a connecting passage between the two main wards on each side containing assistant surgeon's and assistant matron's rooms. The central administrative area was generally associated with domestic offices, including the kitchen, stores, and pantries.

Ib – There should be a means of accessing the various wards without passing through each

Only a handful of the asylums in the sample had this feature, which Conolly believed was necessary to prevent disturbances in the wards.

J – Attendant's should have their own dining hall

Again only a few asylums had this feature. Abergavenny, for example, had a general servant's hall, as did Cheshire.

K – Accommodation should be primarily in the form of single rooms with few dormitories

The asylums showed a range of distributions of single rooms to dormitories and only Abergavenny, Buckinghamshire and Sussex appear to match Conolly's requirement.

DISCUSSION

Table 4 shows that many of the British asylums had a large proportion of Conolly's 17 features, with most falling between 13 and 17. Surrey had the lowest number of matches with only seven, while Carmarthen had eight. There is no particular pattern in the adoption of features. Those asylums built closest to the publication of Conolly's book did not conform most closely to his requirements, and there was no lessening of the matches the further away in time one went from the publication of Conolly's book. The closeness of Conolly's 'ideal' asylum to those actually built may be the product of the copying of existing

Discussion

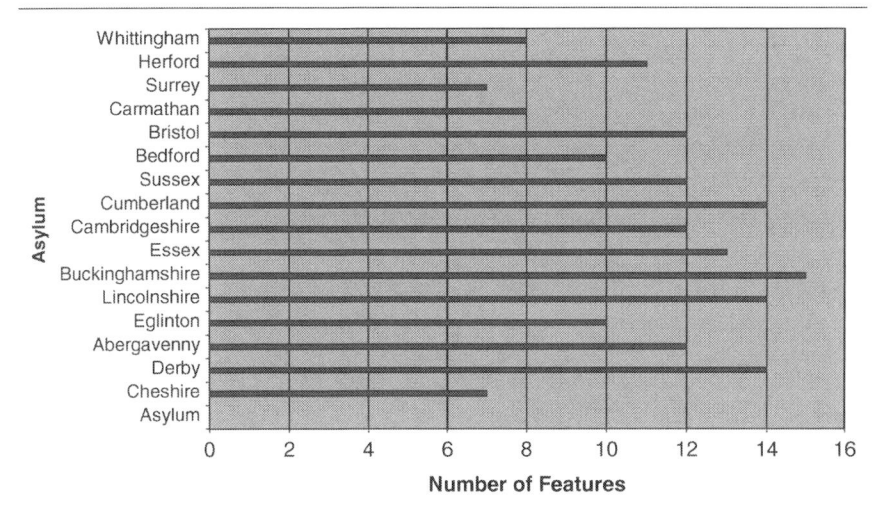

Table 4. The Number of Conolly's Features Found in Each Asylum

Asylum	Number of Features
Cheshire	7
Derby	14
Abergavenny	12
Eglinton	10
Lincolnshire	14
Buckinghamshire	15
Essex	13
Cambridgeshire	12
Cumberland	14
Sussex	12
Bedford	10
Bristol	12
Carmathan	8
Surrey	7
Herford	11
Whittingham	8

asylum designs, combined with a recognition of those features deemed necessary for providing a healthy and viable asylum environment. As can be seen from Table 5, the main variations occurred in size. At the time of construction many asylums would have come under Conolly's requirement, but many also went far beyond it. The late 1850s/early 1860s saw a growing realization that asylums were rapidly filling

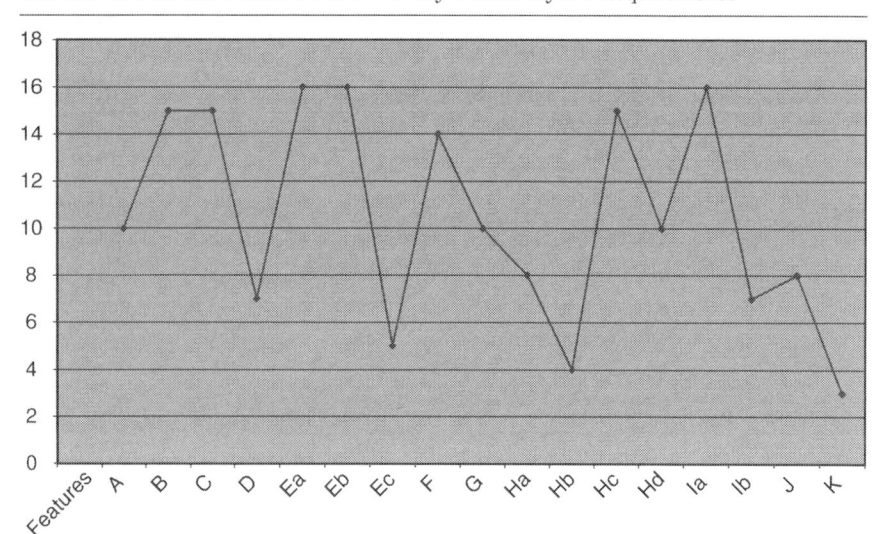

Table 5. Distribution of Matches to Conolly's Ideal Asylum Requirements

Features	
A	10
B	15
C	15
D	7
Ea	16
Eb	16
Ec	5
F	14
G	10
Ha	8
Hb	4
Hc	15
Hd	10
Ia	16
Ib	7
J	8
K	3

up with an apparently ever-increasing number of the insane, and a cycle of additions to existing asylums began. Consequently the original small asylums were rapidly expanded, with the average number of beds increasing to 548.6 by 1870 (Scull 1979: 198). In the case of

Discussion

individual asylums, Surrey County Asylum in 1859 had been enlarged to accommodate 700 additional patients despite opposition (*The Builder* 5/11/1859: 722). By 1866 additions to the Asylum of West Riding of Yorkshire had brought the population of patients to 1,150 (*The Builder* 23/6/1866: 458). With the addition of a 134 bed ward for men in 1871 the County and City Lunatic Asylum at Worcester became capable of taking between 700 and 800 patients. While the County Asylum at Macclesfield opened in 1871 with beds for 250, building work was still undertaken to bring its capacity up to 700 patients (*The Builder* 3/6/71: 424; 8/7/71). Consequently size was to be a large variable, with no standard size, and early matches quickly lost.

A consideration of Table 3 suggests that the features not commonly found were those that were not essential to the effective running of the asylums. Conolly's 'ideal' asylum model had combined features that were essential to create a healthy environment within the asylum and the effective management of the patients, with other features that sought to make life more comfortable for patients and staff. The latter included the rooms for various activities, the separation of day rooms from work rooms for the women, the possibilities of a view from windows and the provision of attendant's dining halls to allow them some time away from the patients. It was these spaces which were the least commonly adopted features of the British asylums.

The absence of school rooms, attendant's dining halls, and open day areas as opposed to day rooms, can be seen as an absence of discretionary spaces. These were not essential to providing healthy, reasonable living areas, and if building to a specific cost, they were the most amenable to being left out. The provision of discretionary spaces also led to variations between the asylums, for example Cambridgeshire had day rooms and water closets in its airing courts, and Lincolnshire had attendant's sitting rooms on the wards. The fact that Medical Superintendents were involved in their design, may have led to the inclusion of spaces that they recognized from their own experience were needed. Robertson's role in planning the Sussex Asylum saw the provision of a range of spaces for patients including a recreation hall, dining hall and library (Robertson 1860: 267). However, only Lincolnshire provided a ward designed specifically for a particular class of patients. The refractory ward had only single rooms, as noisy patients often disturbed each other in dormitories; it had only a bay rather than an enclosed day room allowing easier observation of the patients, and had a padded room (Palmer 1859: 74).

School rooms appear in three asylums, and a central recreation hall in eight asylums, with only two asylums built in the same year having both. An examination of the features of the Buckinghamshire and Essex Asylums shows a similar close correlation of other features. However they were not designed by the same architect (Taylor 1991: 202). Of the sample, only two architects are represented twice, H. E. Kendall who designed the Essex and Sussex Asylums, and David Brandon who designed Bedford and Carmarthen Asylums (Taylor 1991: 202–203). Bedford and Carmarthen shared most of the same features, with the variation being that Bedford (the earlier of the two) had a chapel and external communication corridors. Bedford had enclosed day rooms while Carmarthen had open day spaces. Kendall's two asylums were identical in most points, with Essex having a slightly different arrangement of day spaces and a school room. From this small amount of evidence it is difficult to speculate whether these differences reflected the requests of the County authorities or changing thoughts about the design of the asylums on the part of the architects. However, overall, the consistency of features in asylums designed by a range of architects does suggest some agreement on the need for Conolly's requirements as expressed in the 'ideal' model.

The County Asylums of this period shared another trend that did not meet with the approval of writers on the 'ideal' asylum. This was the linking of work areas with wards specifically for workers. These wards separated these patients in some cases from the rest of the asylum world. At Bristol Asylum dormitories, day rooms, attendant's rooms, baths and water closets were provided adjacent to and above the laundry and workshops on the female and male sides respectively. It appears from the plans that the working patients were physically separated from the other patients in their wards by the lack of any access point to workers' wards from the main wards. They would have to be taken across the airing court to reach the dining hall, but probably ate in the day room provided. Interestingly, while the laundry was internally accessible for the women, the men were required to go outside and around the workshops to enter them. This may have been a means of keeping the male area well ventilated or it may have prevented patients from freely accessing tools, but this must remain speculation.

The question of directly associating patient accommodation with their work area caused some concern for writers on lunatic asylums (Arlidge 1859: 143). It was felt that the workers may not experience the feeling that they were in an asylum recovering; rather they had just exchanged one working life for another. Certainly living directly above the work areas and with no gallery space to use, the patient's lives were considerably restrained in the variety of spaces they could use. This factor gains more importance if we consider that working patients were often those who were chronically ill and likely to remain for the rest of their lives within the asylum. As Conolly indicated, these patients needed more variety in their spaces than short term patients because of the time they were to spend in the asylum (Conolly 1847: 4–5).

Overall, the county asylums from this period showed a marked similarity in their separation of the worlds of the asylum. There was a central administrative world, often with the domestic rooms in close proximity. The wards on either side of this formed separate patient worlds, while the service areas were either separated physically or separated from the wards by points of access, creating a third world. The only time the patient world interacted with the administrative world was on arrival and departure, and when the recreation hall or chapel was centrally located next to the administrative area. At Essex County Asylum this separation was maintained by placing the chapel and school rooms at the back of the asylum between the wards.

LATER COUNTY ASYLUMS – 1870 TO 1880

The idea of the pavilion asylum as recommended by Robertson in 1867 does not appear to have been realized in the two county asylums in the sample dating to this period. The Hereford County and City Asylum, opened in 1871 for 400 patients, continued the linear corridor system of the earlier county asylums and in building layout comes closest to Cheshire. Hereford Asylum comes very close to Conolly's model, providing a range of patient and staff spaces including recreation rooms as well as a central dining and recreation hall (Table 3). There was a chapel and the women were provided with a separate sewing room where the first and infirmary wards met, and there appears to have been attendant's living rooms as recommended by Conolly. The laundry and workshops were provided with their own day room and kitchens, an interesting inclusion allowing the workers to have hot meals. The male side was also provided with a dirty clothing washhouse, suggesting some recognition of the hard labor the women endured in doing all the asylum laundry.

The Third Lancashire County Asylum at Whittingham, opened in 1873, was designed by the Medical Superintendent, Dr. Holland (Taylor 1991: 146). It offered a mixture of pavilions and linear wards in a shape that echoed the horseshoe shape of Devon asylum and the end pavilions of Cheshire Asylum. The asylum consisted of a D-shaped arrangement of corridor wards. The administrative offices and the domestic offices formed the centre. Linking the male and female sections of the asylum was a large recreation hall flanked by male and female dining halls. Of all the asylums, Whittingham reflects the most diverse arrangement with a series of wards and pavilion blocks offering a variety of accommodation and day space for the patients. The ability to provide a diverse range of wards may have reflected Dr. Holland's beliefs about the classification of patients, but interestingly, would have required staff to travel large distances to supervise the patients which should have been a priority for the Superintendent. As with Hereford, Whittingham came close to Conolly's model (Table 3).

THE 'IDEAL' ASYLUMS OF JACOBI, SANKEY AND ROBERTSON

While it has become apparent that many of the county asylums came close to Conolly's 'ideal' asylum, what of the other 'ideal' models? Jacobi's 1841 model falls in the period where there are few examples in the sample. In terms of the asylums that came later in the 1850s and 1860s, a few met Jacobi's requirement of having 200 patients. One of these was Buckinghamshire Asylum. Cambridgeshire and Lincolnshire came close at 252 and 250 patients respectively. All favored a linear layout, but none of the asylums followed Jacobi's suggestion of arranging houses around courtyards. Most met the requirements of a country location with the exception of Essex Asylum which was placed in the urban setting of Brentwood (Manning 1868: 17). While there was a strict separation of the sexes, the linear design meant that the various classes were visible to each other to some degree. Certainly all the asylums offered classification of the patients and small spur wards which could be used to separate the noisy and infirmary patients if necessary. As these asylums were for paupers there was no emphasis in providing different rooms for the various social classes as Jacobi recommended.

To achieve light and ventilation most of the asylums included in this sample used a linear ward system in an open layout. The problem in designing an asylum was to place the various parts in such a way that no part of the wards had the light block by another part. The asylums in the sample often had wards that were arranged at right angles to each other or were offset from each other, such as at Essex asylum, to overcome this problem. The open W shape used at many of the asylums allowed the creation of airing court spaces (Figure 6.2), but this may actually have hindered air flow into the ground floor wards as airing court walls were generally 8 to 10 ft. high to prevent escapes. The placement of rooms on one side of the gallery in the wards allowed for a range of windows to allow light in, but it was up to the architect what size these windows should be. Hence the arrangement did not always guarantee that wards would be filled with light. This led writers such as Conolly to specify the size of windows on the wards (Conolly 1847: 15).

It is clear from the plans that airing courts were provided, but from the documentary evidence of the *Sixteenth Annual Report of the Commissioners in Lunacy* (1862) the presence of an airing court did not mean that it was necessarily useable (16th Report. Comm. in Lunacy 1862). The work areas provided tended to be those that would support the economy of the asylum and their provision would be automatic. The main difference would have been the employment of the patients in place of servants, rather than in the provision of rooms. The asylums from the 1850s and 1860s did provide chapels as recommended by Jacobi. While differently arranged than Jacobi's 'ideal' model, these asylums did embody most of the features of Jacobi's 'ideal'.

In 1856 W. Sankey had offered a different model for the layout of the county lunatic asylum. Sankey had based his model on an asylum for 1,000 patients; unfortunately it is not clear from the sample plans whether the later asylums, such as Whittingham, were approaching this size. Certainly asylums were rapidly becoming larger as a result of additions. Sankey's model echoed Conolly's model in its requirement for the division of the asylum along gender lines, the inclusion of centralized offices, a recreational hall and chapel. However its biggest departures were in the recommendation of the separation of the day and night time rooms to different floors and the placement of officer's rooms in the divisions rather than in the central building. None of the asylums in the sample achieved this separation of day and night spaces and rooms. Wards continued to contain both sleeping and day spaces on the ground floor. While some such as Sussex and the Three Counties Asylum had floors dedicated purely to sleeping accommodation, they retained the dormitory room arrangement rather than moving to the open plan wards suggested by Sankey. Only the Three Counties Asylum had rooms for its officers distributed throughout the asylum. Both Sankey and Arlidge, a few years later, had followed Conolly in arguing for more patient rooms, such as libraries and dining rooms, reflecting the continuing absence of these rooms in the asylums built. Most asylums were, however, to include separate infirmary wards in their designs as recommended by Sankey.

There is no evidence of the rationalization of space and room use as recommended by Sankey and Arlidge, and certainly Arlidge's belief that asylum life should be as home-like as possible was far from being realized with the maintenance of the gallery ward with its day rooms and dormitories. The only exceptions to this were the undated additions to the Essex, Three Counties and Surrey asylums which were more 'home-like'.

The plan of the Three Counties asylum, in the 1862 16th Annual Report of the Commissioners in Lunacy, included two small plans of the proposed asylum cottage. The cottage was composed on the ground floor of a sitting room, a dining room, a kitchen, a six bed dormitory and two attendant's rooms. On the first floor were four dormitories of six, six, eight and nine beds respectively, a single room and a third attendant's room. This was probably as close to normal home life as an asylum patient could find. While not indicated, the cottage may have been for worker patients, chronic or imbecile patients, in which case it provided one to two day spaces for 35–36 patients; effectively offering an existence little different from the wards.

The plans for the additional buildings at Essex Asylum were published in 1868 (Manning 1868) and again it is not indicated whether they were actually built or proposed. The additions consisted of two cottages and a third building that was extended beyond the cottage to include a kitchen, laundry, attendants' rooms and a dining hall for 100 patients. Each cottage had a large ground floor day room and four single rooms opening off this room. Across the passage was a downstairs bath and water closet. Upstairs was a large dormitory and two attendants' rooms. The arrangement of these buildings suggests that they too were probably intended for chronic or working patients. The presence of the laundry and kitchen suggests that the buildings were intended for a self-sufficient group of patients. Women patients would work in the laundry and kitchen, while others were occupied in the day rooms. The only variety in the day was provided by the dining hall, which may have been adaptable as a recreation space. Here, then, was a form of Sankey's and Arlidge's re-organization of the asylum space into separate day and night areas, and also Toller's 1865 idea of the cottage asylum with patients classified into working or type of mental illness groups.

DISCUSSION

This chapter has set out to address several questions. These included: were the county asylums built between 1842 and 1880 copies of Bethlem Hospital as suggested by John Arlidge? Did the designs for these asylums become more standardized under the compulsory County Asylums Act of 1845?

Arlidge had argued in 1859 that the existing county asylums were copies of Bethlem Hospital, which consisted of a linear building with a number of wards composed of single rooms with accompanying day rooms. His argument appears to be valid in two respects. Firstly the wards continued to be composed of single rooms and day rooms, with a few dormitories added. Space was arranged in a similar way in the wards themselves. Secondly the county asylums had not broken away from the pattern of linear wards with a centralized administrative centre. Ward designs show very little adaptation to the varying needs of particular groups of patients and, as Arlidge had argued, bore little resemblance to the homes of the patients. Variations seemed to occur in the placement of dormitories in relation to single rooms and in the discretionary spaces provided for the patients, such as school rooms, dining and recreation halls, rather than in major changes to the layout of the lunatic asylum itself.

Prior to 1845 there was a period of experimentation in the design of lunatic asylums. Layouts included house-like designs, radial plans, modified H-shapes, pavilion and linear designs. These designs saw various arrangements of sleeping spaces, day rooms, and work areas, along with varying provisions in the day time living spaces of the patients. With the passing of the 1845 County Asylum Act this experimentation all but disappeared and for around 20 years there appears to have been a standardization of design that may have reflected a copying of existing designs. These buildings returned to the linear ward arrangement as found at Bethlem Hospital and seen as so successful by Conolly at Derby. Certainly the experimentation found before 1845 did not return until after 1870, when asylums increased in size. The London County Asylum at Cane Hill, completed in 1883, was initially designed for 1,200 patients and the East Sussex Asylum at Hellingly for 1,115 patients (Hine 1901: 175). Asylums designed for such large populations required different arrangements of the wards, such as a linear W shape if they were to successfully distribute the wards over an area manageable to the staff. Designs included pavilion arrangements and different patterns for the placement of wards in connection with each other.

LIFE WITHIN THE ASYLUM

The analysis above gives a beginning point for understanding lunatic asylums, a way of organizing information to understand how asylums were arranged. But to understand life within the asylums we have to look at the impact on life of the provision or absence of rooms and spaces called for in the 'ideal' asylum models. Plans represent a static moment in time when the asylum was planned and built and not necessarily the use a room will be put to when the buildings are filled with people. To understand the room use we need to look at documents relating to individual asylums. In the later case studies of South Australia and Tasmania this approach will be taken. For the British asylums this was not possible, but it is still possible to obtain an understanding of room use at English county asylums through the Commissioners in Lunacy's *Sixteenth Annual Report* of 1862. Several of the plans discussed in this chapter came from this report. The Commissioners in Lunacy, had been charged by the English Parliament with the task of inspecting county asylums, and of making recommendations in relation to them (see Hervey 1985: 103–4), and the question of the provision of rooms and spaces to make life for the patients more comfortable was a matter of concern for them.

The Commissioners' *Sixteenth Report* reveals the flexibility of room use within the asylums and the problems of interpreting room use solely from plans. For example while the plan of Buckinghamshire County Asylum (which was included in the sample) had not shown a central recreation hall, the visitors were happy to note that:

> ... Entertainments, comprising music and dancing, in which the Patients of both sexes associate, are now given weekly, and in these about 100 generally take part.

It appears that a gallery was being used for this purpose as they went on to remark:

> ... we think that the construction of a new and larger chapel, and appropriation of the present to the purposes of a recreation and dining hall, will have soon to be considered (16th Report. Comm. in Lunacy 1862: 106).

So while Buckinghamshire did not have the central recreation recommended by Connolly, this did not preclude entertainments from being held. However the use of a gallery or similar space would have limited the number of patients who could attend; this is reflected in the Report's recommendation of the re-use of the chapel. Chapels at asylums were often unconsecrated to allow a more flexible use of space. By calling for a recreation room to be included in the planning of an asylum Conolly was making sure that space would be available for that purpose and an absence of space could not be used as an excuse not to relieve the boredom of asylum life.

At Abergavenny the visitors anticipated that the new spacious day room over the laundry could be used for amusements for both sexes. At Nottingham County and Borough Asylum they noted that the ironing room had been given a ceiling and could be used as a recreation hall (16th Report. Comm. in Lunacy 1862: 149 & 154). Clearly any large, plain room could be put to a number of purposes, depending on the mobility of the furniture. A room furnished with large tables would be impractical for a range of uses, while one furnished with small moveable tables lent itself to various uses. In terms of the plans considered above, the description of a room as a day room may not indicate its full range of uses, and the lack of a central recreation hall does not indicate that both sexes did not interact. Day rooms could easily be provided with shelves for books and musical instruments and galleries could be used for dances. At Hanwell women had access to a room called the Bazaar, a 'large, lofty, cheerful and well furnished apartment' adjoining the chapel. This apartment was used for three different purposes: firstly as a superior day room for the women; secondly as a fine needlework room and thirdly for parties. Men did not have access to a similar room, reflecting the differences between male and female experience of the asylum (16th Report. Comm. in Lunacy 1862: 143 and 144; see also Piddock 1999).

However, the flexible use of space was not limited to the provision of spaces for entertainments. At Cambridge County Asylum, where there was insufficient female accommodation, visitors noted that it was contemplated to use part of the male wing for the women. The visitors, however, recommended using the space under the roof, if ceilings and windows were put in, for this purpose. At Lancaster, they recommend the practicalities of turning the basement rooms into day rooms. Pressures on accommodation could also lead to the loss of recreation rooms - at Worcester the recreation hall had been converted into an infirmary ward. The visitors recommended its restoration and use for recreation and as a school when the new infirmary was built (16th Report. Comm. in Lunacy 1862: 108, 131 & 175). What is clear from these comments is that the lunatic asylum space was not static, and was responsive most often to the needs of a particular time. Ward accommodation had to take precedence over entertainment rooms. However it is important to realize that the spaces that might be called discretionary in Conolly's 'ideal' model were given primary importance by the Commissioners who were directly concerned with patient welfare. Room flexibility did bring the British county asylums even closer to Conolly's model if individual asylums are considered over a period of time.

Asylums were, in effect, organic in their development with changes to room use and the provision of spaces over time in response to need, funds and annual inspections by the Lunacy Commissioners. The mirror imaging of the asylum plan, which appears quite frequently, can be deceptive as access to various rooms, particularly in the central section of the asylum, and the use of spaces may be based on the associated gender roles of each sex (Piddock 1999). Access to particular day rooms may be answerable by considering passages and access ways for example; a method often used to interpret space in archaeologically based studies (West 1999: Figures 7.2 to 7.3). But the use of the male wing by women at Cambridgeshire Asylum and the use of the ironing room as a recreation space at Nottinghamshire Asylum, which is likely to be marked as 'male' and 'ironing room' on a plan, present clear problems to the archaeologist trying to understand how space was used within the asylum. Only an integrated approach using all possible sources of information makes such analysis viable in terms of lunatic asylums.

The demands to accommodate the patients and the provision of rooms necessary for the economically efficient running of the asylum were likely to take precedence over spaces for recreational activities, even if such recreations were seen as part of the cure of the patient. The visitors, when they found patients who were listless, excited or noisy, often recommended that these patients be allowed more exercise away from the wards, more opportunities for occupation and amusement and that the ward environment be improved (16th Report. Comm. in Lunacy 1862: 130, 138 and 162). Efforts were being made at some asylums to improve life for the patients through changes to the physical environment. The Buckinghamshire County Asylum had built a greenhouse to grow plants and flowers for the wards, while at Cambridgeshire County Asylum, a skittle alley was being constructed and a bowling green established. At some asylums the airing courts were in such a poor state that they were unusable in the winter months. The visitors recommended the creation of gardens within the courts and the provision of sun shades (16th Report. Comm. in Lunacy 1862: 106, 109 129, 140, 145, & 175).

The reports often commented on a lack of furnishings - chairs, tables, seats, prints and carpets - in a number of asylums. At the Middlesex Asylum at Colney Hatch "Everywhere there is a deficiency of comfortable and ordinary domestic furniture; backed seats, chairs, sofas, and small tables, were required for the galleries and day-rooms." (16th Report. Comm. in Lunacy 1862: 139; see also 146, 160 & 161). Others lacked wash basins and stands, combs, brushes and towels for daily use on the wards. Few of the asylums had curtains or blinds on the windows to keep out the cold and the visitors reported that some asylums were making efforts to curtain windows (16th Report. Comm. in Lunacy 1862: 104, 105, 127, 139, & 146, 147).

Many asylums needed the walls painted or colored. These furnishings were needed to provide a basic level of comfort for the patients. As Conolly noted, there was no reason to believe that the insane were not aware of their surroundings (Conolly 1847: 9). Many of the asylums were particularly lacking in the area of amusements. The visitors recommended the purchase of books and newspapers for the wards at the Three Counties Asylum along with other amusements and were happy to note the building of a library at Cambridgeshire. But the presence of a library did not always mean that the books circulated through the wards. At Hanwell, of 436 books in the women's library only 60 to 80 were ever in circulation. The men's library by contrast only contained 180 volumes (16th Report. Comm. in Lunacy 1862: 104, 109–110 & 144). So while the 'ideal' model would indicate that the requirements appear to have been met, in reality the naming of a room did not in fact indicate its use.

The presence of rooms and spaces did not necessarily mean that they were furnished. This may have been a pattern remaining from the time when restraints were used and the insane were seen as less than human, or it may have been an economizing factor in response to the costs of constructing a lunatic asylum. All the authors who wrote on the 'ideal' asylum, from Tuke to Sankey, had not only included the built environment in their models, but included both the internal furnishings and activities available to the patients. Authors such as Jacobi and Conolly recommended the provision of chairs, tables, armchairs, wash basins/stands for patient use, board games, books, curtained windows, birds and animals and so forth to provide a more home-like environment and to break the monotony of the appearance of the wards and life within them (Jacobi 1841: 107; Conolly 1847: 52–4). Connolly and Arlidge recommended the provision of school rooms and libraries for patient use; a chapel and some kind of central dining hall or recreation hall; gardens and airing courts planted with flowers and trees were equally recommended by most authors as basic requirements (Conolly 1847: 52–4). Clearly, from the visitors' reports included in the Commissioners in Lunacy reports there was no uniformity to the recreational spaces and to the internal furnishings of the county lunatic asylum. Rather there were 'ideal's such as those expressed by Jacobi, Conolly, and the other writers on lunacy, whose translation into the real world of the asylum was to vary considerably.

A GENDERED WORLD

If the lunatic asylums were intended to provide a curative environment, they also, through the principles of internal management and classification, created an artificial world where the inmates' daily lives and movement through the asylum reflected ideas about gender. Internal worlds were created within the areas of the asylum inhabited by the men and women that were directly affected by the roles men and women played in the world outside of the asylum. These roles dictated suitable activities, both work and leisure related, for each group and led to different provisions for men and women in the asylum in terms of room allocations and movement through the asylum space.

As seen above, the lunatic asylum was divided into two halves by the central administrative block, this effectively creating two separate worlds, one for men and one for women. Only occasionally did the two worlds meet in the central recreation room if there was one (16th Report. Comm. in Lunacy 1862: 149). The laundry and drying rooms, and possibly a sewing room, were generally attached to the women's side of the asylum. On the men's side a series of workshops were usually found. It is in this provision of work areas that the assumed roles of men and women outside of the asylum find their clearest expression.

One of the basic tenets of moral treatment was the provision of some kind of activity, both to occupy the mind and to retrain it in good moral values (Conolly 1847: 78). This kind of activity was often seen in terms of labor as opposed to recreational activities. In the world of the asylum, work for women was defined as being purely domestic, despite the range of work women did outside of the asylum (Perkin 1995: 169–201). Women were employed predominantly in the laundry or in doing needlework. At some asylums they served in the kitchen but this does not seem to have been a general practice (Conolly 1847: 78–9). While authors such as Conolly recommended the provision of separate sewing rooms, women generally spent the day sitting in the galleries or in the day rooms sewing. The only time they left the ward was when they were taken down to the airing courts for periods of exercise. That this did not always occur is reflected in the *Suggestions and Instructions* issued by the Board of Lunacy Commissioners of Scotland published in 1859, which indicated that "the day rooms and workrooms for the females should be so arranged as to afford ready communication with the grounds," (Comm. in. Lunacy 1871: 480). By this means attendants could more easily ensure that women went outside. In 1861 the Commissioners of Lunacy found that more than two-thirds of the women in the Hants County Asylum never walked beyond the airing court walls. They recommended a reduction in the women's working hours to allow them to exercise and participate in recreations (16th Report. Comm. in Lunacy 1862: 127).

The women working in the laundry led similarly constrained lives, often eating their meals in a room adjacent to the laundry, returning to the galleries at the end of the working day or in some cases sleeping over the laundry (Arlidge 1859: 143). By contrast, the range of activities available to men was far more diverse. Most asylums provided tailor's, carpenter's and cobbler's shops. Men worked on the farm and in the garden producing food for the asylum (Conolly 1847: 52).

They were also employed in maintenance work such as painting and general laboring around the asylum. Men were generally employed in the brew houses and bake houses of larger asylums. At Colney Hatch, one of the largest asylums with over 1500 beds, there was an upholstery shop and printing shop again offering different activities for men (Conolly 1847: 81; Art. 111. 1857: 375; Hunter and MacAlpine 1974: 130).

In an interesting contrast men were often encouraged to learn new skills, woodworking for example, or were allowed to amuse themselves in the workshops (Art. 111. 1857: 371). Women's work was seen more in terms of its economic value, as Conolly noted "The importance of the duties of the laundry being regularly performed may be productive of some disposition to overwork the patients employed in it" (Conolly 1847: 88). In sewing clothes and linen for the asylum the women were also directly contributing to the economy of the asylum (Hunter & MacAlpine 1974: 131).

As even the very sick women were able to sew, there was often a major difference in the number of women and men employed within the asylum. At Colney Hatch in 1857, of 503 women capable of working, 270 sewed, 72 worked in the laundry, and 125 helped in the ward. The value of their work was put at 500 pounds a year. Of the 514 men, only 245 were considered employable, with 180 working in the workshops and 65 farming or gardening (Art. 111. 1857: 372). In 1884 54 percent of women at Colney Hatch were 'usefully employed', compared to 38 percent of men (Hunter and MacAlpine 1974: 130). The monotony of life on the wards becomes most clear when going to the kitchens to fetch meals was seen by the women as a treat, as was being allowed out to participate in hay making (Art. 111 1857: 378).

While an initial examination of the plans would suggest that women and men had similar worlds based on the mirror imaging of the main buildings, a closer examination reveals that women's worlds were much more confined than men's. Their movements were far more limited and they were very much confined to a limited number of areas: the gallery, the day room, the laundry rooms, the airing courts, and occasionally the grounds for walks. Men, while having similar access to the gallery, day room and airing court, also had a variety of workshops and service rooms to use, as well as being able to work outdoors and around the asylum grounds and wards.

It is important that in examining plans we do not make the automatic assumption that the placement of the laundry rooms on the women's side of the asylum was natural. There was no reason that men could not do the laundry. Gender roles about appropriate work for men and women seem to be at their most influential in the asylum and in the workhouse in England. Women in the eighteenth century worked as field hands and in gardens producing food (Hill 1994: 150), so there was no reason for women not to help in the gardens in asylums. Yet Conolly in 1847 clearly states that the men were involved in gardening, while women were simply observers showing an interest in the fruit and vegetables as they passed by on their walks (Conolly 1847: 52). It appears that the strongest influence in determining women's movements and activities was the growing association of women with the home and passive activities, otherwise characterized as the cult of domesticity (Showalter 1981: 320; Welter 1966: 159, 162, & 165).

This narrowness of women's movements through the lunatic asylum was further reinforced by the leisure activities available to them. Women and men were offered different activities, with women's again centered on the gallery and its sitting areas. Activities available to women included cards, reading, dominoes, bagatelle, and draughts (Conolly 1847: 54). If a female attendant was available the women would be taken to the airing courts, and for the convalescent and orderly women the gardens were available for leisurely walks. For men similar ward activities were available, along with cricket, ball games, such as skittles, and lawn bowling which removed them from the wards and allowed them outside. These games were considered masculine activities; women were to be passive onlookers (Art. 111 1857: 377; Showalter 1981: 321). Highlights for both men and women were dances and theatrical or musical events which were held in the recreation/dining hall if one was available or in the wards if one was not. Large balls where men and women danced together appear to have been limited to the largest of the asylums such as Hanwell. This was one of the few times men and women were allowed contact together, although in 1857 at Colney Hatch men and women were being allowed to eat together, but only on either side of the dining hall (Art. 111. 1857: 375 & 376). Through an analysis of the plans and documents relating to the lunatic asylums it rapidly becomes clear that life for men and women in the asylum was entirely different.

Interestingly one male superintendent, T. S. Clouston, believed that women found the restrictive world of the asylum with its dances and 'general liveliness' better than their humdrum lives outside of the asylum and might wish to stay (quoted in Showalter 1981: 321). Yet the artificialness of the world created by asylum life for women was further reinforced by the complete lack of recognition of their role as mothers and wives. None of the lunatic asylum plans so far studied indicates the presence of nurseries or lying-in wards. Women were admitted into the asylum pregnant, became pregnant while in the asylum, or were admitted suffering from what is now recognized as post-natal depression

(Burrows 1828: 146–148; Hunter & MacAlpine 1974: 98; Skultans 1975: 32) but no provisions were made for them to care for their babies and there is evidence that the babies of single women were sent to the workhouse nursery shortly after their birth (Showalter 1981: 320). Women, in fact, were restricted to a very limited and specific role within the lunatic asylum: they were simply mad women, not wives or mothers - a role reinforced by the physical spaces provided for them.

CONCLUSION

Overall, the county asylums came closest to achieving the 'ideal's concerning comfortable and appropriate accommodation, day spaces and a rationalization of the placement of the domestic and administrative offices as recommended by Conolly, even if they were lacking in recreational spaces. More radical ideas for re-organizing asylum space in new ways, such as those proposed by Sankey and Robertson do not seem to have been realized in this major period of asylum building. The reason for this remains difficult to determine. Although tradition and the ease of following what was previously done may have played a part, certainly the increasing uniformity of the county asylums after a period of experimentation suggests that what was seen as a successful design was simply being copied. While there were architects who were repeatedly involved in asylum design, there was a sufficient range of architects to allow for some variation in ideas if a template was not being used (see Taylor 1991: 203–205 for a listing of architects and their asylums).

With this standardization of the layout of the lunatic asylum it becomes easier to see that the asylum was divided into four discrete areas: administrative, domestic, service and patient worlds. The curative asylum had called for direct medical supervision of the patients by the Medical Superintendent, yet the administrative section was always clearly separated from the patient areas. While it would be possible to read all sorts of implications into this separation, clearly it reinforced the division between the patients' world and that of the guiding officers. The officers' only contact with the patients was when they did the rounds of the wards or when cases where brought to their attention. This must have limited their personal knowledge of the patients, which had been the base of moral therapy as practiced at The Retreat. In effect, by trying to provide all lunatics with a curative environment and suitable attention, those working in the field were defeated by their own purpose. The county asylum was required to take more and more patients, and, while the original plans indicated that asylums where to be of a reasonable size, the possibilities of additions broke through any barriers limiting its size.

The curative regime was equally difficult to achieve. As reinforced by notions of the 'ideal', the asylum provided a reasonably comfortable environment and occupations other than work. From the lack of patient spaces beyond the wards and the service areas, this aspect was hardest to achieve. While as archaeologists we are aware, through ethnoarchaeological studies, that room definitions do not always indicate their use by the inhabitants, the lack of music rooms, libraries and recreation rooms does not necessarily mean that these activities were not occurring, although the lack of dedicated rooms may indicate a lack of formalized activity that ensured variety in the daily regime of the asylum. Rather, activities may have rested with the interests and enthusiasm of the attendants on particular wards and the flexibility of the ward space and furnishings, although supervision of activities would have been easier in dedicated rooms. It could ultimately be that the failure to provide these spaces rested with the county authorities, particularly with economics and class based views influencing provisions.

This chapter has highlighted some of the problems of understanding the actual use of spaces within British lunatic asylums. The plans do not allow us to access the realities of the use of space in an asylum. As highlighted above, Cambridgeshire Asylum was designed with beds arranged in what would normally be a gallery or corridor, but was the space actually used in this way or did it prove impractical? Did the limited amount of day space lead to the use of a dormitory as a day room? Were recreation halls converted to dormitories under the pressures of overcrowding? These questions can only been answered if all possible sources of information are considered. The Annual Reports of the Commissioners in Lunacy indicated that room use was far more flexible than indicated on plans, with rooms serving different purposes as required at the time, although there was an overall emphasis placed on returning spaces to recreational uses.

This analysis of British lunatic asylums has two roles: firstly it has provided a test of the descriptive framework using the 'ideal' asylum model; secondly, it forms, in itself, a part of the descriptive framework. For these built asylums formed a further source of information on which the colonists of South Australia and Tasmania could draw. Consequently the descriptive framework is formed by the features of the 'ideal' asylum and of the features of the built asylum where they differ from the 'ideal'. If the British asylums came close to meeting Conolly's 'ideal' model, did the colonial asylums of Australia demonstrate a similar pattern?

South Australia and the 'Ideal' Lunatic Asylum | 7

The first colonists arrived in Australia in 1788 with the establishment of the convict colony of New South Wales. Subsequently other areas of Australia were to become colonies, with some like Van Dieman's Land and Queensland beginning as penal colonies, while others such as Western Australia and South Australia established as free colonies without a resident convict population, although Western Australia later became a penal colony to survive. Each colony had a different history and they were not to join together under a federal Parliament until 1901. Consequently for this study two colonies, South Australia and Van Diemen's Land, were chosen as they reflect fundamental variations in Australia's past. South Australia was unique amongst the other colonies in Australia as its foundation was based on a plan of colonization developed by private individuals rather than the English Colonial Office. South Australia was not a penal colony, unlike Van Dieman's Land (Tasmania) which had a predominantly convict population for many decades.

The founding colonists of the province of South Australia had very clear views of the society they wished to create, and this had a direct impact on early emigration policies. South Australia would be a respectable province, free of the taint of convict populations. The South Australian Act of 1834 specified that the transportation of convicts to the province would never occur, and this was to be a central part of the campaign to encourage migration to the colony (Main 1986: 97). Those who received assisted passages were required to meet strict criteria, with the intention of giving South Australia a young and physically able population (Allen 1847: 21–22). Consequently no provisions were made for the sick or the mentally ill. However, in the face of less than strict selection processes in England, South Australians soon found themselves with a range of people who required assistance on arrival (Nance 1992: 30). South Australia consequently had to provide a destitute asylum and a lunatic asylum, both institutions they had not anticipated providing (Piddock 1996).

Logically, within any group of convicts, there was likely to have been a number of sick or mentally ill persons. Thus it can be expected that Tasmania, which was established both for economic reasons and as a penal colony, would need to provide for these individuals from its first days, and that some institutional provision would be part of the infrastructure of the colony.

With these very different histories it is possible to ask questions that address the social basis of the provision of care for the mentally ill. Did the presence of convicts affect the types of provisions for their care in terms of the built environment of the asylum? Is it possible to detect differences in the provisions made for the free colonists of South Australia and the convicts of Tasmania? Do social attitudes affect the adoption of the 'ideal' asylum features? These questions will form Cleland's third level of questions, as discussed in Chapter Three, which look beyond the individual site, or in this case single asylum, to the wider patterns influencing the built provisions for the insane.

In these two chapters, a range of data sets are used to allow us to access this information. These include a history of the lunatic asylum buildings which reflects room and space use, a building chronology, plans, photographs and primary documents relating to the asylums. These data sets are compared to the 'ideal' asylum models constructed in Chapter Five, not just at the moment in time represented by the plans, but over several decades.

A BRIEF HISTORY OF THE ADELAIDE AND PARKSIDE LUNATIC ASYLUMS

South Australia's first public lunatic asylum was a residential house in the suburbs of the town of Adelaide (Figure 1.2). Opened in 1846, it provided limited accommodation for both men and women (S.A. C.S.O. Letters No. 484 and 1173). Prior to this the insane had been kept in the Adelaide Gaol, but pressures on accommodation led to the Colonial Surgeon, James Nash, being asked to select a site for a new purpose built asylum. Surrounded by the police paddock, the site Nash chose was on the western side of the colonial hospital, on a gentle rise, and sufficiently elevated to catch fresh breezes, with the boundary wall lower down the rise so that the inmates would be able to see over the walls. It was located on a road leading out of Adelaide and was considered far enough from town to prevent annoyance to the inhabitants, yet close enough for the Visitors appointed to the Lunatic Asylum to make their inspections, and for the visits of patient's friends (S.A. C.S.O. Letters 24/6/1343).

The asylum plans drawn up in 1850 indicate that the Adelaide Asylum was intended to accommodate 60 patients, but in practice the building only provided for 40 (S.A. C.S.O. Letters No. 1640 and 1990). The asylum opened in March 1852 and consisted of a single linear building with the kitchen and laundry forming an attached annex to the rear of the main building (Figure 7.1, Figure 7.2). The centre space of the ground floor was given over to the surgeon's rooms, a keeper's room, committee room, surgery and receiving room. On each side of these rooms were the wards. Each ward consisted of 7 sleeping rooms, a day room, with the lavatory, bath and water closet opposite the sleeping rooms. At the end of the ward were three more rooms: two for refractory patients and one for incontinent patients. The first floor consisted of two wards each composed of four dormitories, a corridor ward, and day room, while in the centre space were two infirmaries and the Master's and Matron's rooms (Figure 7.3). These divided the asylum into male and female sides. Originally this floor had a bath and water closets. The original water closets on the first floor opened directly onto the wards, pervading them with an offensive smell. These were eventually removed in 1854, with the creation of more day room space (S.A. Visitors 8/7/1852; S.A C.S.O. Letters 24/1625). The small second floor over the central section had two dormitories and a foyer around the stairs. The yard to the rear of the building was used by both sexes until it was divided into male and female yards in 1854. As can be seen in Figure 7.4,

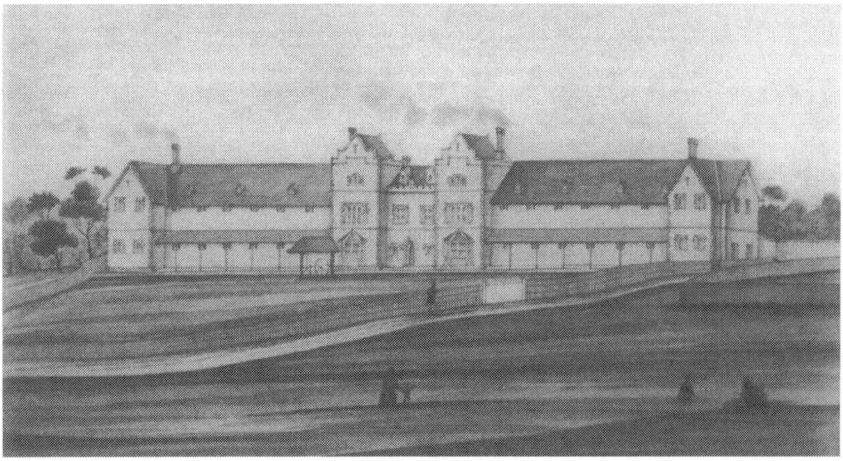

Figure 7.1. Drawing of the Adelaide Lunatic Asylum circa 1852. Courtesy of the State Library of South Australia, B16073.

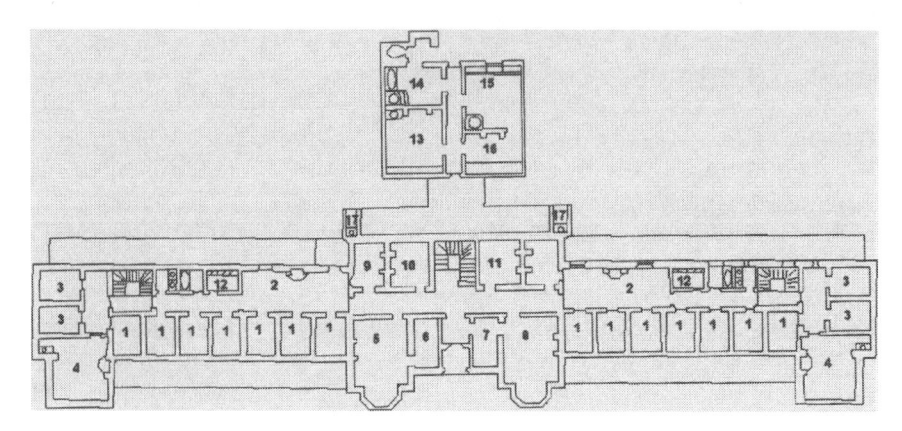

Figure 7.2. Plan of the Adelaide Lunatic Asylum, Ground Floor. Original plan held by State Records of South Australia GRG38/52/1-13. Tracing by author, redrawn by J. Gibb. (1. Cells; 2. Day Rooms; 3. Refractory Patient's Rooms; 4. Wet Patient's Rooms; 5. Surgeon's Living Room; 6. Surgeon's Bedroom; 7. Receiving Room; 8. Committee Room; 9. Keeper's Room; 10. Surgeon's Kitchen; 11. Surgery; 12. Lavatories; 13. Kitchen; 14. Scullery; 15. Washing Room; 16. Laundry; 17. Water Closets; 18. Wards; 19. Infirmary Wards; 20. Master's Living Room; 21. Matron's Rooms; 22. Master's Sleeping Room; 23. Matron's Sleeping Room).

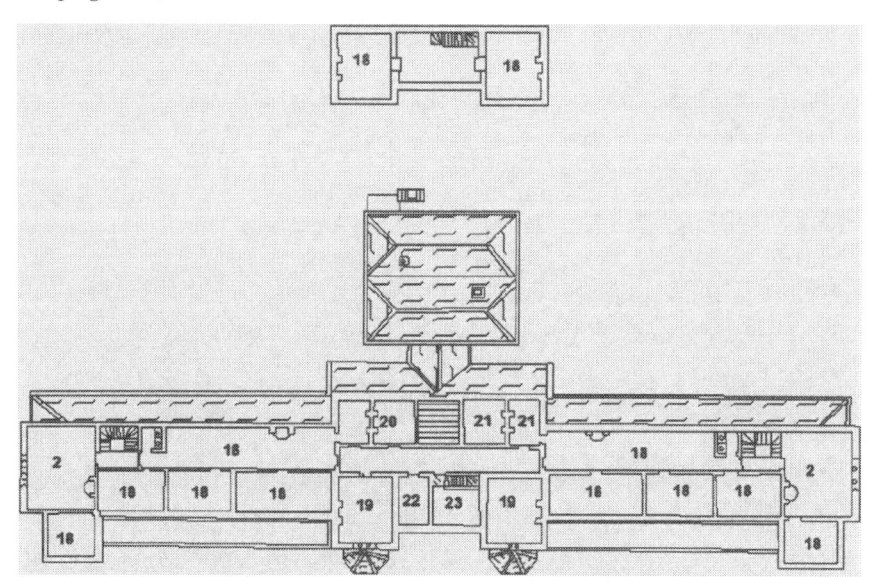

Figure 7.3. Plan of the Adelaide Lunatic Asylum, First Floor. Original plan held by State Records of South Australia GRG38/52/1-13. Tracing by author, redrawn by J. Gibb. (1. Cells; 2. Day Rooms; 3. Refractory Patient's Rooms; 4. Wet Patient's Rooms; 5. Surgeon's Living Room; 6. Surgeon's Bedroom; 7. Receiving Room; 8. Committee Room; 9. Keeper's Room; 10. Surgeon's Kitchen; 11. Surgery; 12. Lavatories; 13. Kitchen; 14. Scullery; 15. Washing Room; 16. Laundry; 17. Water Closets; 18. Wards; 19. Infirmary Wards; 20. Master's Living Room; 21. Matron's Rooms; 22. Master's Sleeping Room; 23. Matron's Sleeping Room).

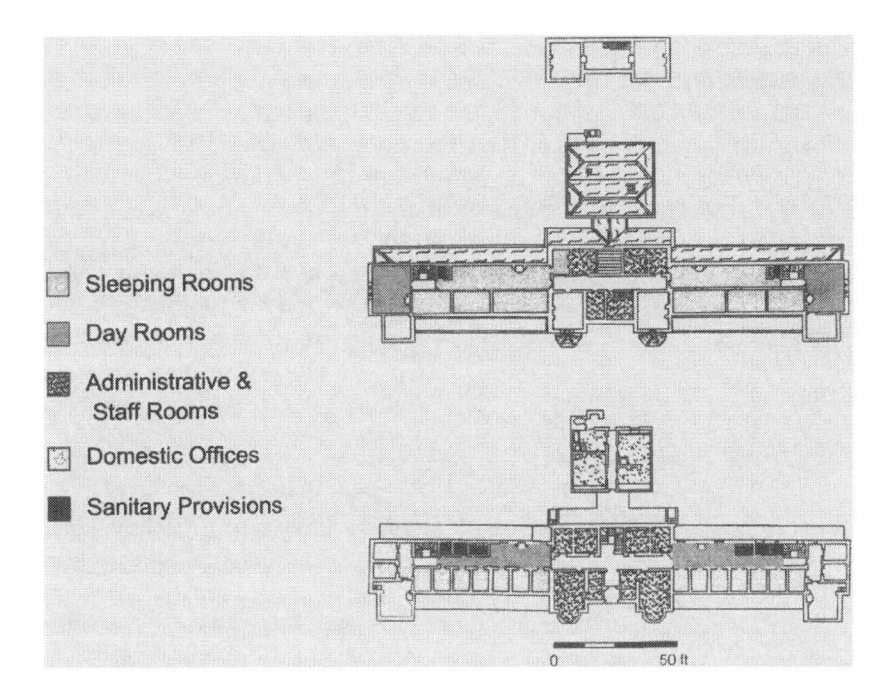

A Brief History of the Adelaide and Parkside Lunatic Asylums

Figure 7.4. Room and space distribution in the Adelaide Lunatic Asylum. Tracing of plans held by State Records of South Australia, GRG 38/52/1-13.

the day spaces of the asylum were spread over both floors with the day rooms directly connected to the wards.

While the opening of the Adelaide Lunatic Asylum was meant to prevent the keeping of lunatics in the Adelaide Gaol, the decision of the Government to use one floor of the new asylum for the overflow of the Destitute Asylum meant that many of the single cells in the male department were accommodating two men and patients were sleeping on the floor (S.A. Visitors 8/11/1852). A consequence of this was that lunatics were still residing in the Gaol rather than in the asylum; this situation was to continue until August 1853 (S.A. C.S.O. Letters 17/1/1852 and 24/6/1990).

Less than two years after the asylum opened its failings had become apparent and in September 1853 plans were drawn up to modify the asylum with additional accommodation for 40 patients, day rooms for both sexes, further exercise yards, a new laundry and kitchen being provided (S.A C.S.O. Letters 24/6/2429). The same year a Select Committee was appointed to consider the plans and the possibilities of building an entirely new asylum. The Colonial Surgeon James Nash thought that this new asylum should accommodate 200 patients, and be located on from fifty to one hundred acres. He believed it should be about two miles from town, which would be convenient for friends and medical attendants to visit while keeping away curious visits from others (Parliamentary Paper (S.A.P.P.) 1853 No. 89).

The Committee favored the option of a new asylum for 135 patients located on fifty acres. The South Australian Parliament agreed that the proposed work on the Adelaide Lunatic Asylum should be suspended, and money placed on the Parliamentary Estimates for 1854 for a new lunatic asylum (S.A.P.P.1853 No. 89). Possibly in anticipation of a new asylum being built, 40 acres of land directly abutting the Adelaide Lunatic Asylum was given over to Botanic Gardens (Votes and Proceedings (S.A. V. & P) 18/10/1854). This limited any expansion of the asylum as the gardens directly adjoined the end of the women's ward and exercise yard.

In 1854 sixty acres of land for a new asylum was bought in the village of Woodforde, at the base of the Adelaide hills, and plans were drawn up by the Colonial Architect, Bennett Hays. The anticipated cost of the new asylum for 228 patients was £80,300. Despite the progress made, it was decided not to go ahead with the new asylum, or even with modifications to the existing asylum. Instead, the Colonial Secretary informed the Colonial Architect that part of the Adelaide Gaol was to be modified and declared a lunatic asylum. At this time the Gaol was already acting as an asylum, taking the overflow from the overcrowded Adelaide Lunatic Asylum with prisoners caring for the lunatics day and night (S.A. C.S.O. Letters 24/6/72, 2/6/984, 24/6/1402, 24/6/2506; S.A. Government Gazette (S.A. G.G.) 8/3/1855; 8/11/1855). While it was originally considered that the lunatic asylum would be separate from the Gaol section, this could not be made to work on a practical level, so modifications were planned to some of the Gaol buildings. However there is no indication that this work was ever begun.

In 1856 a Parliamentary Select Committee was appointed to consider the treatment of lunatics in Her Majesty's Gaol and the Adelaide Lunatic Asylum. At this time equal numbers of lunatics were being housed at the asylum and the gaol. The Committee condemned conditions at both institutions where, in the latter, patients were doubling up in single cells no larger than 10 ft. long and 7 ft. 4 in. wide while many of the available rooms were being used by the staff. The Committee recommended the expansion of the present lunatic asylum as the most convenient and speedy option while recommending that the Resident Surgeon temporarily move out to provide accommodation for 12 to 20 patients. Classification of the patients could be achieved by using the old Adelaide Hospital for "patients whose cases are considered hopeful and temporary, and who are of a quiet and inoffensive disposition;" (S.A. S.C. 1856: iii).

In 1856 work commenced on building new dormitories to the rear of the main building of the Asylum (Figure 7.4). This new wing was to consist of two new wards of single cells with day rooms. The building was completed by March 1857 with the upper floor immediately occupied (S.A. Visitors 6/3/1857). Reflecting possible financial concerns, the accommodation appears to have been limited to 10 single rooms in each of the two wards. Assuming keepers occupied possibly one or two rooms this allowed accommodation for only 16–18 more inmates at cost of £3,500. By July 1857 the Gaol was no longer being used to house lunatics (S.A. P.P. 1859 No. 31; S.A. Gov. Gaz. 3/7/1856, 31/7/1857).

In 1858, reflecting the adaptation of the asylum spaces to fit daily requirements, the sheds in the airing yards, used as ad hoc dining rooms, were converted into proper rooms with fireplaces (S.A. Visitors 12/5/1857, 7/4/1858, 6/10/1858). While funds for additions had been voted in 1859 the Government changed its mind and decided to use the money for a Destitute Free School.

In 1861 accommodation pressures led to the use of the adjacent old hospital building as temporary asylum accommodation as had been recommended in 1856 (Select Committee 1864 (S.A S.C. 1864): Q. 42). Overcrowding continued to be a problem, and work began in 1861 to build a further male dormitory (Figure 7.5). This building was constructed abutting the first addition, providing 18 single rooms, two dormitories, and two small and one medium day rooms over two floors and a partial lower floor. Work appears to have begun on a set of rooms for both men and women at some distance from the main building (Figure 7.6). These rooms included male and female dormitories, three single rooms for refractory patients, male and female dining rooms and one bath for each sex.

Problems with the Adelaide Lunatic Asylum design and overcrowding had caused the official Visitors, appointed by the South Australian Government to inspect the asylum, to call for a commission to consider a new site and design (S.A.Visitors 30/1/1861). This commission was finally called in 1864. They found that the existing asylum did not allow for sufficient classification, and the site had become inappropriate. The expansion of the town of Adelaide and the suburbs on the other side of the Parklands meant that the roads passing the asylum had become main thoroughfares (S.A. S.C. 1864: Q. 277, 365, 431). The present Asylum had become a collection of buildings comprising the original building, the dormitory additions and the old hospital (connected to the asylum by a covered way) accommodating around 150 to 160 patients

Again the question of expanding the present asylum was considered but the limitations of the size of the site and the costs involved meant this was not a practical solution (S.A. S.C. 1864: Q. 892–894, 900–907,

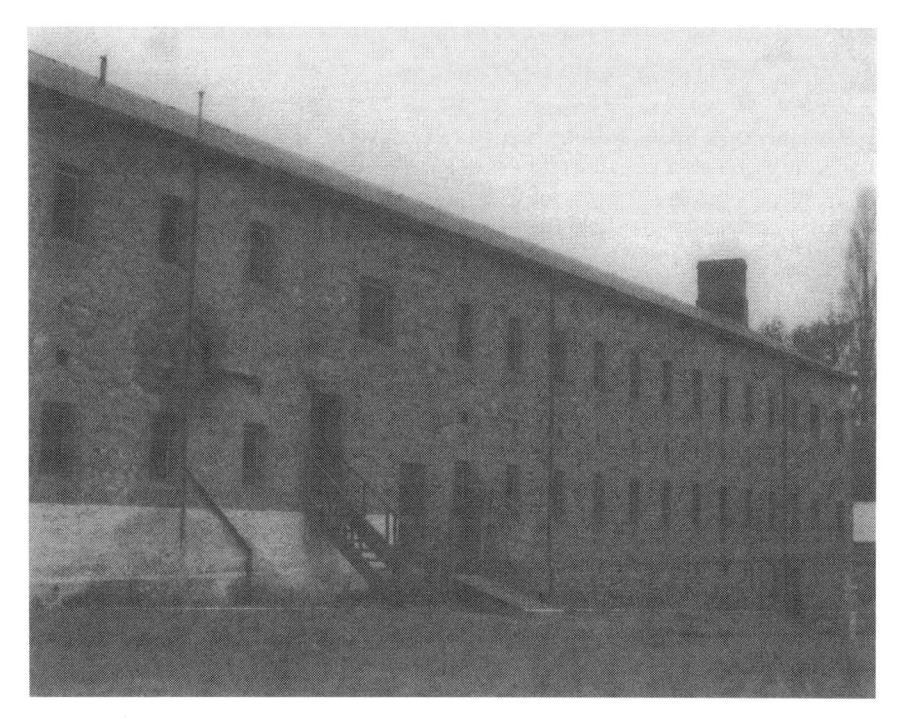

Figure 7.5. Male dormitory, Adelaide Lunatic Asylum. Courtesy of the State Library of South Australia, B16073.

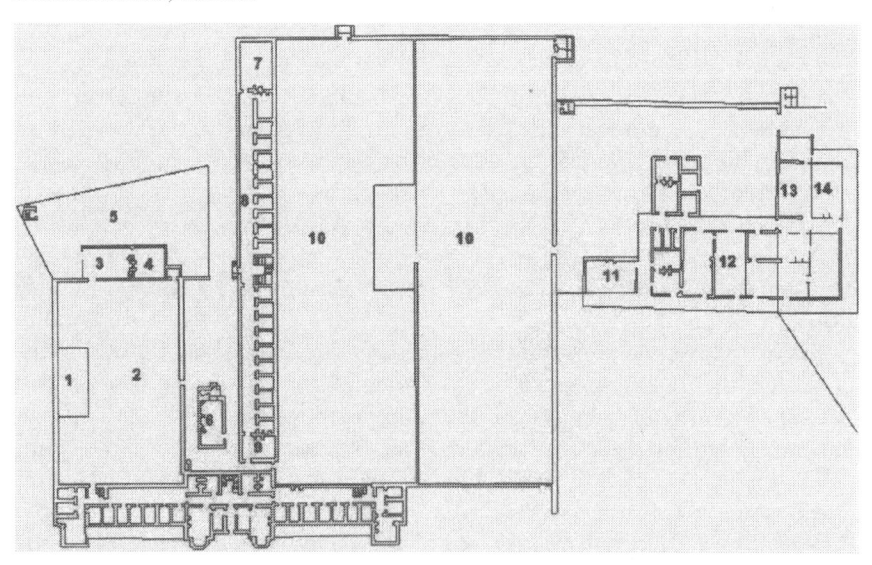

Figure 7.6. Additions at the Adelaide Lunatic Asylum. Tracing by author of a plan held by State Records of South Australia, GRG 38/52/1-13. Redrawn by J. Gibb. (1. Shed; 2. Women's Yard; 3. Washhouse; 4. Laundry; 5. Drying Yard; 6. Kitchen; 7. Day Room; 8. Male Dormitory; 9. Keeper's Room; 10. Men's Yard; 11. Women's Dining Room; 12. Refractory Cells; 13. Men's Bedroom; 14. Men's Dining Room).

A Brief History of the Adelaide and Parkside Lunatic Asylums 115

914–919). Instead the Commission recommended the construction of a new purpose-built asylum for 700 patients along the best European and American lines on a site of not less than eighty acres (S.A. S.C. 1864 Report). They, however, rejected the land purchased at Woodforde as being too far from Adelaide, and recommended the purchase of land within four miles of the centre of Adelaide. While this new asylum was being designed and built the Commission recommended the building of increased accommodation for forty women at the present site at a cost of some £4,000.

The next two years saw a period of activity, with the Colonial Architect, W. M. Hanson, drawing up plans for a new lunatic asylum to house 350 patients at a cost of £50,000. In 1865 a separate residence for the Resident Medical Officer was built at Adelaide Asylum (Figure 7.7) freeing up rooms in the main building for patient use, and in 1866 a

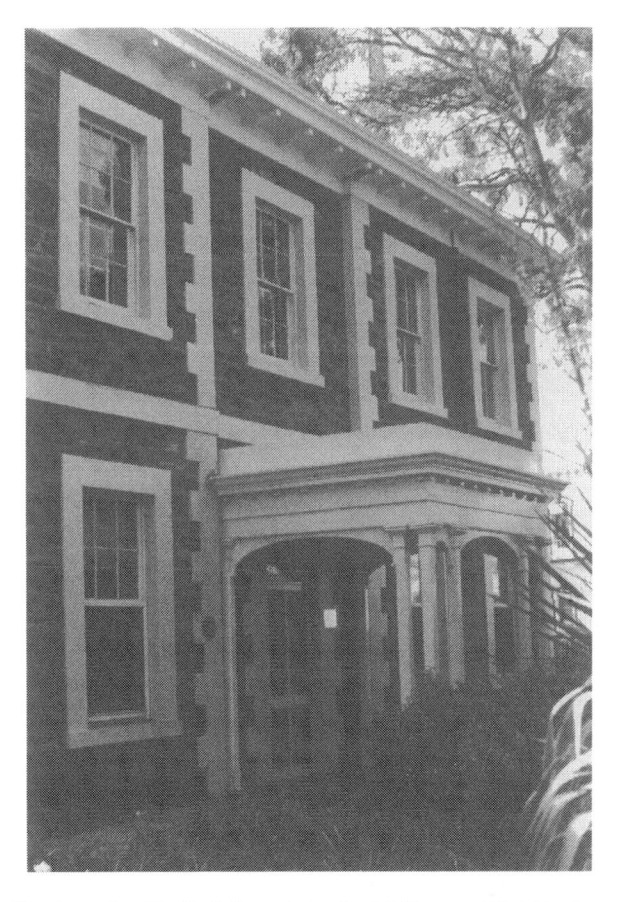

Figure 7.7. Yarabee, the Medical Superintendents' House, Adelaide Lunatic Asylum. Photograph by author 1998.

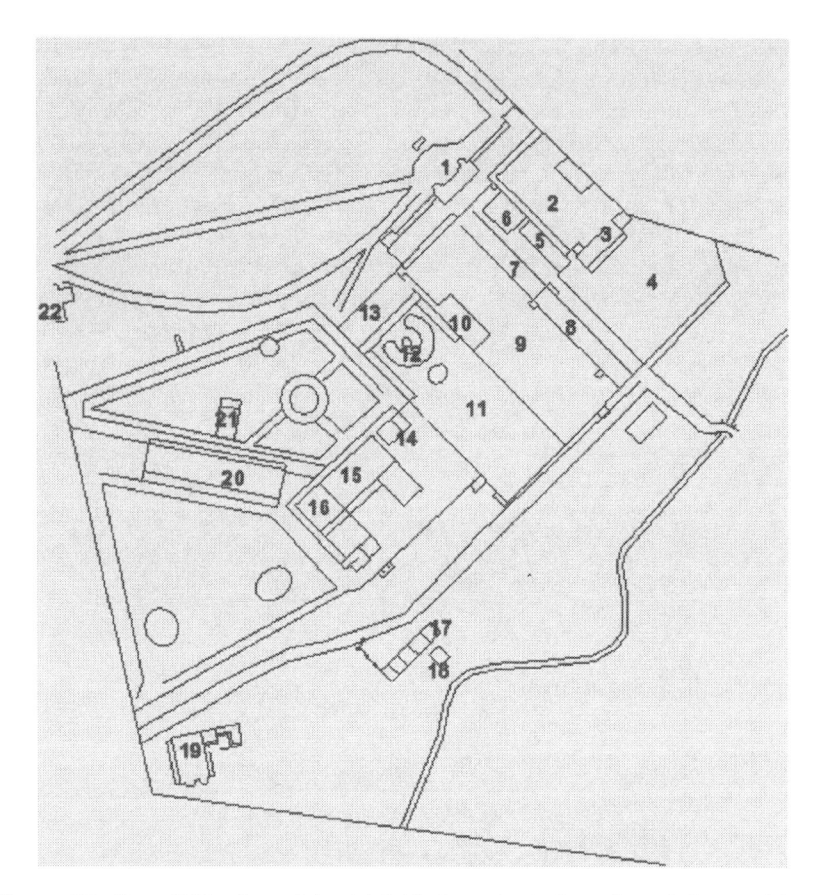

Figure 7.8. Post 1890s plan of the Adelaide Lunatic Asylum. State Library of South Australia, GRG 38/82/1-13. Tracing by author. Redrawn by J. Gibb. (1. Original Asylum Building; 2. Women's Yard; 3. Washhouse; 4. Drying Yard; 5. Fuel Shed; 6. Kitchen; 7. First Male Ward Addition; 8. Second Male Ward Addition; 9. No. 1 Male Yard; 10. Dining Room; 11. No. 2 Male Yard; 12. Aviary and Fountain; 13. A and B Building; 14. Day Room; 15. Female Ward; 16. Male Paralytic Ward; 17. Workshop; 18. Dead house; 19. Superintendent's House, Yarabee; 20. Later Dormitory Addition; 21. Later Dormitory Addition; 22. Lodge).

new female dormitory was added (Figure 7.8). Importantly 1866 saw the purchase of land for the new asylum at Parkside, just beyond the Parklands that surrounded the town of Adelaide. Foundations for the new asylum were laid in December 1866 and the new Parkside Lunatic Asylum opened in March 1870.

The asylum at Parkside was planned as a series of three pavilions housing several hundred patients, but by 1870 only one building had been built (Figure 7.9). This building was designed to copy the shape of

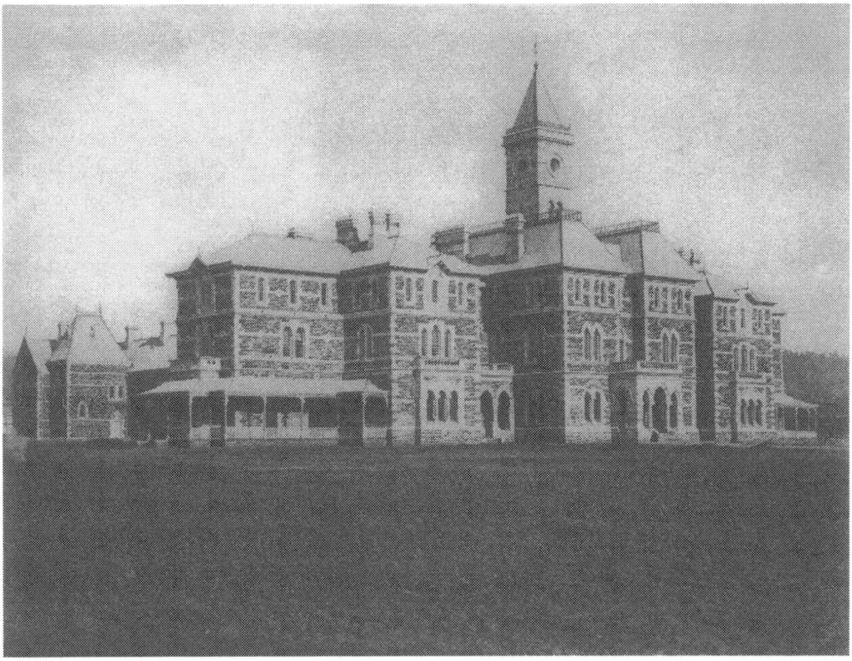

Figure 7.9. Parkside Lunatic Asylum, 1872. Courtesy of the State Library of South Australia, B1903.

the administrative building at the Essex County Asylum at Brentwood, but not its overall layout. The building was T-shaped in plan with a courtyard in the centre.

Of its three stories, the ground floor (Figure 7.10) was devoted mainly to administrative rooms, with the addition of two large day rooms. The centre space was taken up by the Medical Officer's rooms and consulting room, and the porter's room. On either side of these were day rooms. On the men's side an adjoining room was given over to a billiards room, but on the women's side the same space was occupied by a workroom. On the male and female sides respectively were the Matron's and Medical Officer's offices and dining rooms. On either side of the courtyard were the dispensary, service, and food storage rooms. The rear of the quadrangle was given over to the kitchen and distribution room in the centre, and was flanked by a female attendant's dining room and visitor's room on one side, and the male attendant's dining room and a second visitor's room on the other side. This allowed the sexes to be kept strictly separate.

The first floor was given over to a range of sleeping accommodation (Figure 7.11). Along the quadrangle sides were single rooms, with a four

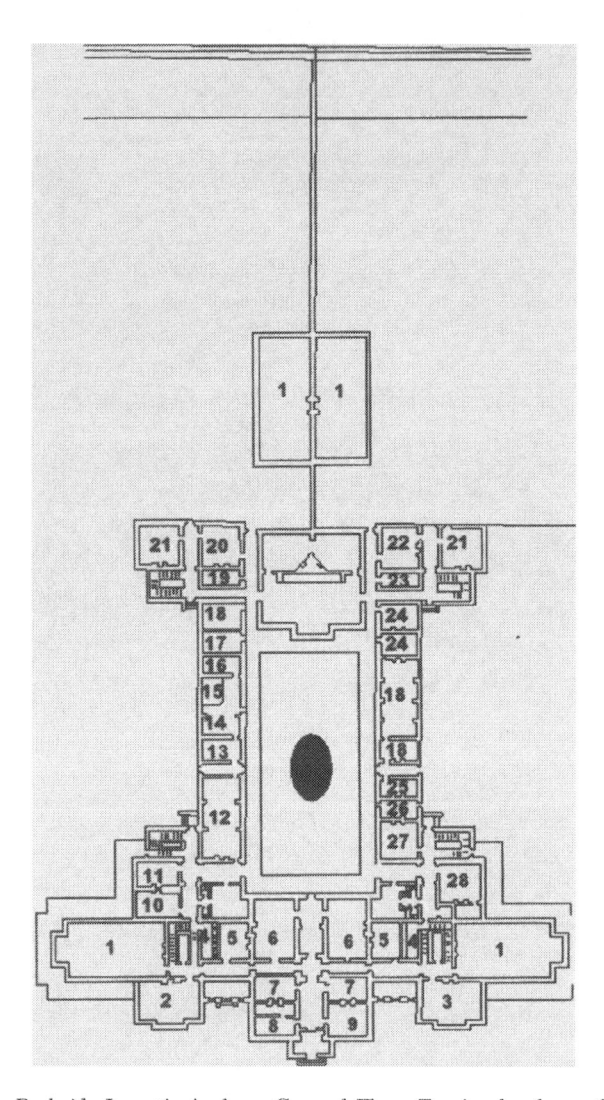

Figure 7.10. Parkside Lunatic Asylum, Ground Floor. Tracing by the author of a plan held by State Records of South Australia, GRG 34/138. (1. Day Rooms; 2. Work Room; 3. Billiards Room; 4. Water Closets and Lavatories; 5. Senior Attendant's Rooms; 6. Visitor's Rooms; 7. Consulting Room; 8. Hall Porter's Room and Bedroom; 9. Medical Officer's Room; 10. Matron's Dining Room; 11. Matron's Bedroom; 12. Clothing Store; 13. Flour Store; 14. Bakery; 15. Oven; 16. Bread Store; 17. Cook's Dining Room; 18. Store; 19. Pantry; 20. Female Attendant's Dining Room; 21. Visitor's Room; 22. Male Attendant's Dining Room; 23. Pantry; 24. Scullery; 25. Steward's Office; 26. Dispensary; 27. Officer's Dining Room; 28. Office; 29. Dormitories; 30. Single Rooms; 31. Attendant's Rooms; 32. Officer's and Matron's Bedrooms; 33. Staff Bedrooms).

A Brief History of the Adelaide and Parkside Lunatic Asylums 119

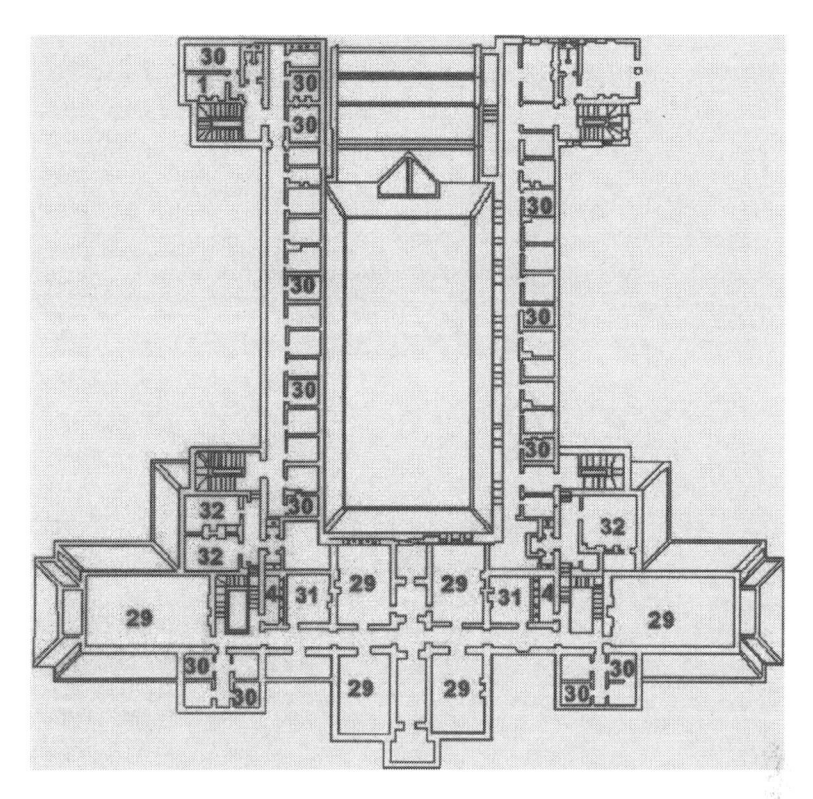

Figure 7.11. Parkside Lunatic Asylum, First Floor. Tracing by the author of a plan held by State Records of South Australia, GRG 34/138. (1. Day Rooms; 2. Work Room; 3. Billiards Room; 4. Water Closets and Lavatories; 5. Senior Attendant's Rooms; 6. Visitor's Rooms; 7. Consulting Room; 8. Hall Porter's Room and Bedroom; 9. Medical Officer's Room; 10. Matron's Dining Room; 11. Matron's Bedroom; 12. Clothing Store; 13. Flour Store; 14. Bakery; 15. Oven; 16. Bread Store; 17. Cook's Dining Room; 18. Store; 19. Pantry; 20. Female Attendant's Dining Room; 21. Visitor's Room; 22. Male Attendant's Dining Room; 23. Pantry; 24. Scullery; 25. Steward's Office; 26. Dispensary; 27. Officer's Dining Room; 28. Office; 29. Dormitories; 30. Single Rooms; 31. Attendant's Rooms; 32. Officer's and Matron's Bedrooms; 33. Staff Bedrooms).

bedroom block at the rear. The corridor in front of these rooms was narrow and was not intended to be a gallery such as was found in British asylums which often became additional living space. The size of this corridor may have been determined by the size of the domestic rooms on the ground floor. Over the day rooms in the front of the building were dormitories, with an adjoining annex of four bedrooms; while in the centre were the Matron and Officer's rooms, the water closest and lavatories, and two further dormitories. Although not clearly forming wards, it appears that there could have been three separate patient areas.

The second floor had the same arrangement of dormitories and bedrooms as the first floor, though there were no further rooms over the quadrangle sides (Figure 7.12). While the plans show two airing courts complete with dining rooms to the rear of the building, these in fact were not built until a few years later. As can be seen in Figures 7.13–7.15 Parkside was clearly divided into day and night spaces with the upper two stories being composed of patient sleeping spaces and attendants' rooms. The day rooms were clearly separated from the wards, unlike at the Adelaide Asylum.

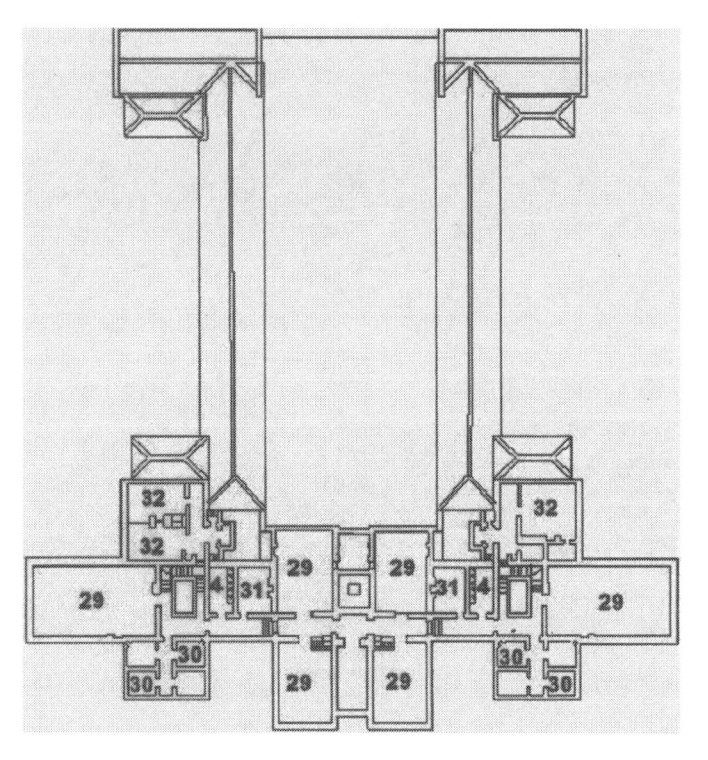

Figure 7.12. Parkside Lunatic Asylum, Second Floor. Tracing by the author of a plan held by State Records of South Australia, GRG 34/138 (1. Day Rooms; 2. Work Room; 3. Billiards Room; 4. Water Closets and Lavatories; 5. Senior Attendant's Rooms; 6. Visitor's Rooms; 7. Consulting Room; 8. Hall Porter's Room and Bedroom; 9. Medical Officer's Room; 10. Matron's Dining Room; 11. Matron's Bedroom; 12. Clothing Store; 13. Flour Store; 14. Bakery; 15. Oven; 16. Bread Store; 17. Cook's Dining Room; 18. Store; 19. Pantry; 20. Female Attendant's Dining Room; 21. Visitor's Room; 22. Male Attendant's Dining Room; 23. Pantry; 24. Scullery; 25. Steward's Office; 26. Dispensary; 27. Officer's Dining Room; 28. Office; 29. Dormitories; 30. Single Rooms; 31. Attendant's Rooms; 32. Officer's and Matron's Bedrooms; 33. Staff Bedrooms).

A Brief History of the Adelaide and Parkside Lunatic Asylums

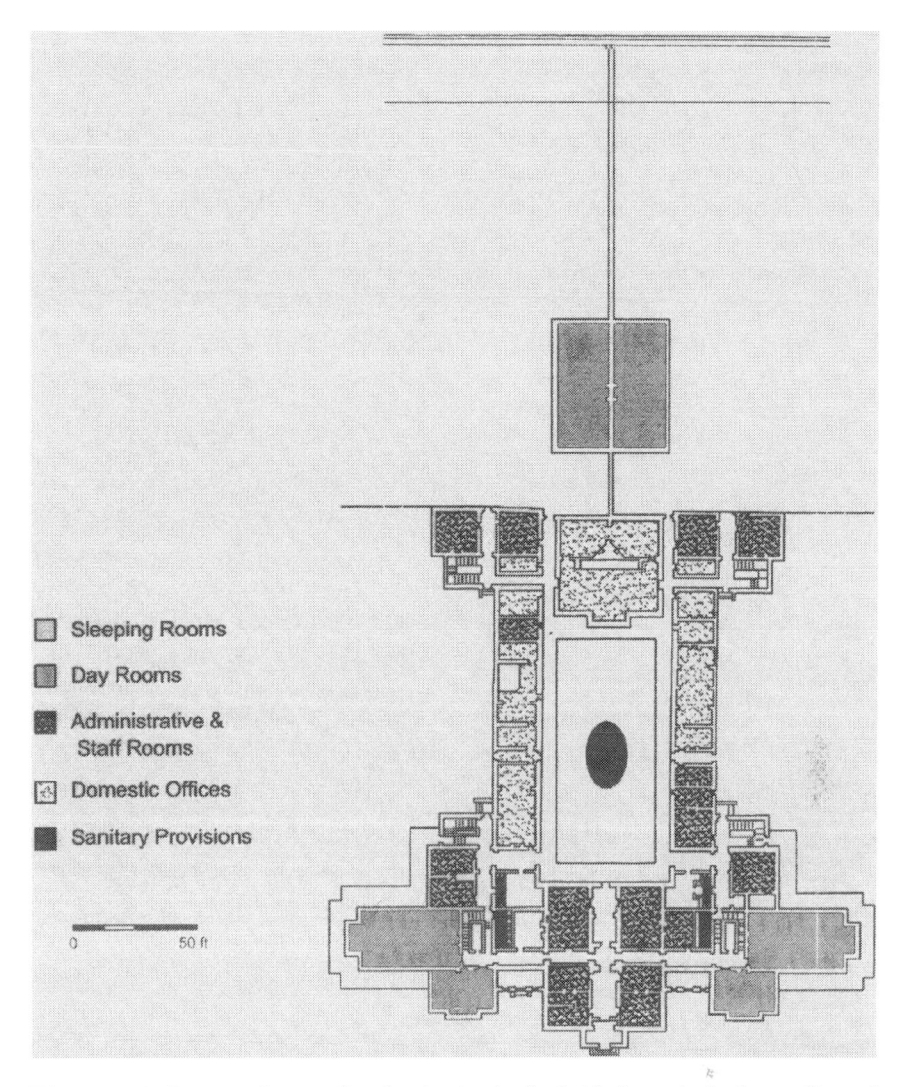

Figure 7.13. Room and space distribution in the Parkside Lunatic Asylum – Ground Floor. Tracing of plans held by State Records of South Australia, GRG 34/138.

Initially, only men were moved to the new asylum, where they could be employed in laboring tasks. The presence of only one airing court prevented the movement of the women to Parkside. The Parkside Asylum remained incomplete for a number of years and the front rooms of the building remained empty. It was anticipated the front offices could be used as additional dormitories to ease the overcrowding of the male wards at Adelaide if the necessary airing courts were built.

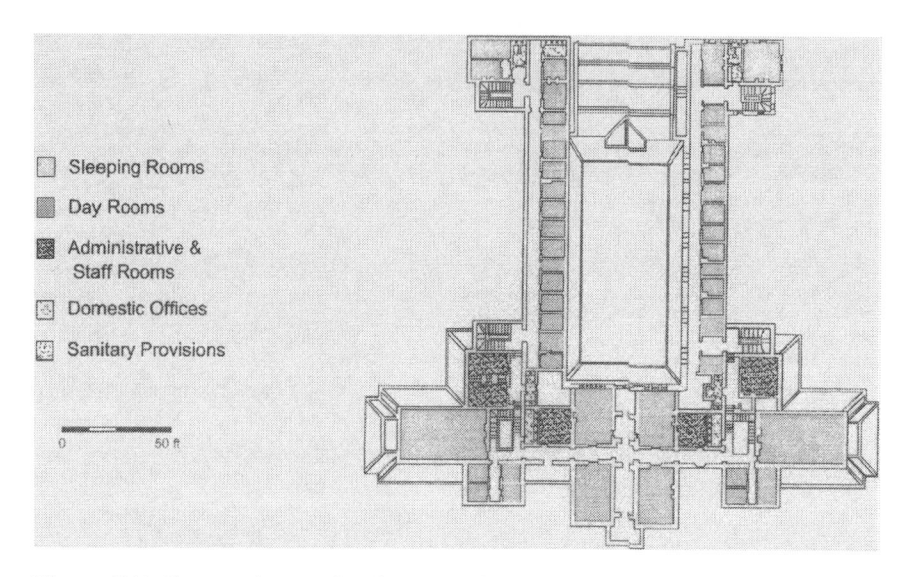

Figure 7.14. Room and space distribution in the Parkside Lunatic Asylum – First Floor. Tracing of plans held by State Records of South Australia, GRG 34/138.

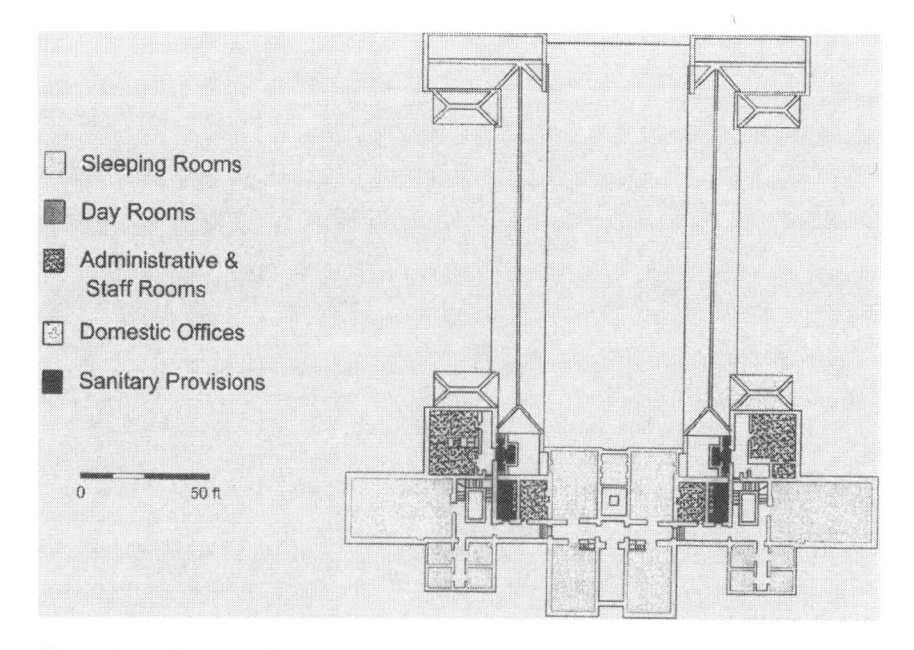

Figure 7.15. Room and space distribution in the Parkside Lunatic Asylum – Second Floor. Tracing of plans held by State Records of South Australia, GRG 34/138.

Day rooms would need to be provided in these new airing courts (Figure 7.16). Work did not begin on the airing courts until 1877, as did work on a laundry (Annual Report (S.A. A.R.) 19/4/1877). Consequently for seven years the rooms remained empty.

In 1871 a further Commission recommended the provision of a ward for criminal lunatics at the Gaol but this was never realized (S.A. Visitors 13/11/1871). In 1878 a criminal building was opened at Parkside to the right of the main building, along with a male dining room in the airing court.

Overcrowding continued at Adelaide Lunatic Asylum on both the male and female sides. The women could not be moved into Parkside Asylum, as despite the existence of an airing court which would allow them to exercise, there was no separate dining room for them to eat in (S.A. A.R. 30/1/1879). The lack of ground floor rooms suitable for acute cases meant that Parkside could only take chronic cases and Adelaide remained the admitting institution. The problem lay with the fact that Parkside had not been completed with male and female pavilions as intended. The central administrative building was intended to provide only limited patient accommodation (S.A. A.R. 19/2/1880).

Eighteen eighty to eighty one saw a flurry of work. Work began on the Residential Medical Officer's Residence at Parkside, which would free up his rooms for patient accommodation, a new pavilion block for 150 female patients (Figure 7.17), and on a multifunctional room in the women's airing court which was to serve the triple purpose of dining room, chapel and general recreation hall (S.A. A.R. 19/2/1880).

There are no surviving plans of the women's pavilion; however it was described as having spacious corridors large enough to form a general dining room on the ground floor and dormitories if necessary on the other floors. This would suggest that accommodation was arranged in the usual fashion with corridors flanked by sleeping rooms. Cottages were built to house hospital cases and 'imbecile' children or harmless patients.

In terms of the layout of Parkside Asylum, the original building housing the administrative offices was centrally placed with the women's pavilion and criminal pavilions symmetrically aligned on either side. The male dining room was placed along the back of the airing court in line with the rear of the main building, while the women's dining hall was placed in the middle of the airing court and slightly off centre to the administrative building. The cottages and laundry were behind the administrative building.

In 1884 work began at Parkside Asylum on a new criminal ward on newly purchased land at the rear boundary of the asylum grounds. A considerable distance from the main building (but directly in line with it), it was to be bounded by high walls.

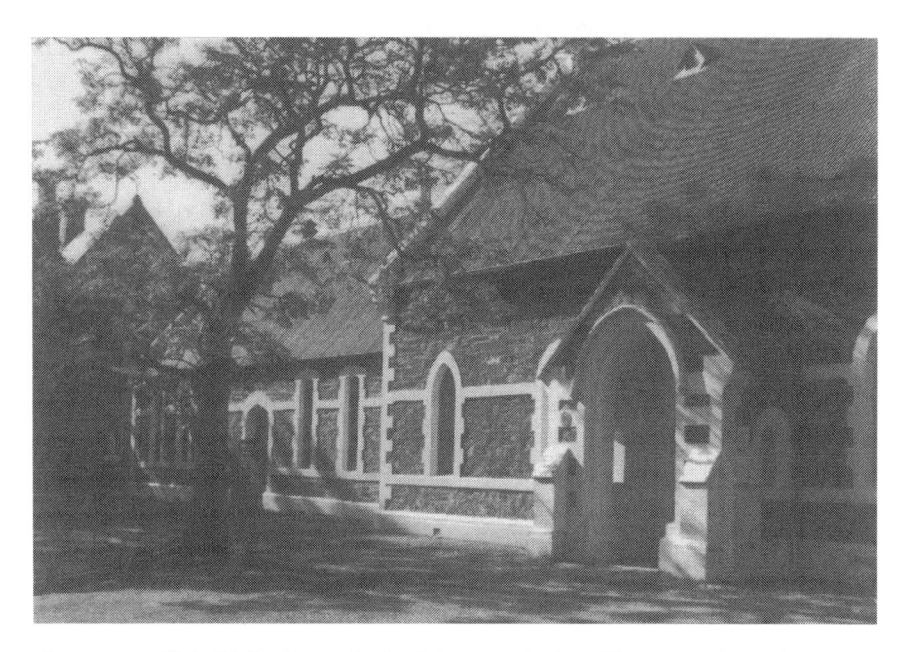

Figure 7.16. Male Dining Room, Parkside Lunatic Asylum. Photograph by author 1998.

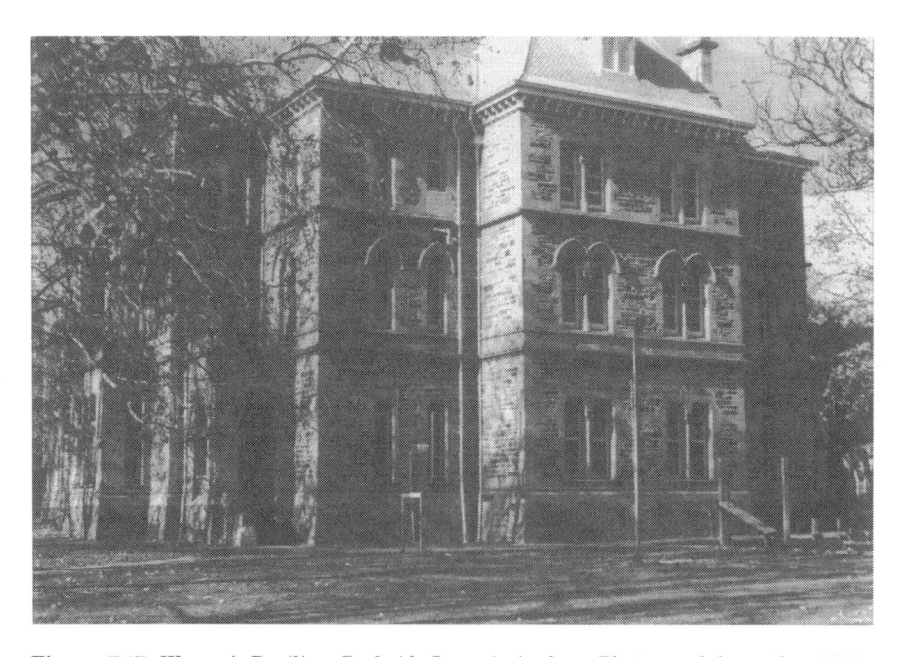

Figure 7.17. Women's Pavilion, Parkside Lunatic Asylum. Photograph by author 1998.

The South Australian Asylums and the 'Ideal' Asylum Model

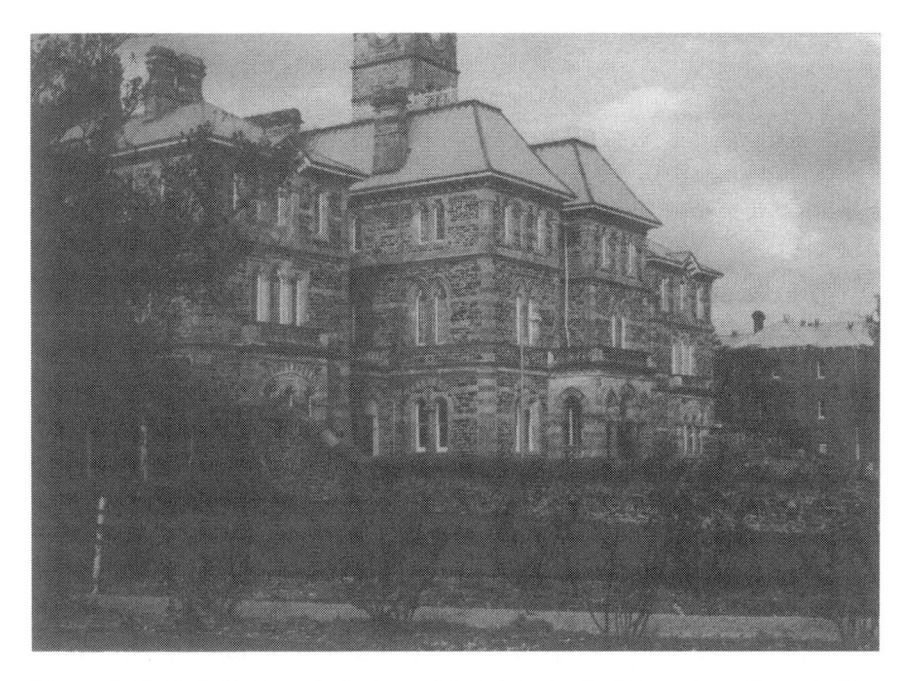

Figure 7.18. Parkside Lunatic Asylum – Administrative Building today with part of the front airing court wall visible. Photograph by author 1998.

Overcrowding continued to be a problem in the 1880s (S.A. Comm. 1884: Q. 8067), but no major building work was undertaken, and presumably with the opening of the new criminal ward, the old one would have been given over to the male division. In 1883 men were using the women's rooms in the main administrative building. Interestingly, despite being opened for 13 years, the patients of the Parkside Asylum were limited to their airing courts as there were no boundary walls. Strangers would often talk to patients over the ha-ha (sunken) walls of the front airing courts and steal fruit and vegetables from the Asylum grounds. Adelaide Asylum similarly lacked privacy, with youths climbing trees and taunting women in their exercise yard (S.A. A.R. 19/2/1880; Comm. 1884: Q. 390–1, 1244). In the 1880s other small additions were made to both Adelaide and Parkside Asylums, including six single rooms with a bath room at Adelaide for feeble and aged women in 1886 and a ward for violent women at Parkside in 1888. A library was also opened in both asylums and estimates prepared in 1885 for a recreation hall at Adelaide, although there is no evidence this was ever was built.

The Adelaide Lunatic Asylum remained open until 1902 when all the patients were transferred to Parkside Asylum, which remains open today as Glenside (Psychiatric) Hospital.

THE SOUTH AUSTRALIAN ASYLUMS AND THE 'IDEAL' ASYLUM MODEL OF JOHN CONOLLY

As in Chapter Five, the asylums are considered here firstly against the model of Conolly (Table 6) and then against the other models; this will be followed by a discussion of the impact of the provision or absence of rooms and spaces on life in the asylums.

A - An appropriate site with some form of scenery

The Adelaide Asylum initially met these criteria. It was placed in an area of open land with the town of Adelaide relatively close, allowing easy access for visitors and relatives. However this site was close to the Adelaide Hospital and was rapidly encroached upon. The possibility of views was prohibited because the walls of the exercise yards were 12 ft. high (S.A. C.S.O. Letters 24/6/2429). As the site was elevated on a knoll, views from the front gardens would have been possible, but the placement of the windows almost directly under the eaves prevented any views from the sleeping rooms. These problems were solved by placing the new Parkside Asylum on an estate of over 600 acres, by the use of ha-ha walls for the airing courts, and the use of paired windows. The Parkside Asylum was located just beyond the Parklands surrounding the town of Adelaide and remained close enough to allow easy access for visitors and inspection. These features would probably have formed part of Conolly's idea of an "appropriate site".

B - An arrangement of the buildings that allowed light in and cross ventilation, with no building overshadowing another or the airing courts

In terms of Conolly's second factor, Adelaide Lunatic Asylum failed miserably. The building was poorly designed with small high windows that let in little light and air. There was no system of ventilation, instead a few air bricks and the windows were relied upon (S.A. S.C. 1864: Q. 929). Given the hot summers of Adelaide, with temperatures often above 35 degrees Centigrade, this building would have been suffocatingly hot and the trapped air would have been highly offensive. The placement of the wards across from the day space allowed no cross ventilation. This problem was resolved in later additions, which featured larger windows, and in the new male wards rooms were placed along only one side of the building to allow more air flow. Parkside Asylum, however, fulfilled this second requirement, having large windows and an open design and layout.

The South Australian Asylums and the 'Ideal' Asylum Model

Table 6. Conolly's Ideal Features and The South Australian Asylums

Lunatic Asylum	A	B	C	D	Ea	Eb	Ec	F	G	Ha	Hb	Hc	Hd	Ia	Ib	J	K	L
Adelaide	X		X		X	X								X				
Parkside	X	X			X	X		X		X		X	X	X	X	X		

Key

A - An appropriate site with some form of scenery
B - An arrangement of the buildings that allowed light in and cross ventilation, with no building overshadowing another or the airing courts
C - A linear form to the layout
D - It should accommodate no more than 360 to 400 inmates
Ea - A building that offered a range of wards for classification
Eb - Each ward should have its own attendant's rooms
Ec - There should be open areas as opposed to day rooms for patients
F - Each ward should have access to a bathroom, lavatory and water closets
G - Each ward should have a wide gallery furnished as a day room with windows low enough to allow a view outside
Ha - There should be a large recreation room
Hb - School rooms
Hc - Work rooms and workshops
Hd - A chapel for the use of patients
Ia - The offices should be centrally located
Ib - There should be a means of accessing the various wards without passing through each
J - Attendant's should have their own dining hall
K - Accommodation should primarily be in the form of single rooms with a few dormitories
L - Above all the asylum should be light, cheerful and liberal in the space it offere

C - A linear form to the layout

Adelaide Asylum's main building did have a linear layout, as did later ward additions for the men. However other additions for the women took the form of clusters of cells. Parkside was designed as a pavilion asylum.

D - It should accommodate no more than 360 to 400 inmates

Adelaide Asylum was originally designed for 40–60 inmates. Over time it was to expanded and by the late 1870s the number of patients accommodated was generally in the mid 200s, peaking at 339 in 1872 (see Piddock 2003 for more details). So, Adelaide was below Conolly's figure, Parkside, however went beyond it, being designed when complete to accommodate 700 patients (S.A. S.C. 1864; *S. A. Register* May 28th 1868). The administrative building erected first was designed for 200 patients.

Ea - A building that offered a range of wards for classification

What is striking about the Adelaide Lunatic Asylum is how little it resembled Conolly's 'ideal' asylum in that most basic feature - classification. The original design of two wards for each sex with their associated day rooms on the main floor, meant only two classifications were possible during the day: acute and convalescent. The attic dormitory only allowed further classification at night, while a single room was provided for infirmary cases on each side. There was no means for physically separating the noisy from other acute cases. There was certainly not a range of wards at Adelaide suited to the needs of particular classes; those available were small and inflexible. The later additions of male dormitories allowed greater classification, although accommodation for the women remained limited. However the documentary evidence indicates that due to overcrowding, even the separation of acute and convalescent was impossible at various times (S.A. S.C. 1856: iii; S.A. Visitors 4/12/1869, 3/8/1870, 15/10/1870, 6/1/1877; S.A. Comm. 1884: iv).

While the main building at Parkside was designed for 200 patients it, too, offered little in the way of classification. This may have arisen as a consequence of the completion of only one of the three intended buildings. If Parkside had been built as a pavilion asylum, the central building may only have been intended to accommodate one class of patients, chronic patients who would live in the asylum for long periods. The possibilities of classifying patients remained problematic at Parkside due to its internal layout. The space appears to have been divided into three wards on each side. On the first floor these wards were composed of a corridor ward of single rooms ending with a water closet and two bedrooms facing each other, and a second ward composed of the dormitories and single rooms in the front section. On the second floor the third ward was composed of identical central rooms. What is particularly interesting about the wards in the front of the buildings was the placement of the central dormitories. This arrangement certainly did not allow for the effective separation of the sexes, as was indicated by the division of the asylum into male and female sides. This suggests that one floor was for women and another for men, or that the central section was given over to men and women on separate floors. Some separation of the patients along classificatory lines was possible through the use of small dormitories and single grouped bedrooms in the small blocks. The separate bedrooms at the end of the corridor wards would also have allowed a noisy patient to be separated, the toilet and wall acting as a sound barrier. There was insufficient space to allow any real classification, as achieved in British asylums, as patients would remain in contact with each other in the front rooms. There was only one day room for each sex in the main building, again allowing no separation of the patients.

Eb - Each ward should have its own attendant's rooms

Originally Adelaide did have separate attendant's rooms as recommended by Conolly, as did Parkside. Overcrowding at Adelaide may have led to their later re-designation as sleeping space for patients.

Ec - There should be open areas as opposed to day rooms for patients

Adelaide Asylum had both enclosed and open day rooms. The latter were on the ground floor and in fact formed part of the corridor. Further day rooms were erected in the airing courts. Parkside similarly had enclosed day rooms and further day rooms in its airing courts.

F - Each ward should have access to a bathroom, lavatory and water closets

In terms of water closets and baths, Adelaide Asylum originally had water closets on the wards. Quickly becoming offensive they were moved outside, and later additions also placed them in the yards rather than on the new wards. The original baths were also removed with the water closets. A bathroom appears to have existed on the ground floor of the main building in later periods but its location is unclear.

The second male dormitory added in 1861 had the bathroom and lavatories adjacent to a day room in a sub floor. These, however, were only accessible from the outside and were not directly accessible from the wards above (S.A. Visitors 8/7/1852, S.A. C.S.O. Letters 24/1625).

The problems with the water closets at Adelaide were solved at Parkside by placing them in open shafts within the buildings and continuing the open space through the upper floors. There were, in fact, limited provisions for the number of patients. Interestingly there are no baths marked on the plans and there is no other evidence of where they might have been located, which raises questions about how the patients were kept clean.

G - Each ward should have a wide gallery furnished as a day room with windows low enough to allow a view outside

Conolly had envisaged this space in terms of the linear gallery ward arrangement found in English lunatic asylums such as Derby. Neither Adelaide nor Parkside were designed with linear wards and wide galleries. There is no evidence that the corridors were used as living space, such as in the male ward additions at Adelaide or the wards of Parkside that flanked the courtyard.

Ha - There should be a large recreation room

Adelaide Asylum was never provided with a large recreation room, although one was proposed in 1885 (S.A. P.P. 1885 No. 60). From documentary evidence it appears that a ward was used on some occasions for entertainments, and possibly one of the front offices as well (S.A. S.C. 1869 Q. 27, 29, 32, 34).

It is unclear whether the completed design for Parkside would have included a purpose-built recreation hall. In 1880 work began on the multifunction room on the women's side of Parkside, which would serve as chapel, recreation room and dining room (S.A. A.R. 19/2/1880).

Hb - School rooms

Neither asylum provided school rooms.

Hc - Work rooms and workshops

Adelaide was not originally provided with workshops and workrooms. Documentary evidence suggests that one room was modified from its original purpose to serve as a workshop. The tailor had been using a room near the front entrance until 1869, when he moved into the new workshops at the rear of the asylum. The women sewed in the day rooms. Parkside had no workshops but did have a workroom adjoining the women's day room. (S.A. S.C. 1869 Q. 43 and 1503; S.A. S.C. 1864 Q. 60, 201; S.A. S.C. 1864 Q. 305, 349)

Hd - A chapel for the use of patients

Adelaide was not provided with a chapel. However, documentary evidence suggests that an office was used for Divine Service (S.A. S.C. 1864 Q. 60, 201). Parkside was similarly without a chapel until 1880.

Ia - The offices should be centrally located

Adelaide had the central offices, but, as indicated, their use was multifunctional and not purely used as office space. At times of overcrowding staff rooms were used for patients (S.A. S.C. 1856: iii). Parkside also had centralized offices, which in the pavilion system occupied the centre of the asylum.

Ib - There should be a means of accessing the various wards without passing through each

The relatively small size of the original Adelaide Asylum meant that it was not necessary to provide access corridors, as the two wards on each side were accessible via the central offices and staff rooms. Additions took the form of small buildings with external access or, in the case of the male additions, a central staircase between the two additions. This allowed ready access to the wards on either side. Parkside similarly used centralized staircases to allow access to the front and side sections of the building.

J - Attendants should have their own dining hall

Adelaide did not provide separate halls; rather staff had their own table in the patients' day room (S.A. S.C. 1864 Q. 167). Parkside provided two attendants' dining rooms, one for each sex.

K - Accommodation should primarily be in the form of single rooms with a few dormitories

From the plans it appears that accommodation was primarily in the form of single rooms at Adelaide, while at Parkside accommodation appears to have favored the dormitory.

Overall, the Adelaide Asylum possessed only a few of Conolly's features, while Parkside Asylum had slightly more. Adelaide lacked both spaces that would have made patient life more bearable, and a basic design that would have supported the effective use of space and allowed for ventilation. Later additions only partially brought the asylum closer to the Conolly model, in that the male dormitory additions had larger windows and a separate day room rather than using corridor space for this purpose.

The Adelaide Lunatic Asylum had opened in 1852, only five years after the publication of John Conolly's seminal work. Given the normal building period of one to two years, it is unlikely that Conolly's work could have directly influenced the design of the original asylum. Maximilian Jacobi's treatise would seem more likely to be expressive of ideas that might have influenced the design of the Adelaide Lunatic Asylum. However much of what constituted the model asylum, in Browne's and Connolly's view, was concerned with providing the insane with a more comfortable life and supporting their daily management. So, to a degree these could be considered common sense provisions. Works such as Conolly's were a crystallization of these ideas, expressed as a coherent system of accommodation and management. Consequently if not all of the ideas about the provision of an environment to support moral management and non-restraint were known by South Australians, some ideas might have been public knowledge. Certainly, the introduction of full non-restraint in 1858 (see Appendix 2), should have given rise to requests for modification to the original asylum to support this regime.

The fundamental point, which arises from the comparison to Conolly's model, is that despite its opening 18 years after the Adelaide Asylum, Parkside Asylum repeated many of its failings. There was a distinct lack of spaces for the intended number of patients to be housed there, and, while one set of water closets were provided, they had to service a large number of patients. There was also no apparent provision of baths. This was despite the experiences gained from the day-to-day management of the Adelaide Asylum. For example, as originally opened, the Parkside Asylum offered only a female work room for the employment of patients, despite the fact that the employment of the men had always been an issue at Adelaide (see for example S.C. 1864:

Q. 10–11, 16–17, 76). Similarly the lack of a recreation room or dining hall is not readily explainable. Clearly, by the time Parkside was designed and constructed, ideas about what was required to provide a healthy and reasonable environment for the insane should have been readily accessible in a variety of forms, and Parkside should have come much closer to Conolly's 'ideal'.

From the brief description of the intended Woodforde Asylum (228 patients) provided by the Colonial Architect (S.A. C.S.O. Letters 24/6/2506; Piddock 2003 Appendix A), it appears that this would have been closer to the Conolly model. It was planned to have centralized offices, linear wings with detached buildings for paying patients at the ends of each wing, a chapel and infirmaries. The asylum was intended to have workrooms for the men and a laundry for the women in the rear of the airing courts. The plan supported self-sufficiency principles with a dairy and farm included, and gardens would have been available for the men to work in. The site was large (60 acres, 3 rods and 4 perches) and sufficiently far from Adelaide to provide a peaceful environment and scenery of the foothills (S.A. C.S.O. Letters 24/6/172; 24/6/984; 24/6/1402). The description of the asylum suggests that it would have followed the design of the linear asylums found in England.

If the South Australian lunatic asylums only partially met Conolly's model were there any similarities to the other models discussed or to the lunatic asylums actually built in England?

THE 'IDEAL' ASYLUMS OF BROWNE, JACOBI, SANKEY AND ROBERTSON

Two models predate the opening of the Adelaide Asylum - those of Browne (1837) and Jacobi (1841). In terms of Browne's 'ideal' model (Table 7), Adelaide had a reasonably healthy site, but was not located in the country. The boundary between country and town in the 1850s in South Australia was not as strictly defined as one would find in Europe. Adelaide was at this point a town, with a number of surrounding villages on the plains between the sea and hills and the country was only a short distance from the Adelaide Asylum. The development of suburbs just beyond the Parklands surrounding Adelaide may not have been predictable at the time the site was chosen. With respect to the building features (Table 7) there are no matches to Browne's model, apart from the provision of a bath room and water closets.

Similarly, there are few matches with Jacobi's asylum model (Table 7). Classification was clearly being attempted, with the assignment

Table 7. Ideal Asylums and the South Australian Asylums

Browne's Features found in the Adelaide Asylum

1) A healthy site with a dry cultivated soil, and an ample supply of natural water
2) A country site, elevated or on a slope, near enough to a town for supplies and activities
3) There should be free access to airing courts for exercise
4) There should be baths, showers and water cleansing privies

Browne's Features found in the Parkside Asylum

1) A healthy site with a dry cultivated soil, and an ample supply of natural water
2) A country site, elevated or on a slope, near enough to a town for supplies and activities
3) Windows should be placed low on the walls to allow a view out
4) There should be free access to airing courts for exercise
5) There should be baths, showers and water cleansing privies

Jacobi's Features found in the Adelaide Asylum

1) It should allow classification, in particular the separation of the sexes, and the noisy and violent patients from the convalescent
2) It should be placed in the country and close to a town
3) There should be a good water supply

Jacobi's Features found in the Parkside Asylum

1) It should allow classification, in particular the separation of the sexes, and the noisy and violent patients from the convalescent
2) It should be placed in the country and close to a town
3) There should be a good water supply
4) That there be a chapel attached to the asylum
5) That the building be sufficiently lit and ventilated

Sankey's Features found in the Adelaide Asylum

1) A separate infirmary ward should be located on both male and female sides

Sankey's Features found in the Parkside Asylum

1) The officers for the male and female divisions would have their rooms in the divisions themselves rather than in the central building
2) Each division would have wards divided into two classes, those for day time use and those for night time use
3) The day and night areas were to be completely distinct and separate to the point of having separate sets of staff
4) All should freely communicate with each other

Robertson's Features found in the Parkside Asylum

1) Series of blocks dedicated to a particular class of patient
2) The provision of single rooms and dormitories in a percentage reflecting the classification (acute and chronic)
3) Ground floor day rooms and sleeping rooms on first and second floors
4) Division of the floors into day and night roles
5) The provision of the separate recreation hall, attendant's rooms and chapel recommended by Conolly

of different rooms to different patient groups on the original plans (refractory, acute and wet on the ground floor, convalescent and sick on the first floor), but there was no way to actually separate the patients, and the physical dimensions of the original building did not allow any barriers to noise passing between the wards. Separation of the sexes was maintained in the original building by having stairs located in the wards. Unfortunately, it is not clear who was using the second floor dormitories, although it is possible as suggested above for Parkside Asylum, that one sex only may have been using these rooms. Adelaide Asylum matched Jacobi's recommendations in its size and scraped through in terms of storeys, as the second floor was only partial. There is some evidence of the adaptation of the rooms for the various groups of patients based on class, but this was apparently only in the 1880s, and the windows did not support the rooms being well lit (S.A. Comm. 1884 Q. 390–1, 1244). There were no work areas, and access to the garden was severely limited for the women (S.A. S.C. 1864 Q. 458–459).

As would be expected, a comparison of the Adelaide plans with the British asylum designs finds no echoes. Certainly, the building did not copy the linear ward pattern of Bethlem Hospital. However, the documentary evidence available gives no indication of whether Adelaide Asylum was based on any particular design from England or Europe.

Parkside Lunatic Asylum had some of the features of Sankey's 1867 'ideal' asylum model (Table 7). Sankey had advocated the provision of separate day and sleeping accommodation on different floors, which was found at Parkside, but not the ward arrangement he recommended. Similarly, Parkside originally lacked the chapel and entertainment room of Sankey's model. It originally had the centralized residence for the superintending officer as Sankey recommended, but a house was later built for the Superintendent on the asylum grounds. However, the senior staff were provided with their own bedrooms on each side of the Asylum on the upper floors, making them readily accessible at night if needed. It is unclear from the plans whether there was a separate infirmary ward as recommended, but there may have been a separate dormitory for them. The lack of a boundary wall for many years meant there was no accessibility to the grounds for the patients, and there were no gardens for patient use. As indicated above the patient living spaces were very limited, with the dining rooms not being built until a number of years after the asylum opened.

In 1863 C. L. Robertson recommended the use of pavilion blocks in association with middle class asylums[1] and later in 1867 with asylums

---

[1] See Robertson 'On the want of a Middle Class Asylum in Sussex, with Suggestions how it may be established.' *The Journal of Mental Science* 1863 Vol. VIII No 44: 465–482.

in general (Table 7). The main difference between his proposed plan and Parkside Asylum was that sufficient blocks would be built to allow classification of the pavilions even for a small asylum. The original design of Parkside had allowed only three blocks: one each for men and women, and the administrative block which included some accommodation.

The possible uses of the corridors in the women's pavilion as day space and wards suggests that the building design followed the traditional pattern of arrangement, rather than the splitting of day and night spaces suggested by Sankey and Arlidge, and further recommended by Robertson. Certainly Robertson's model had retained the separate recreation hall and chapel of earlier models, along with male workshops - spaces that were lacking in the design for Parkside. The pavilion system aided ventilation and helped with supervision, as patients were localized in fewer spaces than was found in the gallery wards. Yet Parkside was lacking in so many ways. There was limited day space, insufficient accommodation for the Resident Medical Officer, no workshops, recreation hall or chapel, and initially no laundry or airing courts.

Parkside Asylum was constructed after a period of intense consideration of the 'ideal' asylum by lunacy reformers, but still only reflected a few ideas about the 'ideal'. Rather, its innovation rested with its pavilion form and cottage additions. The modified pavilion form was not adopted for British asylums until the 1870s/1880s, which instead continued the linear ward layout discussed in Chapter Six. Certainly, it is possible to speculate why the pavilion was chosen over the linear system. It may have reflected a familiarity with the written ideas of Robertson, who had proposed the block system as early as 1863, three years before work began on Parkside, or it may have reflected a choice based on climate. The gallery design allowed extra exercise space if the weather was inclement or too cold. With South Australia's climate of long periods of fine, warm weather it may have been assumed that patients would spend large amounts of time in the airing courts. This, of course, failed to recognize the additional role of the gallery as recreational space for entertainments and dances, and for the separation of the patients.

There are no ready matches to Parkside among the British asylums, and the failure to provide either a recreation room or separate dining hall was not in keeping with the trend in British asylums. These asylums, again, generally provided workshops for those activities that benefited the asylum economy, as well as separate chapels.

In terms of the rooms found in the British County Asylums (Table 8), Parkside comes close in only a few areas, such as the patient, administrative and domestic rooms. However, it lacked many of the service rooms and many of the discretionary spaces, with some aspects being

Table 8. Rooms Found in British County Asylums Compared to the South Australian Asylums

Room Type	Adelaide	Parkside
Patient	X	X
Single rooms	X	X
Dormitories	X	X
Day rooms	X	X
Attendant's rooms	X	X
Bath	X	Not known
Water Closet	X	X
Lavatory (wash room)	X	
Administrative		
Visitor's room	X	X
Assistant Surgeon's room(s)		X
Matron's room(s)	X	X
Surgery/Dispensary	X	X
Porter's Room		X
Committee/Board room	X	X
Waiting Room	X	
Medical Superintendent's Rooms	X	
Domestic		
Bakehouse		X
Brewhouse		
Kitchen	X	X
Flour Store		X
Bread room		X
Dairy		
Beer cellar		
Scullery	X	X
Stores		X
Pantry		
Larder		X
Matron's Store		
Steward's store		
Service		
Carpenter's shop	X	
Smith's shop		
Matmaker's shop		
Painter's		
Plumber's shop		
Cabinet shop		
Shoemaker's shop		
Tailor's shop	X	
Laundry	X	X
Ironing and folding room		

(continued)

Table 8. (continued)

Room Type	Adelaide	Parkside
Drying room		
Washhouse	X	
Foul linen washroom		
Engine house		
Boiler room		
Coals	X	
Gas works		
Chapel		
Discretionary		
Chaplain's room		
Dining hall		
School room		
Workrooms		
Servant's hall		X
Post mortem room		
Dead house	X	X
Lodge	X	
Total	22	23

met by later additions. Adelaide Asylum exhibited a similar pattern, being composed primarily of accommodation, some day space, a kitchen and laundry. It lacked the domestic rooms of Parkside, but had slightly more service rooms. Any closeness to the discretionary areas came from the multi-functionality of some spaces, while later additions probably returned some of the administrative rooms to their intended purpose.

LIFE IN THE ASYLUMS

It is possible to understand what life was like within the South Australian asylums from the comparison to the 'ideal' models, and with additional information from the available documents. From the patient's perspective the asylums offered a life dominated by the ward and the airing court. For the Medical Superintendent, it presented ongoing challenges to the effective supervision of patients and attendants, and limited spaces for the classification and separation of patients based on their mental illness and treatment regimes. It further offered limited opportunities, in terms of its spaces, to control the behavior of inmates through regimes such as moral treatment.

Life in the Asylums

Moral treatment and the non-restraint regime had both focused on the provision of an appropriate built environment to aid patient management and bring about a cure. Their key features of kindness towards patients, classification, religious consolation, a clean environment, exercise and some kind of activity to occupy the mind, required the provision of the necessary spaces and rooms to support this. Thus, it is possible to understand life within the asylums through the absence or provision of these rooms and spaces.

As indicated above, the Adelaide and Parkside Asylums each had limited ward accommodation which prevented any extensive classification, and due to overcrowding even the most basic of classifications was impossible to maintain. What were the implications of this? The nineteenth century asylum patient had no access to the chemical restraints of modern medicine. Those experiencing the acute or fully-blown attack of mental illness were thus likely to be agitated, noisy, possibly unrestrained in their physical movements, panicky, and desperate even to cope with the sensations, feelings, hallucinations, and physical manifestations of their illness. For those recovering from their illness, these unrestrained patients provided reminders of their illness, disturbed the quiet of the ward, and made it more difficult to behave in a restrained manner that indicated one's return to sanity which ultimately led to release from the asylum. Hence a basic level of classification was essential for the effective management of the patients. The separation of epileptics allowed for closer observation of these patients who could die during a fit if they choked or fell against furniture and injured themselves. Acute or epileptics wards could be differently furnished to meet the needs of these particular patients. Adelaide appears to have had a padded room on the male side for these patients; the women had to make do with a few mattresses of the floor of a sleeping cell (S.A. Comm. 1884 Q. 4292). The overcrowding at Adelaide directly impacted on the material culture of the asylum, at one time the mixing of acute and convalescent patients meant that spoons had to be used, as knives and forks represented possible weapons or implements of self harm for the acute patients, and thus could not be used. The reality of overcrowding meant equally cramped sleeping accommodations with two patients housed in a cell 7ft. 4in. wide and 10ft. long with the possibility of one patient disturbing the other (S.A. Visitors 15/5/1860, S.A. S.C. 1856: Q. 80–6, 31).

Classification was generally extended to the airing courts for the same reasons as the wards, and access to a nicer airing court could be a reward for appropriate behavior. At Adelaide the men had two airing courts, and there is evidence that by the 1880s, airing court No. 2 was a nicer court having a garden and fountain. The plainer airing court was used for acute and refractory patients. The women only had one yard which housed the laundry, and later, cells for wet and dirty patients (S.A. Comm. 1884 Q. 1740, 4050 & 5608). There is no evidence that the airing court was landscaped. Access to decorative gardens, often in front of the asylums, could also be a privilege granted to convalescent patients. Photographic evidence indicates the front of the Adelaide Asylum was extensively landscaped with trees, plants and ponds. Beyond these small attempts at landscaping, the airing courts must have been bleak with their high enclosing walls offering no views or contact with the outside world.

Parkside Asylum presented similar problems to Adelaide, as a result of the design of its wards and the problems of getting airing courts built. Classification was again problematic as there was only limited separation of the sleeping areas, and the lack of accommodation on the ground floor meant that acute patients could not be accommodated there. Accommodation for acute patients needed to be physically secure to prevent escapes, and required access to an airing court without the problems of getting patients up and down stairs. These problems resulted not from a fault with the original design of the asylum, but rather from the incompletion of the original design with its three pavilions. The wards in the main administrative building would have been intended for convalescent or chronic patients who would have lived for many years in asylum. This may have also been the reason for the limited day space. In the British asylums these patients would have been employed most of the day and effectively away from the wards. Parkside, however, did not have these workshops, nor the dining hall found in some British asylums which would have provided additional day time space for the patients. The one day room provided for each sex rapidly became insufficient and the lack of space meant that meals could not be eaten in these rooms. Consequently additional day rooms had to be constructed in the airing courts as a necessity.

The original design of the Adelaide Asylum had offered limited day space and within a year of their erection in 1857, the shelter sheds in the airing courts were converted into day rooms complete with fireplaces. It seems likely that for the men, the day was spent in the airing courts with meals taken in the day rooms. This would have allowed for easier supervision. The women's world was probably similarly limited, with the main variation being their employment in the laundry and kitchen, or in sewing tasks in the day rooms. The limited ward day space may have led to patients being put in their cells or dormitories quite early in the evening due to the crowded conditions. The same may have occurred at Parkside, although for a number of years only the men were accommodated there, and they may have used the work and day rooms on the women's side.

One of the basic elements of Conolly's model had been the provision of a range of discretionary spaces for patient use, including a chapel, school rooms and a recreation hall, as well as workrooms and workshops. These were designed to support the application of moral therapy and/or non-restraint. As was indicated in the comparison, Adelaide lacked all of these spaces. This did not mean, however, that these activities were not pursued. Non-restraint was not introduced into the Adelaide Asylum until 1858 (see Appendix 2) and prior to that time there were certainly no religious services and activities for the men were limited to board games, cards, and reading (S.A. S.C. 1856 Q. 91, 93, 126–7; S.A. S.C. 1864 Q. 305, 349).

In the 1860s things had improved slightly and religious services were irregularly held in a room in the front of the asylum. Capable of holding 40 to 50 worshippers, it was possibly the Committee Room that was being used for this purpose. Patients were also given prayer books and Bibles. Services relied on the goodwill of a clergyman, as there were none assigned specifically to the asylum (S.A. S.C. 1864 Q. 5, 60, 201).

While in terms of amusements for the men, there was bagatelle, cricket, walking expeditions, newspapers, books, and backgammon, for the women, Dr. Paterson found it was more difficult to find amusements. They had walking expeditions, the *Illustrated News*, and 'a great deal of needlework'. Again the border between amusement and work was blurred for the women. If Dr. Paterson wished to give a bazaar, female patients would be employed in making goods. Dances were now being held, along with concerts, theatrical entertainments, 'Christy Minstrels', and other entertainments. These were attended by all but the sickest inmates, and appear to have taken place in either a front room or a ward (S.A. S.C. 1869 Q. 27, 29).

What is particularly interesting about this change in the life of the Adelaide Asylum is that there were no requests for dedicated rooms for these purposes, and their original absence at Adelaide may be seen as reflective of the original treatment regime based on restraint. However their absence at Parkside is more difficult to explain, as Dr. Paterson, who had instigated a wider range of activities for the patients, was employed to give advice on Parkside's design (S.A. V. & P. 28/7/1864). A recreation hall may have been included in the original design of the asylum, which did include a workroom for the women and a billiards room for the men, spaces not found at Adelaide. This perhaps reflects Paterson's influence or an increased awareness of British asylum designs.

The absence of a chapel is easier to understand than the absence of workrooms/workshops and a recreational hall, as South Australia had been established under the provision that it had no state religion.

Religious freedom and freedom of worship was to make Adelaide the city of churches, with a diverse range of religious practices (see Hilliard and Hunt 1986). Hence a Church of England or Roman Catholic Chapel would not be appropriate at the asylum.

While the employment of the men had always been an issue at Adelaide, where they were sporadically employed in such tasks as matmaking and sewing bags (S.A. S.C. 1864 Q. 10, 11, 16, 17, 76), Parkside lacked workshops for the men. There is no clear reason for this omission, as in England tailors, smiths and carpenter's shops were common provisions in the asylums built during the preceding decades (Conolly 1847: 81). It is unclear whether some undetected assumptions about the skills of the men admitted to the asylum were at work, with most being seen as unskilled laborers (S.A. S.C. 1864 Q. 71–2). Women on the other hand were constantly employed as their tasks related to the laundry or could be done in the day room and did not need specifically designed spaces, though Conolly had recommended work rooms to diversify the experience of daily life.

There is virtually no evidence about the interior furnishing of the asylums in the documents. The only evidence comes from the Parliamentary Inquires of 1864 and 1883. Dr. Moore had introduced caged birds and rabbits onto the wards to brighten them in 1864 (S.A. S.C. 1864 Q. 77, 80). Dr. Paterson, in 1883, indicated that the paying patients had carpets in their rooms and better furniture. This by implication suggests that the general wards were relatively bare (S.A. Comm. 1884 Q. 390–1, 1244).

Overall, then, for the patients at Adelaide and Parkside, there was little variation within their days, and only with the walking parties of the late 1860s were they to be relieved of the sight of the enclosing walls of the asylum. At Adelaide room use was dependent on need, with rooms being modified to meet immediate requirements. The recognition of the need for religious worship and recreations, even though they were being held at Adelaide, did not see the immediate provision of the necessary spaces at Parkside, instead a multifunctional room was provided ten years after its opening. This would indicate that in the 1870s, despite being in a newer building, life was probably even more limited for the residents of Parkside than Adelaide.

Interestingly, there is little evidence that the Adelaide Asylum was built with the South Australian climate in mind. No shades were provided in the airing courts until 1857, five years after the asylum's opening. The small windows and closely confined spaces would have led to a build up of heat within the buildings. The limited day space and the absence of galleries may, in fact, have reflected a belief that the patients would spend a larger portion of their time outside in the yards due to the climate. The harsher climate of England made additional indoor living space essential. Neither Adelaide nor Parkside Asylums had the galleries furnished as day space. As can be seen from the plans, the original building at Adelaide did not even have corridors, as the spaces were occupied by day rooms on the ground floor and wards on the first floor. The additional male dormitories again only had a narrow corridor that does not seem to have been used as a living area. Parkside Asylum when it opened again did not provide galleries for its wards. Although from the later description of the new women's pavilion, it appears that gallery sized corridors may have been provided, as the ground floor gallery could act as a dining room if needed (S.A. A.R. 24/2/1881). There is no evidence of the planting of shade trees and the patients must have spent a considerable amount of time in the summer sun. A similar situation existed at Parkside where sun shades and shade trees were not put in place until 1880 (S.A. A.R. 19/2/1880). As was indicated above, with respect to recreational space and workshops, the problems of Adelaide, which directly impacted on the lives of patients, did not lead to solutions being realized at Parkside on its opening.

Similarly, there was an absence of thought about the maintenance of a healthy environment within the Adelaide Asylum. The water closets had proved so offensive that within a few months of the asylum opening, they and the baths were removed. It seems likely that, as they were later placed outside at the rear of the yards, buckets or something similar must have been resorted to. The waste appears to have been disposed of on the ground to the rear of the asylum as by 1883, when the asylum was attached to deep drainage; the ground was so saturated as to be unusable and must have smelt (S.A. A.R. 22/2/1883). The writers on the 'ideal' asylum had turned their minds to the question of toilets and provided options including self-cleansing water streams that operated when the door was opened (Conolly 1847: 42). Consequently there was a pool of information that could have been drawn upon to improve the sanitary situation. Parkside provided equally limited sanitary provision including an apparent lack of baths. Many patients in their illness were not in control of their bodily functions and the lack of a laundry at Parkside until 1877 suggests that laundry was sent to Adelaide, an impractical option.

The lack of a healthy environment and adaptations to the climate must have impacted on the lives of the attendants. In effect, the attendants were as much confined to the asylum as the insane, with only occasional nights and days off. They lived and slept with the patients, hence the importance placed by Conolly on the provision of separate dining rooms for attendants to give them time away from the ward. Parkside did provide these rooms. Supervision of the patients must have been relatively straight forward as the men appear to have spent their days in the airing courts or in their associated day rooms. The women shared equally confined lives and their supervision must have been straightforward.

For the Medical Superintendent the Adelaide Asylums' nature as a collection of buildings without an organizational pattern had to prevent any effective supervision of the attendants. He was required to pass in and out of several buildings spread around the grounds when doing his rounds. While the Superintendent had been originally accommodated in the main building where he was readily available, in 1865 a residence was built for him on the boundary of the asylum grounds. This placed him a considerable distance away from the buildings erected over the 1860s including the main building (Figure 7.7). The question of this remoteness and how often Superintendent Paterson visited the wards was to be one of the focuses of the 1869 Select Committee (S.A. S.C. 1869 Q. 19–22, 259, 1866, 1873, 1876, 1881, 1904–5, 1942, 1945). A similar pattern occurred at Parkside with the Superintendent originally housed in the asylum, until a later residence was built.

Clearly, the lack of discretionary spaces and the overcrowding of the wards must have affected the implementation of treatment regimes by the various Superintendents as much as it impacted on the lives of the asylum patients.

A GENDERED EXPERIENCE

For women the asylum world offered little distancing from the cares of everyday life and the world of work. The association of women with domesticity ensured that they were almost constantly employed in the asylum laundry, and in sewing and knitting. The non-specialized nature of sewing meant that an ordinary day room could be used for such work, again providing little diversification in women's day-to-day lives. This and the placement of the laundry at the end of the women's airing yard at the Adelaide Asylum meant that the women were constantly reminded of work. Interestingly, women's work was also class-based with the *coarser* class of women being employed in the laundry and the more refined in sewing (S.A. S.C. 1864 Q. 130 191, original italics). There is no information, however, about how these classes were decided.

Reflecting perhaps the more constant employment of the women or a perception of women as being less active, their airing court was a quarter of the size of the men's two courts. Even when additional dormitories were built for the women, their exercise space was not apparently expanded. The lack of employment of the men meant that they also were given greater access to the front gardens. The separation of the sexes meant that the women could not go into the main garden at the same time as the men. Consequently, Sunday afternoon was the only time they were permitted access, and this came to be seen as a privilege (S.A. S.C. 1864 Q. 458–459).

The placement of the Botanic Gardens directly along the side of the women's ward and airing court had the most impact on the asylum experience for the women patients and staff. The placement of the garden alongside the women's yard meant that they were more vulnerable to the public gaze and women experienced taunts by individuals climbing adjoining trees (S.A. A.R. 19/2/1880). Its placement further limited the expansion of the women's sections and later additions were placed at the other end of the asylum's main building. This required the Matron to cover considerable distances to supervise the female attendants. The placement of wet and dirty women in cells adjoining the laundry effectively meant that these women received less supervision when they probably most needed it. Again there is no clear reason for their placement, and in fact they were more vulnerable as there was a charge of sexual molestation bought against a male attendant by one of the women occupying these remote cells (S.A. Comm. 1884: Q. 5440–5449).

The rooms provided in the Parkside Asylum reinforced the separate experiences of men and women. In the original plans the men were provided with a day room and billiards room, the women with a day room and adjoining work room. Interestingly Dr. Bayer, one of the official Asylum Visitors, noted in 1864 that the women had no amusements apart from hard physical labor, while the men certainly had access to playing cards, dominoes, board games, books and papers from as early as 1856 (Select Comm. 1856 Q. 91, 93, 126–7; Comm. 1864 Q. 305, 349). It is unclear why women did not have the same access to these recreations.

The role of women as mothers was also not acknowledged in the spaces provided of the South Australian asylums, with no nurseries being provided. Similarly, both men and women were denied their role as family members by the apparent lack of visiting rooms for family and friends in Adelaide Asylum, except when it was originally opened. Parkside Asylum did appear to have visiting rooms on each side of the asylum for gender separation, however it may have been the case that the reception and visiting rooms were used for purely official business and were not available for family visits.

DISCUSSION

The Adelaide Asylum was from the beginning of its existence a custodial institution. It is clear from the documentary evidence that the primary form of treatment practiced from 1852 to 1858 was based on physical restraint of the patients and the use of baths as a means of punishment for difficult patients[2] (S.A. S.C. 1856: Q. 40, 50, 52, 97–8, 511–525, 773, 776). The apparent lack of knowledge of moral treatment and non-restraint, which had been practiced in England since the turn of the century and more widely from the 1830s, also appears to have directly affected the design of the asylum. The asylum was built with few patient spaces, the main focus being the provision of wards and limited exercise space. The provision of day rooms seems to have been a secondary factor, as the use of a corridor for day space on the ground floor must have created disturbances and with overcrowding may have been turned into sleeping accommodation. There were no provisions to aid the cure of the patients or any provisions for activities or employment. This custodial aspect was reinforced when the issue of bars for the high windows to prevent escapes and inspection plates for the doors was raised shortly after the asylum's occupation (S.A. Visitors 30/3/1852). The patient was effectively a prisoner to be observed. The custodial nature of the treatment was reflected in the support given to the modification of the Gaol as an asylum rather than the building of a new one on the 'best English principles' (S.A. C.S.O. Letters 24/6/2506; S.A. S.C. 1856: Q. 40, 50, 52, 97–8, 511–525, 773, 776).

The introduction of full non-restraint to Adelaide by Dr. Moore in 1858 was not welcomed by all the attendants and some refused to work under the regime and were dismissed (S.A. S.C. 1864 Q. 6, 20–22, 34–5). Dr. Moore appears to have introduced activities to the wards and attempted to employ the men. In 1864 at least two visitors found the Asylum was prison-like and one noted "It is so different from what we read of places of the kind in England" (S.A. S.C. 1864 Q. 822, 880). These later observations may have arisen because there were no attempts to physically modify the main building beyond the insertion of air bricks and some ward additions. There was no large recreation hall or dining hall, workshops or workrooms, or real space to allow classification.

Parkside Asylum, opened 18 years after Adelaide, moved away from custodial care of the insane and provided an environment closer to Conolly's model. But Adelaide, with all its faults, continued to be used

---

[2] Once a patient was placed in the bath a constant stream of water was poured over his head for prolonged periods such as an hour.

alongside Parkside for a further 32 years. While Dr. Paterson extended the activities available to the patients, he did not ask for additional recreational spaces until the mid 1880s - more than a decade after his employment. He does not appear to have given value to these spaces nor appeared to object to the inconveniences of re-arranging office and ward spaces for entertainments etc. Thus, the levels of care for the patients represented by the features of Conolly's model are not realized.

Within the concepts of domination and paternalism, the Adelaide Asylum buildings can be seen as being expressive of a dominating regime, where patients were controlled and accommodated. Parkside Asylum, with its improved environment and increased range of patient spaces over a period of time, is more expressive of a caring paternalistic regime where the environment was more supportive of patient comfort and welfare. In this context the earlier dominative regime sought to simply remove the insane from society and hold them. Under moral treatment the Superintendent had a paternalistic role, as the central figure in the life of the patients; he sought through his skill to bring them back to sanity. Moral treatment and non-restraint were different from the earlier regimes as they focused on the well-being of the patient as an essential aid to curing the patient. This well-being came directly from the diet, care and treatment prescribed by the Superintendent.

Tasmania and the 'Ideal' Asylum | 8

If South Australia, a free colony, was to struggle to realize the provisions required by the 'ideal' asylum models of John Conolly and later asylum reformers, what then was to be the fate of the insane in Tasmania where a portion of the colonists were convicts serving out their sentences in Australia and not the prisons of England? This question leads to other important questions such as did the social and class based judgments about the perceived inmates of the lunatic asylum affect the type of buildings provided and the treatment regime undertaken? Was the treatment of the convicts more punitive? South Australia had provided purpose-built asylums for its colonists; did Tasmania provide similar institutions for its convict population? Were there separate institutions for convicts and free colonists?

A CONVICT COLONY

It was to forestall continuing French interest in southern Australia that the English decided to establish a settlement on an island just off the mainland to be called Van Diemen's Land. On January 4th 1803 David Collins was commissioned the first Lt. Governor of a colony to consist of convicts, marines and free settlers (Townsley 1991: 3). The town of Hobart was established in 1804 on Sullivan Cove, on Van Diemen's Land's southern coast. Due to perceived problems with the colony, in 1813 the administration of the colony was placed under the control of Governor Macquarie in Sydney, New South Wales, for the next 12 years. Macquarie subsequently sent the worst of New South Wales' convicts to Van Diemen's Land (Townsley 1991: 5–6, 37).

Initially, the transportation of convicts was slow, with only 500 sent to the colony between 1810 and 1817, but steadily increased. Meanwhile, in England the social turbulence arising from the French Wars and growing industrialization led tradesmen, small merchants and yeomen farmers to seek a new life in the colonies (Townsley 1991: 7). Consequently the population of Van Diemen's Land grew quickly from 4,300 in 1820 to 7,185 in 1821, of which 4,380 were convicts (Townsley 1991: 7).

From 1820 to 1840, the colony continued to thrive, with the British Commissariat directly controlling the institutions that dealt with convicts. The percentage of convicts in the general population gradually dropped as the number of free settlers increased. In 1820 convicts represented 54 percent of the population; by 1851 this had dropped to 29 percent, or around 20,000 people (Townsley 1991: 18). This figure did not include the emancipists and their families. In 1853 transportation ceased and in 1856 Van Diemen's Land was given its own Constitution and changed its name to Tasmania.

A BRIEF HISTORY OF THE NEW NORFOLK HOSPITAL FOR THE INSANE, PORT ARTHUR AND CASCADES LUNATIC ASYLUMS

The New Norfolk Hospital for the Insane grew out of the Convict Invalid Establishment, which most probably opened in mid to late 1830 (Tas. C.S.O. Letters 29/1/1829). Situated on the River Derwent, the town of New Norfolk was accessible by boat and road and 22 miles from what was to become the capital of Tasmania, Hobart Town (Figure 1.3).

In June of 1831 the District Surgeon in charge of the Invalid Establishment, Dr. Robert Officer, drew up plans, probably at the request of Governor Arthur, for a building suitable for housing lunatics at New Norfolk costing £604 0s. 6d. Work began in 1832. The new lunatic buildings were to be placed directly behind the existing invalid buildings, to form an enclosed courtyard, with the rear of the original building forming one wall. Intended only for convicts the New Norfolk Invalid Hospital and Lunatic Asylum was funded by the Imperial Government in England.

By 1836 accommodation pressures became apparent, when Robert Officer, in a letter to the Colonial Surgeon, indicated the need for additional buildings (Tas. C.S.O. Letters 1/811/17340). He argued that it was particularly difficult to achieve any classification among the lunatics based on their malady or constitution of mind "under such circumstances, the chance of recovery is greatly lessened and their domestic comforts (a most necessary part in their treatment), sadly diminished" (Tas. C.S.O. Letters 1/811/17340).

One of the few surviving plans of the Hospital, dating to 1829 and including the proposed additions of 1836, shows it to be composed of

A Brief History of the New Norfolk Hospital for the Insane

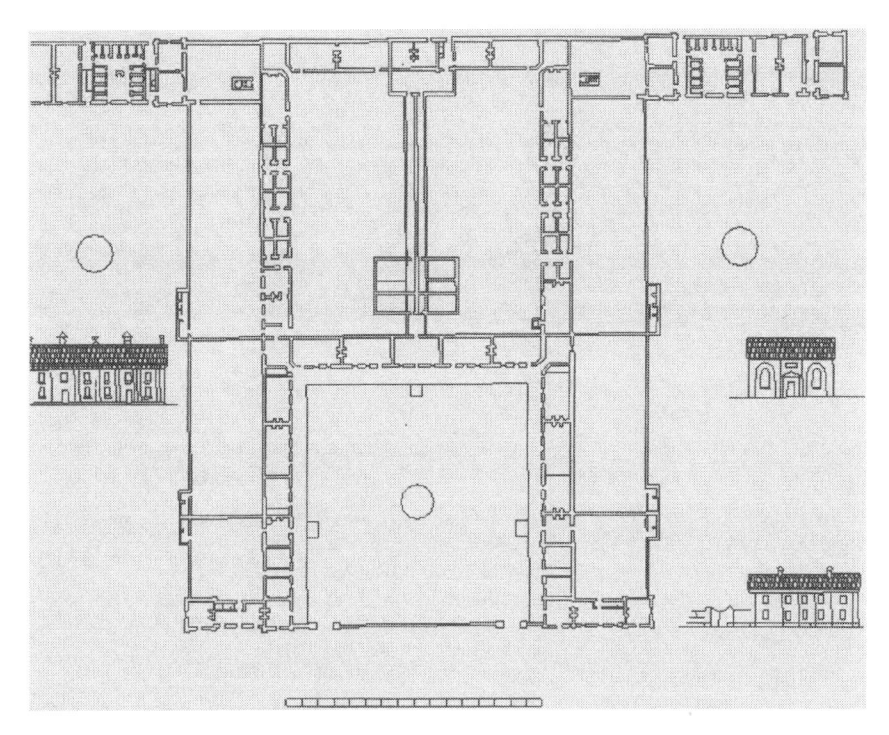

Figure 8.1. Roger Kelsall's Plan of New Norfolk, 1836. Archives Office of Tasmania, PWD 2666/1432/2. Redrawn by J. Gibb.

two squares with the invalids occupying the front section and the lunatics the rear (Figure 8.1). This rear quadrangle was divided into male and female sections. Roger Kelsall's plan and elevation shows a modified H plan with extensions to the right and left of the back building line. Some rooms are identifiable, while on others the legend is not clear. On the left hand side of the front quadrangle were two wards in a two storey building extending out from an overseer's room (sic). Moving upwards on the plan there was a store room, office, dead room, wash room, two wards, a store, two wards in the dividing section, with the kitchen in the centre, and then another two wards with a store in the corner. Down the right hand side were three wards, an unidentifiable room, the surgery and dispensary, an overseer's room (sic) and the two wards extending to the right. The left side of the back quadrangle had two rooms, then 12 pairs of cells, a ward and a store in the corner. Along the back were a washhouse, kitchen, Superintendent's Quarters, a second kitchen, and a store in the corner. The right side of the back

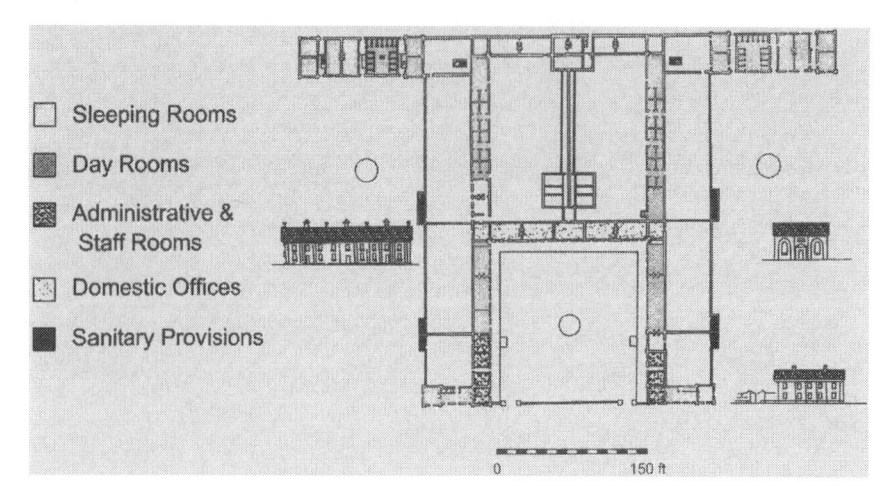

Figure 8.2. Room and space distribution in the New Norfolk Hospital for the Insane, 1836. Archives Office of Tasmania, PWD 2666/1432/2. Redrawn by J. Gibb.

quadrangle was composed of a ward, 14 cells, and then a second ward. The interior space was divided into male and female divisions with a chapel near the kitchen. From available documentation it appears the chapel was never built.

Two extensions formed a continuation of the back wall. The buildings (identically arranged) were composed of two rooms marked 'overseers', a passage containing a staircase, a large lunatic ward which appears to have some form of open partitions dividing the space, a second staircase passage, two large wards, another staircase passage, and two wards again. These extensions were separated from the original building by small yards, with privies located in the yards. Along the outside of the main buildings were six yards of different sizes equipped with privies.

From the extant buildings of Willow Court which formed the front courtyard, it appears that there were rooms above the centre block (Figure 8.3), and at the corners and ends of the building range (Figure 8.4). It is possible that the centre rooms may have been accommodation for one of the Superintendents (there were two Superintendents, a medical one and one for the insane asylum). It is possible to speculate the other rooms may have been additional wards. There is certainly no indication of day rooms on the plan. The accommodation was basic in the extreme. There were no bathrooms and water closets were only placed in the yards. The centre wall through the yard along with the Superintendent's quarters divided

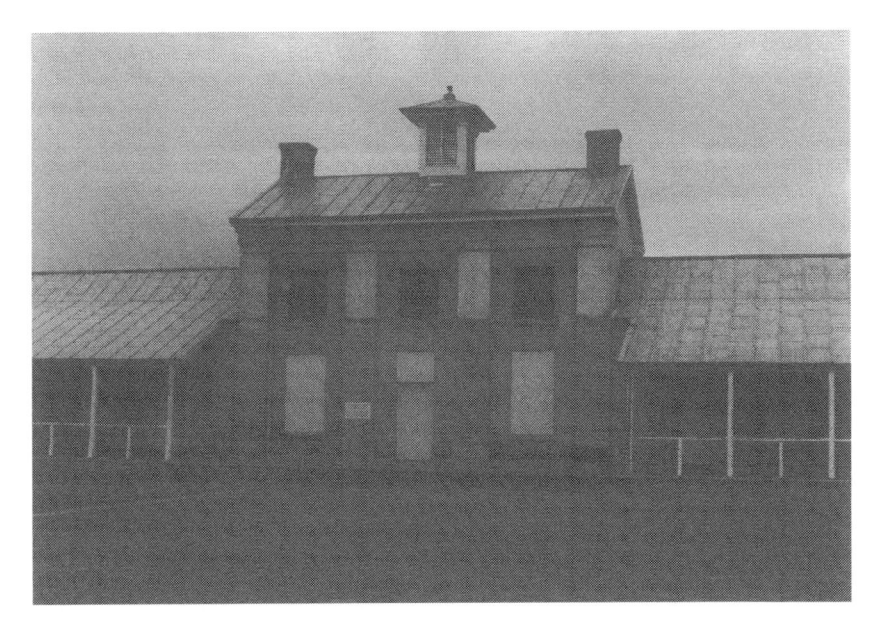

Figure 8.3. The building housing domestic offices, New Norfolk. Photograph by author 2001.

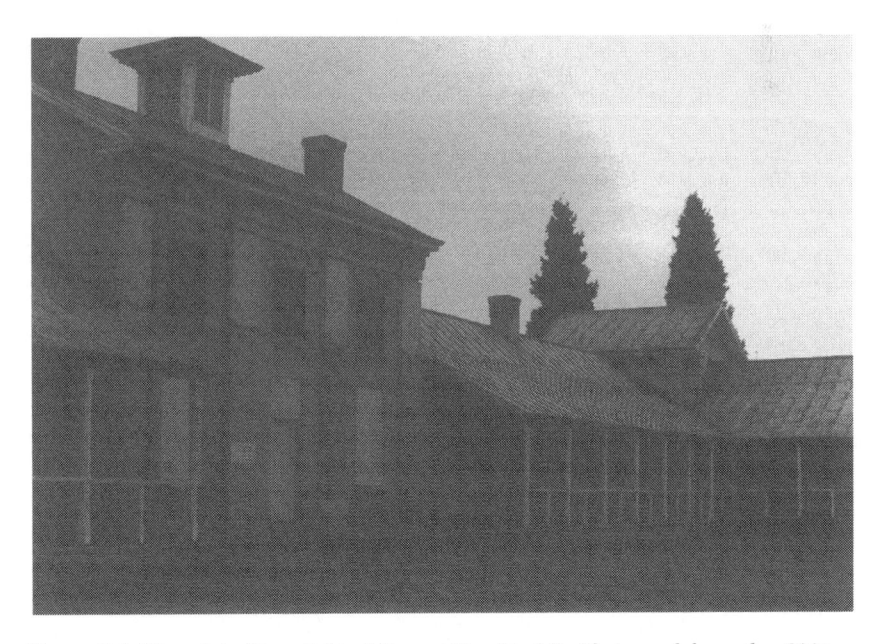

Figure 8.4. The original hospital buildings at New Norfolk. Photograph by author 2001.

the back quadrangle into male and female divisions. The provision of two kitchens took this separation to the extreme and, interestingly from a gender perspective; the washhouse was on the male side rather than the female. The separation of the invalids and lunatics was maintained through the dividing building only opening onto the front quadrangle.

There is scant information about the New Norfolk Hospital while it remained in the hands of the Imperial Government. New Norfolk was a closed establishment. This changed on October 18th 1855 when control passed to the colonial authorities. It is not clear from surviving nineteenth century documents when the Hospital became purely a place for the accommodation of the insane, but certainly by 1855 it had become so.

With the change in responsibility came the establishment of a Board of Commissioners, who were given charge of the New Norfolk Hospital, and with this change came the first snapshot of conditions within the Hospital. The Commissioners were to find much wrong as indicated in their initial report to the Governor: "its condition is very far behind that of similar institutions in the Mother Country. The internal accommodations of the several buildings were small, badly constructed, ill ventilated, dark, dismal, while the day rooms, so called, afforded very inadequate convenience for the purpose intended."(Quoted in Gowlland 1981: 50). The yards and grounds were divided into smaller spaces by high walls and allowing little room for exercise and outdoor recreation. The 100 women resident in the Hospital had the use of two small yards of less than a quarter acre each. The adjoining three acre paddock was forbidden to them. The male division had a walled garden of a quarter acre. Two small enclosed yards of a quarter acre each were in use for unquiet patients and a small area in front of the Hospital was used by quiet and convalescent patients. There was no classification of the patients.

In response to these conditions the Commissioners began a cycle of requests that sought to reshape the Hospital. The first priority was the replacement of the cells, particularly the wooden ones. The second priority was the provision of separate accommodation for those of a 'superior' rank, 12 of each sex, in a secluded part of the grounds. Unfortunately there is no precise evidence as to how they defined 'superior' in this context. Certainly the Commissioners saw New Norfolk as accommodating all the insane, not just convicts as probably occurred when it was an Imperial establishment. The Commissioners further recommended that an area be enclosed to allow the separation of the "worst" females from the quiet, and that verandahs be built to offer shade and exercise areas in wet weather

(Quoted in Gowlland 1981: 50–51). The New Norfolk Correspondence book indicates an almost immediate response by the Colonial Government to the problems at New Norfolk as extensive repairs were undertaken (Tas. N.N. Corresp. 14/1/1856).

While Tasmania was facing bankruptcy in 1857 (Townsley 1991: 98–100), work began on building the cottage for 'superior' male patients in 1858 and the female division additions were in plan form in early 1859 suggesting that this work was considered important even in a time of financial restraint (Tas. N.N. Corresp. 14/9/1858, 2/2/1859, 1/2/1859). In late 1859 plans had also been drawn up for the new laundry and store in the female ward, and the proposed additions to the male division cells, as well as improvements to the ventilation and heating in the Hospital overall (Tas. N.N. Corresp. 8/12/1859, 21/12/1859). By 1861 changes had been made to the female refractory addition and male division, and the extension of the central building was underway. The plans for the lodge and female division kitchen had been drawn up.

In understanding the history of building work at New Norfolk it is important to realize that the New Norfolk Commissioners continually asked for improvements to the Hospital, but only some of these were realized. As an example, in 1856 the Commissioners indicated that they wished for a residence for the under keepers, a chapel, suitable accommodation for six males and six females of the 'inferior rank of life', a lodge at the front gate, a further house in the female division and a new kitchen (Tas. N.N. Corresp. 14/1/1856, 12/5/1856). Of these, however, only the lodge and kitchen were ever realized. Priority rested with improving sleeping accommodation, which was composed of small cells opening directly onto the courtyards, followed by domestic and service areas, with living spaces coming last.

Not everybody saw the re-modeling of New Norfolk as the best option. In 1859 the first Roman Catholic Bishop of Hobart, Robert William Willson, was appointed to the New Norfolk Board of Commissioners. Willson was an experienced lunacy reformer having served seven years on the Board of Management of the Nottinghamshire County Lunatic Asylum in England (1830–1842), and was licensed to care for lunatics privately (Southwood 1973: 140). He began a letter campaign calling for a new asylum to be built close to Hobart and on a site of not less than 50 acres (22/10/1858 Tas. P.P. 1859 No. 10; Piddock 2003 Appendix D for full details). Willson roundly condemned New Norfolk for failing as "a '*Curative Hospital*' or one at all suitable for affording that comfort even the incurable have a right to receive" (8/3/1859 Tas. P.P. 1859 No. 10). Having experienced the humane and successful change in the treatment of the insane in England, he felt that much more could be done to improve conditions at New Norfolk. New Norfolk resembled nothing more than a prison. Gloomy, ill-ventilated, dark cells, prison-walled yards, swarms of vermin in the wooden buildings, no classification at all with the noisy and offensive mixed with the 'delicate and tranquil', the 'congenital idiot' with the recently admitted, and the 'imbecile' with the neat in habits.

Willson argued in the strongest possible terms that not even the leading non-restraint reformers, Robert Gardiner Hill and John Conolly (discussed in Chapter Four), could redeem New Norfolk, it fell so far short of British lunatic asylums (8/3/1859 Tas. P.P. 1859 No. 10). Instead, a new institution should be erected offering "those advantages and comforts of a well-conducted establishment with airing grounds, garden, &c." (8/3/1859 Tas. P.P. 1859 No. 10). An establishment closer to Hobart, he felt, would be visited more frequently and proper supervision would occur. With an eye to the economic advantages, the Bishop also believed a 'proper Hospital for the Insane' would attract upper class patients (presumably paying) to the asylum.

In his reply the President of the New Norfolk Board of Commissioners, E. S. P. Bedford, reflected the ambiguity towards New Norfolk that at the same time appears to have been affecting attempts to improve it. While he despaired of ever achieving perfection due to the inherent defects of the building, the lack of classification and the poorly ventilated cells, Bedford felt the dangerous character of many of the lunatics meant that security precautions would always give the Hospital the nature of a prison house (6/7/1859 P.P. 1859 No. 10). However the Commissioners welcomed a new purpose-built asylum along the best English lines but its anticipated cost (£65,000) seemed to preclude the possibility of it ever being built, instead they felt that much could be done to improve New Norfolk, principally because it was on a good site and far enough in the country to prevent disturbing casual visits by curious strangers (6/7/1859 Tas. P.P. 1859 No. 10).

Bishop Willson launched another volley on August 6th 1859: the buildings had been designed with convicts in mind and those in the Hospital who were not convicts should not be experiencing these conditions. He further challenged the cost of a new asylum, believing it would cost no more than £35,000 based on land prices in the colony. As the number of convicts were diminishing, the new asylum needed only to accommodate 200 patients and if built along pavilion lines it could be built in installments (6/8/1859 point 11, 17/8/1859 Tas. P.P. 1859 No. 10). A further option proposed by the Board of Commissioners was to build a smaller curative institution, with New Norfolk acting solely as an incurable Hospital (Tas. P.P. 1860 No. 12: 4).

A Brief History of the New Norfolk Hospital for the Insane

A Joint Committee was appointed in 1859 in response to Bishop Willson's letters. They were asked to decide between a new asylum or continuing modifications to the existing hospital. New Norfolk, they found, was situated on only 10 acres and exhibited a great many deficiencies with respect to its position, its accommodation, the health, classification, occupation and recreation of the inmates (Tas. J.C. Report 1859: 3). The original nature of the Hospital as an infirmary had resulted in a number of buildings that were unsuited to their purpose (for full details see Piddock 2003 Appendix D). In brief, the Joint Committee found overcrowding, and some attempts at classification through the creation of many small yards. Sleeping accommodation was poor and needed redesigning and rebuilding, and there were no day rooms, with verandahs being used instead. Patients spent their time in small yards, never going beyond these walls. Some men were employed in workshops but it is unclear where these were located. There was a need for baths, day rooms, large workshops, gardens, and staff rooms, as keepers presently lived outside of the Hospital (Tas. J.C. Report 1859: 5).

The Committee found the women's division was in a worse state than the men's, with only two classifications and one day room, and even the new plans for a women's building did not allow for exercise or recreation space (Tas. J.C. Report 1859: 5). Baths and a new laundry were required. Most significantly the Committee found:

> ... from the original plan and structure of the buildings, and their present condition there exists an innate difficulty, amounting to an impossibility, of converting the Asylum into an efficient curative establishment (Tas. J.C. Report 1859: 6).

This conclusion is important for two reasons: firstly there was a clear intention to have a curative lunatic asylum in the colony, with its implications for the built environment; and secondly the New Norfolk Hospital was entirely unsuited to this purpose. A curative establishment would have provided spaces for classification, exercise, work and leisure activities, and appropriate levels of sanitation to maintain the health of the patients.

However, the Committee was divided over its recommendations. Five members argued for a new asylum closer to Hobart, provided with modern quiet dormitories, sleeping cells, and day rooms for a range of pursuits. Using the Cumberland and Westmoreland County Lunatic Asylum as an 'ideal' asylum model, they anticipated a new asylum would cost £30,000. Failing this a long list of alterations to New Norfolk was required (Table 9) (Tas. J.C. Report 1859: 8). Four members of the Committee, while recognising the problems with

Table 9. Recommendations of the Joint Committee 1859

1. The purchase of the house and grounds now occupied as tenant by the Superintendent.
2. The purchase of the Nine acres of land between the Asylum and the Lachlan Creek, and its enclosure. The enclosure of the paddock of about six acres on the north.
3. The lowering of the present north and south walls, and placing iron railings on the top.
4. The removal of the dividing walls running north and south across both the Male and Female Compartments, and the laying out of those grounds.
5. In the Male Compartment the removal of the interior of the whole of the cells and dormitories, and reconstructing them with corridors.
6. The erection of additional dormitories, which would be rendered necessary by the enlargement of the old ones.
7. Providing pleasure and recreation grounds for the Second class, which can only be done by a removal of the Third class ward, and re- erecting it with a like provision of grounds for exercise and enjoyment.
8. Providing day-rooms for the Three classes Building capacious workshop.
9. Building enlarged kitchen for the general body of the inmates.
10. The like for the detached building for the Patients of the better class Building baths.
11. Accommodation for Attendants, to include quarters for Three married families and some single men.
12. *In the Female Compartment.*-The removal of the interior of the whole of the cells and dormitories, and reconstructing them with corridors.
13. The erection of additional dormitories which would be rendered necessary the erecting of at least one ward for Females of the better class, with kitchen and other apartments distinct from the other inmates; and additional means of classsification for others, as recommended in the evidence.
14. Providing day-rooms for the Female inmates.
15. Providing recreation ground and enclosures for the class of violent and refractory patients.
16. Building capacious wash-house.
17. Ditto laundry.
18. Ditto drying-room.
19. Ditto accommodation for Attendants.

Source: Parliamentary Papers 1859 No. 91. *Report of the Joint Committee on the Accommodation of the Hospital for the Insane.* Parliamentary Papers of the Legislative Council.

New Norfolk, felt more consideration was required firstly of the costs of bringing New Norfolk up to English standards, and secondly the cost of building a new asylum. They felt that conditions had to be improved even while construction of a new asylum was being undertaken, requiring a further review of costs (Tas. J.C. Report 1859: 9).

There was little or no response to this Report, and the next ten years saw continuing requests, through the Annual Reports, as the New Norfolk Commissioners sought to improve conditions at the Hos-

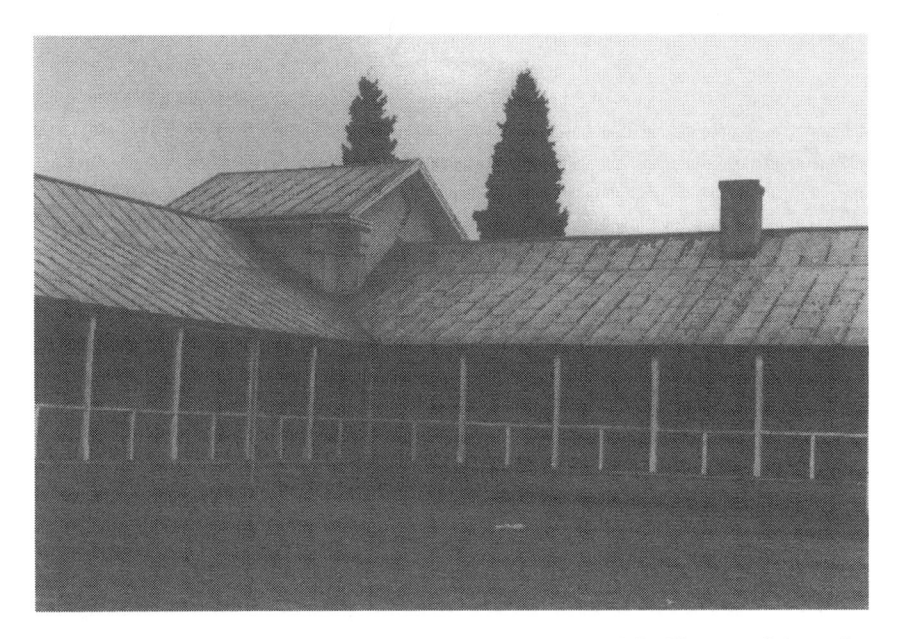

Figure 8.5. Possible day room and sleeping rooms, New Norfolk. Photograph by author 2001.

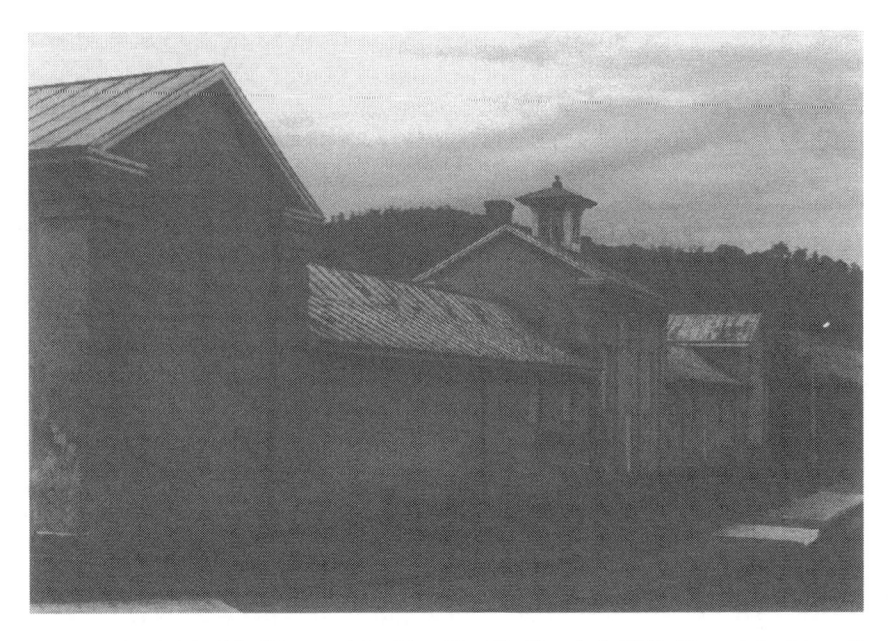

Figure 8.6. Original buildings of the New Norfolk Hospital, 2001. The original lunatic hospital section has been demolished and this view shows the dividing wall originally between the Invalid Hospital and the Lunatic hospital. Photograph by author 2001.

pital (see Piddock 2003 Appendix D for full details). Eighteen sixty one saw the building of a large day room, a new dormitory and six sleeping cells in the female division as well as a Matron's cottage. Only the Matron was resident in the Hospital, the Superintendent living in a leased house which the Commissioners purchased in 1861.

During 1861 several building works were undertaken, including the addition of a verandah to the female division, a day room and airing court to the women's refractory building, and the conversion of the Head Keeper's quarters to accommodate the 'idiot' boys. Despite these small improvements the Hospital still lacked proper baths and water on tap; there were no staff rooms, and the kitchen was too small (Tas. A.R. P.P. 1863 & 1864). In 1865 the new kitchen was underway, and in 1867 a Ladies Cottage was finally approved. With the purchase of further land, the farm yard abutting the main buildings was finally removed (Tas. N.N. Corresp. 7/1/1867; Tas. A.R. P.P. 1866). There were few requests for building changes over the 1870s. The only additions to New Norfolk were a new female dormitory completed in 1880, and a further six rooms, two sitting rooms and a bathroom added to the Gentlemen's cottage (Tas. A.R. P.P. 1880, 1881).

In 1869 a lunatic asylum was opened at the former penal colony of Port Arthur, to house lunatics maintained by the Imperial Government in England (Figure 8.7). The asylum was designed as a cruciform and came complete with dormitories, single rooms, a central hall, baths, cook house, and laundry (Brand 1998: 185, 187). This was followed by the proclamation of the Hospital for the Insane, Cascades, in 1877. The Cascades Asylum housed the former inmates of the Port Arthur Asylum after it closed. The Cascades had been a female factory and sections were minimally converted to house lunatics. The men were divided into two classes: the refractory and the remainder. Accommodation was in the form of barred cells with some wards, a lavatory, water closets, cook house and exercise yards (Tas. A.R. P.P. 1878, 1881).

In 1882 a Royal Commission was appointed to consider the character of the lunatic asylums in Tasmania and to enquire into the safe keeping and treatment of the insane in Great Britain, Europe and the neighboring colonies. The witnesses before the Commission indicated that New Norfolk was far from perfect, and the focus of the evidence was on what should be provided in a curative asylum built along modern lines. Dr. Macfarlane, the Superintendent of New Norfolk, envisaged the Hospital being rebuilt as a series of pavilions and cottages. He felt that some buildings, like the Ladies' and Gentlemen's Cottages, could be retained if thoroughly renovated. Macfarlane envisaged a rolling cycle of building and demolition to replace the existing buildings,

A Brief History of the New Norfolk Hospital for the Insane 161

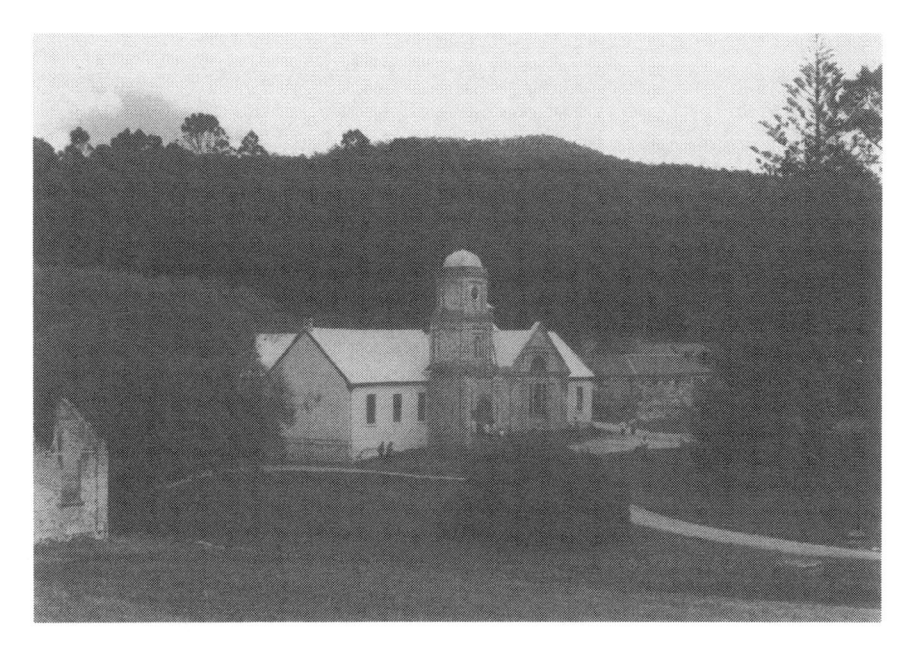

Figure 8.7. View of the remaining buildings that formed the Port Arthur Lunatic Asylum. Photograph by author 2001.

with airing courts being landscaped as gardens (Tas. R.C. Report 1883: 38, 40).

The Commission concluded that, while the site of New Norfolk was healthy, with a good water supply, drainage, and cheerful scenery, the buildings were lacking. Housing 300 patients, the buildings offered little opportunity for classification. The male division needed complete rebuilding, while the female refractory division needed remodeling. Offices and staff accommodation were needed, along with new stores and repairs to the laundry and kitchen (Tas. R.C. Report 1883: ix). The Cascades Asylum was equally ill-adapted to its purpose and was felt to induce mental illness rather than cure it (Tas. R.C. Report 1883: ix).

Having weighed the options, the Commissioners recommended increasing the New Norfolk grounds by at least 100 acres; building new pavilions and cottages for a further 100 patients, including new administrative offices, waiting rooms and store rooms. As can be seen from Table 10 their recommendations would have made substantial improvements to the environment experienced by the patients, with an emphasis on new or improved sleeping and living accommodation including pleasant exercise spaces and better sanitary provisions. Again no action was taken with respect to the Royal Commission's

Table 10. Recommendations of the Royal Commission of 1883 with respect to the Buildings.

1. That the site of the Hospital for the Insane at New Norfolk be retained for the purposes to which it is now applied.
2. That about 62 acres of land adjacent to the present Hospital grounds be procured; and we that the authority of Parliament be sought for closing up Burnett-street recommend between George and Grey streets; for closing that portion of Grey-street as far as Humphrey-street, and for closing the whole of Charlotte-street; and also for the purchase of the following blocks of land, coloured red on the plan annexed, and numbered A. to H:-A., 15a. 3r., 14p.; B., 2a. 0r. 20p.; C., 5a. 1r. 14p.; D., 2a. 2r. 1 0p.; E., 5a. 2r. 6p.; F., 2a. 3r.; G., 18a. 1r. 24p.; W, 9a. 2r. 33p.; total, 62a. 1r. 1p.
3. That the erection of new buildings to accommodate 100 patients be undertaken, in proximity to the present buildings at New Norfolk, without delay. In such new buildings the Pavilion and Cottage Systems be combined, and to be so disposed, and of such a size and character, as to afford every provision for the classification and the comfort of the patients, for the reception of visitors, and the general administration of the Institution. Each Pavilion should provide accommodation for about 20 patients.
4. That the grounds generally be rendered more attractive by planting ornamental trees, shrubs, and flowers.
5. That the refractory yard for females be extended and improved in appearance, and that it be more securely and neatly fenced.
6. That in the back male division the yard be extended, and otherwise improved by planting trees &c.
7. That the refractory wards for females be immediately improved by better lighting and necessary repairs.
8. That the main building for females be placed at once in thorough repair and better adapted to the requirements of the patients.
9. That the corridor in the male division be extended and its roof elevated, to afford better day accommodation.
10. That all other wards in the back division should cease to be used for the accommodation of patients as soon as better quarters can be provided for them, and that some portion of these buildings should be entirely removed to afford the needful space tor the extension of the recreation ground in that division.
11. That improved bath-rooms and better kitchen and laundry arrangements and appliances should be provided for, partly perhaps in some of the present buildings, but chiefly in the new buildings which we recommend should be erected.
12. That temporary improved store accommodation he provided at once, which may be done most inexpensively by transferring the criminal lunatics at New Norfolk to the Cascades thus relieving the pressure on space in the wards, a portion of which could, in that case, be utilised for store purposes pending the completion of the new buildings, when more permanent store arrangements could be effected.
13. That more comfortably situated quarters be provided for the Matron of the Hospital.
14. That provision be made for the residence and board of the Assistant Medical Officer within the Institution.
15. That some additional buildings at the Cascades be devoted to the purposes of the Asylum for the Insane, so that proper provision may be made there immediately for the reception of the criminal and Queen's-pleasure patients now at New Norfolk.
16. That two padded cells for males and two for females be constructed at New Norfolk.

Of these recommendations we specially note Nos. 5, 7, 8, 9, 12 and 15 as requiring immediate attention, there being no necessity to defer dealing with them until the new buildings shall have been erected.

Parliamentary Papers 1883. *Royal Commission on the State of the Lunatic Asylums in Tasmania. Report*

A Brief History of the New Norfolk Hospital for the Insane

Report and the New Norfolk Commissioners' request for £1423 5s. to undertake necessary repairs was not funded (Tas. A.R. P.P. 1883).

Amid accusations of incompetence, a second Select Committee was called in 1883 to consider the management of New Norfolk (for details see Gowlland 1981: 76–81). The Committee was composed of Dr. Frederick Manning, the Inspector of Insane in New South Wales and a leading lunacy reformer, Dr. Alexander Paterson, Superintendent of the Adelaide Lunatic Asylum and Dr. Dick of Melbourne. The Doctors found much wrong with the asylum buildings and an inexperienced elderly staff. More importantly, they found the Board of Commissioners lacked the power to authorize repairs and alterations to the buildings and the requests for funding had fallen on deaf ears (Gowlland 1981: 87). Like the Royal Commissioners, they recommended a remodeling of New Norfolk, even though they felt this would still leave it short of modern standards. The best option was a new asylum near Hobart. The latter option was considered too expensive, and the new Official Visitors, who replaced the Board of Commissioners in 1885, began drawing up a series of recommendations to improve New Norfolk (Piddock 2003 Appendix D). A plan drawn in 1886 shows New Norfolk as the Official Visitors envisaged it, with new buildings and the demolition of parts of the male division containing the original 1830s cells.

From this plan it is possible to understand the arrangement of the Hospital. The original design of New Norfolk consisted of two squares: the back one completely enclosed and the front square – Willow Court – open on the eastern side. In 1858–9 the Gentlemen's Cottage had been erected to the south of Willow Court, and in 1861 the Matron's Cottage had been erected some distance from it in the north-east corner of the grounds. This placed the Matron's Cottage directly in the centre of the women's area, with the Female Refractory Building to the west on the northern side. Unfortunately there is no indication when this building was erected, although it was being modified in 1860. The Ladies' Cottage, which continued the northern line of buildings, was completed in 1869. Again there is no precise date for the two storeyed women's building on the eastern boundary along Humphrey Street, although the room arrangement does match the 1836 planned extensions, while the day room marked 'recreation room' on the plan appears to have been added in 1861. This suggests the building dated to quite early in the Hospital's history. The laundry and wash house appear to have been located to the back of the rear square of buildings. It is possible that the planned extension of 1836 was only undertaken on the women's side because this allowed the two squares to be totally given over to the men, making a male addition redundant.

However, a problem exists with using this plan for room identification and use, as it is unclear whether the room designations reflected how the

Royal Commissioners envisaged the rooms being used, or their actual use at the time. It seems likely that the description of the Ladies' and Gentlemen's cottages was more accurate.

The Ladies' and Gentlemen's cottages were similarly arranged around a central passageway. The Ladies' Cottage had four large rooms. Two of which appear to have been a drawing or dining room and a sitting room, nine dormitories, a kitchen, bathroom and possibly a lavatory or water closet. The Gentlemen's Cottage had a drawing room, sitting room, ten dormitories, a kitchen, bathroom, and three unidentifiable rooms.

Despite the Commissioner's plans outlining what needed to be done, change was slow and work did not begin until 1889, with a new female building and a male building opening in 1893. New Norfolk continues today as a psychiatric Hospital, with Willow Court surviving but not in use.

METHODOLOGICAL ISSUES

Some problems were highlighted in compiling this history of the New Norfolk Hospital which ultimately affects any interpretation of the data. The largest problem was the differing survival rates of the various nineteenth century documents. There are no record books from the Colonial Architect's Office, such as can be found in South Australia, which detail the various building works and repairs made to the Hospital. Parliamentary records are incomplete and there are no debates surviving. In effect, the documentary record consists of the Commissioners' Reports, Bishop Willson's letters, and the two Parliamentary Inquiries from which only one set of Minutes of Evidence survived, and a few Colonial Secretary Office letters. While these form a rich source of information, they were of only limited use for this study. It proved impossible, for example, to chart expenditure on the lunatic asylums, or to lock down the specific nature of changes to New Norfolk. The other problem which affects the comparison of New Norfolk to the 'ideal' asylums lies in the contradictory views of New Norfolk which appear in the Parliamentary Inquiries, Bishop Willson's letters and Commissioner Bedford's responses. The most problematic was the site of the Hospital. Where necessary all views are considered in the interpretation that follows.

Of the three plans of New Norfolk, the 1836 plan shows proposed additions (Figure 8.1), and as discussed above, it is possible that only some of these rooms were added; the 1886 plan shows the proposed redevelopment of New Norfolk (Archives Office of Tasmania JJJP48/1886), and consequently provides only limited evidence of room use; and the final plan from 1888 shows no room designations, only space divisions (Figure 8.8). There are no photographs of New Norfolk until the early

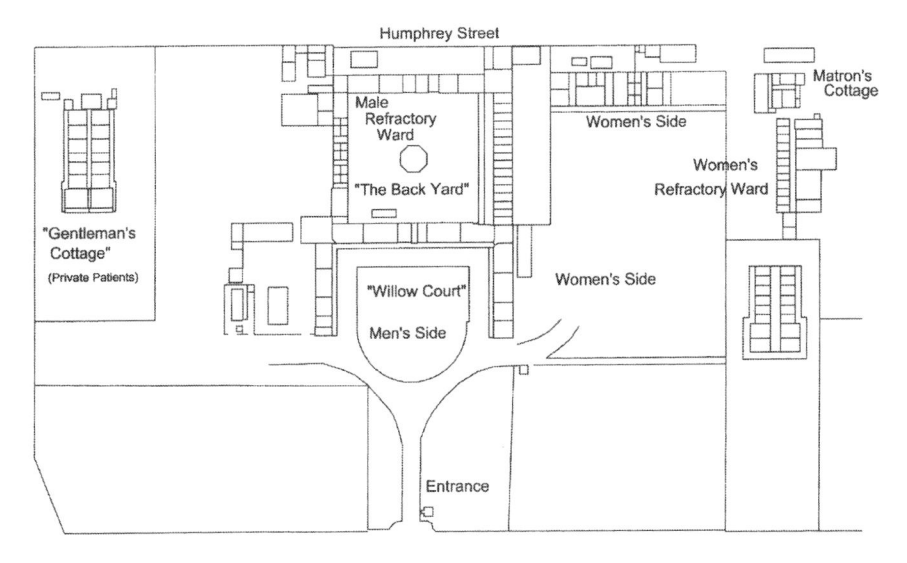

Figure 8.8. Plan of New Norfolk, 1888.

twentieth century. Similar problems exist for the Cascades and Port Arthur Asylums. For the former, there is one plan (Archives Office of Tasmania PWD 266/410) and for the latter, one photograph. Consequently, it is difficult to gain a real understanding of room and space use, and the main evidence comes from the limited written evidence, which is in turn limited to what the New Norfolk Commissioners or the Parliamentary Inquiries thought were important enough to discuss or which served their arguments. Effectively the New Norfolk Commissioner's Annual Reports were the only record of building changes.

To partially overcome these problems both the reality of New Norfolk as it was, and the vision of New Norfolk as it was intended to be, as held by those directly involved with the Hospital, will be considered in the following discussion. This will allow us to better understand the reality of provisions made at New Norfolk.

PORT ARTHUR AND CASCADES ASYLUMS AND THE 'IDEAL' MODELS

The information about these two asylums is extremely scant, and their role as asylums for criminal lunatics was entirely different from the intentions of the 'ideal' model asylums. There are no plans of the Port Arthur Asylum. It appears from modern observations to have

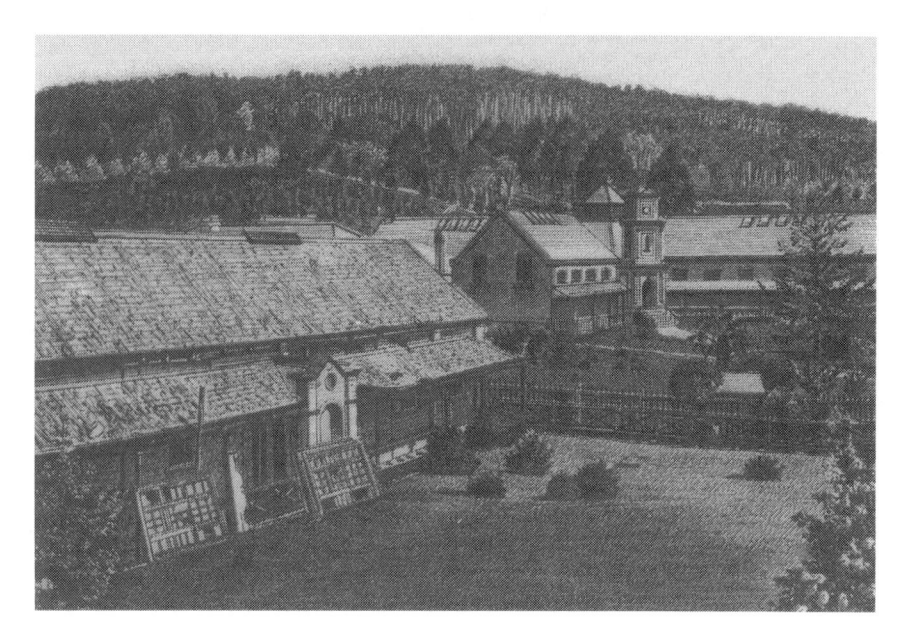

Figure 8.9. Drawing of the Port Arthur Lunatic Asylum 1890. Courtesy of the Archives Office of Tasmania, PH30/1/1720.

been designed with the panopticon principle of central observation as its key rather any classification of the patients. This is supported by the inclusion of a central hall which probably fulfilled the dual roles of day room and dining room. The provision of baths does suggest some inclusion of sanitary considerations. There is no information about the ventilation, windows and attendant's accommodation that could provide some detail about life within the asylum or about the adoption of the principles of patient care that informed the 'ideal' model.

The use of the Female Factory at the Cascades as a lunatic asylum perhaps reflects a stop-gap measure to treat the criminal lunatics after Port Arthur's closure as a penal colony. Two parts of the Factory were used for lunatics. There was a series of cells for the refractory lunatics in one yard, separated by a considerable distance from a set of wards in another yard. The provision of both a day room and a mess room suggests that some classification may have been possible. The keeper was provided with his own quarters and there was a lavatory and water closets, but no indication of a bath house. Exercise space was extremely limited and the refractory patients had even less living space. Both the Cascades and the Port Arthur Asylums were as far removed as possible from the 'ideal' asylum. It is possible to speculate that this arose from the nature of the lunatics being confined. As both criminals and convicts, their accommodation may have been seen in terms of punishment. Certainly the use of the Female Factory at Cascades provided the cheapest option for providing for a small number of criminal lunatics after the closure of Port Arthur.

NEW NORFOLK AND THE 'IDEAL' ASYLUM OF JOHN CONOLLY

Conolly had described his vision of the 'ideal' lunatic asylum in 1847, eight years before the New Norfolk Commissioners took charge. The scant evidence about the Hospital while it was an Imperial Establishment does not allow for much comparison to the 'ideal' model, instead any comparison must look across the history of New Norfolk (Table 11).

A – An appropriate site with some form of scenery

From the documentary evidence it is clear that the site was considered healthy, it had a good water supply, and was surrounded on at least two sides by open country. However the Hospital grounds were severely limited, amounting only to 48 acres in 1883, being "10½ acres on which the buildings stood, 5½ acres for recreation grounds, and about 31½ devoted to farm and grazing ground" (Tas. R. C. Report 1883: viii). It was 22 miles from Hobart. There was much disagreement over whether this distance was appropriate. Bishop Willson felt that it was too removed from Hobart Town for visits by interested people and family members, yet the Commissioners believed the distance was protective, preventing idle visitors from passing time. New Norfolk was accessible by steamer, horse and cart and later by train. In terms of whether New Norfolk had an appropriate site, the answer was probably yes, although the limited grounds available to the Hospital for expansion and to the patients for exercise were a problem.

B – An arrangement of the buildings that allowed light in and cross ventilation, with no building overshadowing another or the airing courts

New Norfolk failed to meet this requirement. As originally designed the Convict Establishment and Hospital for the Insane was based on two quadrangles. The quadrangle for the insane was completely enclosed

Table 11. Conolly's Ideal Features and the New Norfolk Hospital for the Insane

Lunatic Asylum	A	B	C	D	Ea	Eb	Ec	F	G	Ha	Hb	Hc	Hd	Ia	Ib	J	K	L
New Norfolk as Built	X			X					X	X		X			X			
New Norfolk – 1856	X	X				X		X	X	X		X	X		X	X		X

Key

A - An appropriate site with some form of scenery
B - An arrangement of the buildings that allowed light in and cross ventilation, with no building overshadowing another or the airing courts
C - A linear form to the layout
D - It should accommodate no more than 360 to 400 inmates
Ea - A building that offered a range of wards for classification
Eb - Each ward should have its own attendant's rooms
Ec - There should be open areas as opposed to day rooms for patients
F - Each ward should have access to a bathroom, lavatory and water closets
G - Each ward should have a wide gallery furnished as a day room with windows low enough to allow a view outside
Ha - There should be a large recreation room
Hb - School rooms
Hc - Work rooms and workshops
Hd - A chapel for the use of patients
Ia - The offices should be centrally located
Ib - There should be a means of accessing the various wards without passing through each
J - Attendant's should have their own dining hall
K - Accommodation should primarily be in the form of single rooms with a few dormitories
L - Above all the asylum should be light, cheerful and liberal in the space it offerered

by buildings which allowed little ventilation; a problem worsened by the division of this quadrangle into two by a high wall. The verandahs added later, by their design, would have hampered the flow of air into the rooms. Throughout its history, even into the late 1880s, the buildings were frequently described as dank, dark, gloomy and ill-ventilated – a problem exacerbated by the retention of part of the original 1830s cells in the male division of the 1880s Hospital. The women's buildings were separate and placed so that their ventilation may have been slightly better.

C – A linear form to the layout

New Norfolk was not linear in the way that Conolly envisaged.

D – It should accommodate no more than 360 to 400 inmates

As can be seen from Table 12 the Hospital generally accommodated fewer than 300 inmates.

Ea – A building that offered a range of wards for classification

In terms of Conolly's fifth requirement, New Norfolk failed miserably. The buildings never allowed true classification as envisaged as part of a curative regime; a factor which the Royal Commissioners of 1882 believed was the primary cause of the failure to achieve speedy cures (Tas. R.C. Report 1883: x). It appears from the 1859 Annual Report of the New Norfolk Commissioners that no classification had been attempted before they took charge. By 1859 they had classified the men into three classes and the women into two, but the subsequent remodeling of the yards and the increasing number of patients probably left two classes – refractory and ordinary – in both the female and male divisions.

The designs of the two male division quadrangles and the two women's buildings meant that the only possible physical separation of the patients, beyond that allowed by the two women's buildings, was created by points of access. On the plan of 1886 the building designated 'Women's Hospital' is a series of sections that do not communicate with each other, which may have supported a little separation of the women. But this was entirely artificial as there was only one day room and, prior to its addition in 1861, the verandah would have been

Table 12. Return of the Number of Patients in New Norfolk

	Free		Convict		
Date	Male	Female	Male	Female	Total
1845	26	17	56	37	136
1846	31	21	67	40	159
1847	34	23	79	36	172
1848	37	22	75	45	179
1849	38	23	99	54	214
1850	36	24	77	56	193
1851	40	28	86	63	217
1852	49	30	62	55	196
1853	47	36	60	47	190
1854	53	33	111	42	239
1855	54	38	46	35	173
1856	90	74	15	9	188
1857	92	75	16	10	193
1858	96	79	16	12	203
1859	114	96	5	3	218
1860	119	94	3	7	220
1861	127	105	5	2	239
1862	105	96	5	2	208
1863	110	100	5	2	217
1864	109	109	4	1	223
1865	114	110	4	1	229

	Persons who are or have been convicts		Persons who have not been convicts		
Date	Male	Female	Male	Female	Total
1866	71	63	48	47	229
1867	62	59	49	52	222
1868	64	56	54	56	230
1869	71	60	61	58	250
1870	71	59	62	59	251

used instead. It seems likely that part of this building formed one of the 1836 additions to the back quadrangle, as the placement of the staircases match in the plans.

The original design of the male quadrangles did not allow communication between the two halves, and the use of the different sides of the quadrangles may have created a similar type of artificial classification. Unfortunately the limited day space meant that, once again, the men mixed together. The 1836 addition on the left side of the back quadrangle shown on the plan appears never to have been built (Figure 8.1), even though this would have allowed further classification.

One important classification was maintained however: the separation of 'Gentlemen' and 'Ladies' from the other patients with the opening of the Gentlemen's Cottage in 1859 and the Ladies Cottage ten years later (after many funding requests). The terms 'Ladies' and 'Gentlemen' are the ones used by the New Norfolk Commissioners, and while there is no definition given it seemed to be used for anyone who was not a convict or of convict origin.

Eb – Each ward should have its own attendant's rooms

There were no attendants' rooms.

Ec – There should be open areas as opposed to day rooms for patients

In terms of day rooms, in 1860 there was one eating room for the whole male division, which the Commissioners felt was unsuitable for indoor activities, and there was one small room in the female division (Tas. J.C. Report 1859). The Refractory women used the corridor in their building as a dining room. A large day room was added to the female division between 1861 and 1862, while the male day room was replaced in 1860. In effect there appears to have been only three day rooms in the whole Hospital throughout the period discussed. From the evidence available it is not clear whether all the men and women had access to these rooms or only some. All these rooms appear to have been enclosed.

F – Each ward should have access to a bathroom, lavatory and water closets

There were no internal lavatories or water closets, these appear to have been outside in the male yards, and in the female division there may have been no external water closest at all. In 1882 the Matron, Miss Laland, indicated that the women had no place to wash themselves and a wooden tub served as a toilet (Tas. R.C. Report 1883 Q. 238, 251). Bathing patients was an ongoing problem and the Commissioners sought funding for bathhouses from the beginning.

G – Each ward should have a wide gallery furnished as a day room with windows low enough to allow a view outside

While Conolly saw the arrangement of the wards in terms of the familiar linear ward system which he had worked with, the original design of New Norfolk was very different. There were no galleries or even corridors, rather it was formed of paired cells, and later, dormitories. Only the refractory women's building had a corridor which was less than seven feet in width, and was used as living space. In 1860 one side of the back quadrangle of the male division was remodeled to allow a 12 foot wide corridor, bringing one section slightly closer to Conolly's seventh requirement, but this was not a consistent design principle throughout the Hospital. There is no evidence with respect to the placement of windows in the Hospital, but the repeated references to dark, gloomy cells and the sleeping room layout would suggest small, possibly high windows.

Ha – There should be a large recreation room

While there was a request by the Commissioners for a dedicated recreation hall in 1862, none was built, and in 1882 the large women's day room (60 ft by 32 ft) was being used as dining room, recreation hall and chapel.

Hb – School rooms

There were no school rooms.

Hc – Work rooms and workshops

There is evidence that there were workshops at the Hospital throughout most of this period, as the men were employed in maintaining and building the Hospital. In 1883 there is mention of a female dormitory being used as a work room, but there was no dedicated space.

Hd – A chapel for the use of patients

While a chapel was on the original plan this appears never to have been built. As indicated above a day room was used as a chapel.

Ia – The offices should be centrally located

There is little evidence about the offices at New Norfolk. There was probably an office for the Medical Officer but the rest remain speculative. Only the Matron lived within the Hospital, and her quarters were located in the women's division.

Ib – There should be a means of accessing the various wards without passing through each

New Norfolk was composed of a series of buildings so there was no need for this requirement.

J – Attendants should have their own dining hall

Conolly had envisaged this as a necessity when attendants spent all their time with the patients. However, at New Norfolk the attendants lived outside of the Hospital, and either ate with their charges or went home for meals.

K – Accommodation should primarily be in the form of single rooms with a few dormitories

In terms of the ratio of dormitories to single rooms, there is no clear evidence of how many patients were accommodated on their own in single rooms. The original paired cells were, however, generally turned into dormitories and the 1883 plan would suggest that there was a range of single rooms and dormitories of various sizes.

Overall New Norfolk only met two of Conolly's requirements for an asylum over the entire period discussed from 1850 to 1890: the appropriate site and a limited size. In respect to other features it barely scrapes through. It had three day rooms at varying points in time, and it had workshops but no proper workroom. There were not even basic facilities for maintaining patient health, such as bathrooms and water closets.

How, then, does the reality of New Norfolk compare to what the Joint Committee of 1859 envisaged for New Norfolk, if sufficient money had been made available by the Tasmanian Parliament? A consideration of the Joint Committee's recommendations (Table 9) with Conolly's requirements for the 'ideal' asylum (Table 11) shows that if these had been followed through, New Norfolk would have been brought much closer to the 'ideal'. The expansion of the Hospital grounds would have made the site more appropriate, while the removal of dividing walls in the exercise yards and the lowering of the external walls would have let in more light and air as Conolly recommended (*A* and *B*). The rebuilding of the male and female 'compartments' with new sleeping accommodation and corridors would have met Conolly's seventh requirement (*G*) of a gallery that could be used as day space. While Conolly does not include airing courts in his recommendations, an essential part of non-restraint was ready exercise for the patients. So, the enlarged exercise areas recommended by the Joint Committee are, in spirit, a part of his model. The recommended day rooms for *all* (sic) classes of men and women, and capacious workshops follow Conolly's fifth (*Ec*) and eighth (*Hc*) requirements in general terms. In addition, the building of baths in both the male and female divisions met part of his sixth requirement (*F*). In recommending that more dormitories be built, the Joint Committee saw this as a means to ease overcrowding and of increasing classification and separating the social ranks within the Hospital (Table 9 points 8 and 17). While the Joint Commissioners did not include it, the New Norfolk Commissioner in 1861 asked for funding for a large hall for recreations and religious services (Tas. A.R. P.P. 1862). This would have fulfilled a further part of Conolly's eighth requirement (*Ha* and *Hd*).

Before going on to consider the possible reasons for the divide between what New Norfolk was and the vision of what New Norfolk should have been, it is worth considering New Norfolk in light of the other 'ideal' asylum models.

NEW NORFOLK AND THE MODELS OF BROWNE, JACOBI, SANKEY AND ROBERTSON

As can be seen in Table 13, New Norfolk failed to meet these other models. Of Browne's requirements only that of a healthy site was really met to any degree. Although in a small settlement, it was partially countrified. New Norfolk was not large enough to provide the activities Browne envisaged as part of this requirement for a site. In 1883 the Matron, Miss Laland, recommended the removal of the Hospital closer to Hobart so that the patients could go out to church and for outings, suggesting that these options were not viable in the town of New Norfolk (Tas. R.C. Report 1883 Q. 250). Five of Jacobi's 1841 requirements were met: there was a separate building for refractory patients, and the access points of the original buildings used by the men may have

Table 13. Ideal Asylums and the New Norfolk Hospital for the Insane

Browne's Features found at New Norfolk

1. A healthy site with a dry cultivated soil and an ample supply of water.

Jacobi's Features found at New Norfolk

1. It should allow classification, in particular the separation of the sexes, and the noisy and violent patients from the convalescent.
2. It should be placed in the country and close to a town.
3. The building should not go above two stories or to an excessive length.
4. That there should be appropriate rooms for each group, and if necessary rooms should reflect the social class of the inmates to a degree.
5. The building should not go above two stories or to an excessive length.

Sankey's Features found at New Norfolk

1. The officers for the male and female divisions would have their rooms in the divisions themselves rather than in the central building.

---

allowed a separation of the noisy and violent men physically, if not audibly; it was in the country; there were particular efforts to maintain social ranking within the Hospital to the extent of providing separate cottages furnished appropriately; and no building appears to have extended above two storeys.

By contrast, New Norfolk met only one of the requirements of Sankey's 1856 model: the Matron's cottage was in the female division, but there was no matching provision in the male division. Similarly there are no matches for Robertson's model, although the suggested 1883 plan of rebuilding New Norfolk was based on pavilions and cottages.

Fundamental problems with New Norfolk appear to have arisen from the practice of re-modeling sections of a Hospital that was not designed with the insane in mind. There was a clear knowledge of what was required for their treatment and cure, as indicated by the comparison of the 'ideal' model to the 1859 Joint Committee recommendations. Why, then, was New Norfolk not turned into a Hospital that would meet Conolly's 'ideal'? This will be discussed in the next chapter.

LIFE IN THE HOSPITAL

It is possible from the documents and plans to build a picture of life within New Norfolk. Unfortunately it is a picture of cramped and badly designed sleeping areas, equally cramped exercise yards, limited living space, and a very basic level of sanitation and cleanliness which continued throughout a substantial part of the nineteenth century.

Information about the Hospital from its beginnings in the 1830s until it was handed over to the Tasmanian Government in 1855 is scant, but it is possible to understand what life was like from the New Norfolk Commissioners' descriptions of what they found on taking charge of the Hospital.

From the beginning New Norfolk appears to have been considered by those in charge as a place where treatment was based on some form of moral discipline, and removal to the Hospital was intended to bring about the recovery of the insane person (Tas. C.S.O. Letters 7th Feb. 1832 pg. 141–2). Restraint was practiced, and the buildings, despite this curative intention, were small, dark, badly constructed and ill-ventilated (Gowlland 1981: 50; See Appendix 3).

The buildings appear to have been constructed of wood, and they were infested with vermin, and some rooms may have had skylights rather than windows (Tas. C.S.O. Letters 18th June 1831 pg. 111; Tas. P. P. No. 10 8/3/1859). Accommodation in the rear square, built with the lunatics in mind, was considered in 1859 to be worse than that of the Hobart Gaol (Tas. J.C. Report 1859: 4). The patients were kept in very small yards with high walls that offered no views of the world outside, and only men employed as labourers ever went outside of these yards (Gowlland 1981: 50). The buildings lacked verandas and patients probably spent their time in the cells when it rained or was too cold to go outside, as the corridors, where they existed, were too narrow to be used as living space. The New Norfolk Commissioners found there was no classification of the patients based on their treatment requirements and there was no recognition of the needs of those who were not convicts in terms of domestic comforts (Tas. C.S.O. Letters 1/811/17340). Some day rooms appear to have existed at times but there were no amusements for the patients, and religious services may have been the only diversion from the monotony of the days (Tas. A.R. P.P 1865). Life for the patients of New Norfolk was bleak in the extreme.

This life did not immediately change with the handing over of control to the New Norfolk Commissioners, as reflected by the evidence of the Joint Committee Report of 1859. The initial focus of the Commissioners was improving sleeping accommodation and providing verandas as additional living space. The Committee found that New Norfolk was divided by high walls into a number of small spaces. The men were broken down into three classes, but there is no indication of what these classes were. Each class had access to a small exercise yard, some external to the buildings and one formed by the rear courtyard. These divisions meant some men had access to a day room for meals, while others did not. The dormitories designed to house six inmates were housing between 10 and 15 men (Tas. J.C. Report 1859: 4). The exercise yards appear to have consisted entirely of a gravelled surface.

The women's section was considered to be even more defective by the Commissioners, with only two classifications, 'a wretched and small day room', and even more limited exercise space, despite the fact, they noted, that an adjoining dairy paddock could have been used to provide further exercise space (Tas. J.C. Report 1859: 5).

There was no provision of attendants' rooms and all the staff lived beyond the Hospital walls until the Matron's Cottage was built in 1861. There is no evidence with respect to baths, although they appear to have been absent. The Hospital did have a wood yard, garden, tailor's and shoemaker's shops in which a few men were employed. Life for the patients of New Norfolk must have centred on their sleeping accommodation with access for some to a day room. Exercise was still taken in relatively limited yards and there appears to have been little to break the monotony of the day, apart from when the men were employed in helping rebuild parts of the hospital. There is no evidence that the women were employed in any way, although they may have done clothing repairs etc.

Importantly at this point in time the physical environment of New Norfolk directly affected the treatment regime applied. Restraint was practiced until 1860. By 1860 the Commissioners had made progress in changing the environment of the Hospital. They had removed dividing walls from the yards, they had rebuilt parts of the buildings creating living space in the form of day rooms, corridors, verandas, and planned new buildings and airing courts with views. Consequently they noted in their Annual Report for 1860 that these changes had directly affected the patients, who were improved in conduct and demeanour, and mechanical restraint had been abolished (Tas. A.R. P.P. 1861).

From 1860 the treatment regime was based on moral treatment and the best European practices. Moral treatment required the provision of an appropriate environment, patient management based on kindness, classification, a clean environment, exercise, religious consolation and some kind of activity to occupy the mind. As indicated in Chapter Six, by looking at New Norfolk in terms of these factors it is possible to understand life within the asylums through the absence or provision of rooms and spaces to support this management.

From the documentary evidence it appears that classification was never achieved to any degree at New Norfolk. There were simply not enough buildings to support classification given the number of patients accommodated. In 1883 the women remained unclassified, except for the separation of violent women in the refractory building. Consequently there were no opportunities to provide accommodation adapted to the needs of particular classes such as epileptics or perhaps those of different social classes. The provision of the Gentlemen's and Ladies' Cottages had allowed some separation of the social classes, based on the ability to pay a fee. The separation of the non-paying patients, free of 'moral' taint, from convicts in the main buildings had been a real issue for those involved with New Norfolk. The issue had been raised by Bishop Willson in 1859 and by the New Norfolk Commissioners in 1863, who had found 'virtuous' women mixed with those of 'notorious careers' (6/8/1859 Tas. P.P. 1859 No. 10; Tas. A.R. P.P. 1864). The limited accommodation provided by the cottages, however, raises the interesting issue of the perception of the nature of the patients by the New Norfolk Commissioners, for it would suggest that most were seen as coming from the lower classes. This will be discussed further in the following chapter.

The physical environment of the Hospital appears to have remained poor despite the modifications made by the Commissioners and there is little evidence that a healthy or clean environment was maintained. In 1863 there was no workable bathhouse and there was no apparatus for hot or cold water, which must have made cleaning and bathing major undertakings. The male bathhouse was created by the conversion of the old kitchen in 1866, while the women had to wait until 1871 for a bathhouse to be built by the male patients (Tas. A.R. P.P. 1866, 1872). The plan of 1888 indicates that the bathhouse of the Women's Hospital was located near the earth closet in the yard and the male bathhouse in the male refractory yard. This inconvenient arrangement must have been difficult in the cold Tasmanian winter and has implications for the level of cleanliness among the patients. Presumably the men in the front court were taken around the building to access the bathroom in the rear court. As late as 1883 the water closets consisted simply of wooden tubs which were emptied every morning (Tas. R.C. Report 1883 Q. 51–2). The problems with the provision of bathhouses reflect the New Norfolk Commissioners overall lack of power, they were unable even to authorise repairs to the Hospital, and relied upon Government funding for repairs which was rarely forthcoming. Consequently the buildings fell into a state of disrepair, and in 1886 it was reported that the poor condition of the buildings and lack of sanitary provisions "induces us to think that an unwise parsimony has for some time been exercised in the control of the institution" (Tas. Official Visitors Report P.P. 1886). The poor state of the buildings and the lack of proper baths and water closets must have directly impacted on the patient's experience of the Hospital.

Efforts were made from 1859 onwards to improve day to day life for the patients with the introduction of indoor amusements and outdoor activities, and the continuation of daily prayers and Divine Service.

In 1859 the Joint Committee had noted the lack of amusements with some surprise as these were "universally dwelt on in England as forming an essential part of a curative system" (Tas. J.C. Report 1859: 5). Later that year the Commissioners introduced books, draughts, dominoes and magic lantern shows. By 1863 domesticated birds and other animals had been introduced for the patients to care for; dances, music nights, visiting entertainments enlivened the Hospital, and patients left the high walls of the Hospital behind to embark on walking parties and summer picnics (Tas. A.R. P.P. 1860, 1864). There is no evidence about where the entertainments were held or who attended them, but it seems likely that they were held in the large women's day room. The Commissioners had requested funding for a large recreation hall in 1861 but funding was never realised (Tas. A.R. P.P. 1862). It seems likely that a multi-functionality of rooms continued at the Hospital. The women who were employed in sewing may have used a day room for this purpose, although pressures on accommodation in the 1880s saw what Dr. Macfarlane, the Superintendent, called a 'work room' being used as a dormitory (Tas. R.C. Report 1883 Q, 27). The weekly religious services were probably held in day rooms where available.

Moral treatment included employment and there is clear evidence that the majority of the patients were employed from the mid-1850s. Both men and women were employed in making and repairing clothes and footwear, presumably this activity took place in the day rooms and later possibly a work room. Those men with trade skills and those capable of labouring were used in building and repairing the Hospital, and in 1883 there were tailor's, shoemaker's, painter's, blacksmith's, glazier's, plumber's and carpenter's shops. Men were employed to fulfil the double function of attendants and tradesmen, and there was a farmer and a bricklayer, along with the other tradesmen (Tas. A.R. P. P. 1870; Tas. R.C. Report 1883 Q. 8, 27, 45, 66). This suggests that a curative regime may have been sacrificed to economic pressures, with more emphasis being placed on the patient's value as a worker than on a break from the pressures of a working life that may have caused the illness in the first place. Unfortunately there is no information about where these workshops were.

The women were employed in the laundry and here there is the only evidence of class-based differentiation of work. In 1883, the Matron indicates that the penal class did the washing and when they no longer entered the Hospital there would be no one to do it (Tas. R.C. Report 1883 Q. 46). There was no proper laundry, which would have been composed of washing, drying and ironing rooms. Rather, only two single washhouse rooms are marked on the 1888 plan. One adjoined the male refractory ward, and the other was located to the rear of the male division near the Women's Hospital. The former washhouse may have been used for foul or heavy linen, using the male patients for the heavy physical labour. As indicated above there were no formal workrooms for the women and instead the ward formed both work and sleeping space.

Exercise options also appear to have been very limited. Though the New Norfolk Commissioners expanded the exercise yards, they were restrained by the small size of the Hospital grounds and by the arrangement of the buildings. While there was some mention of gardens, there is little evidence of landscaping of the yards, and the gardens may have been associated with the Ladies' and Gentlemen's Cottages only (Tas. R.C. Report 1883 Q. 38). A garden that may have been accessible to the patients was converted in 1881 or 1882 into a grassed area suitable for cricket, croquet, lawn tennis and rounders (Tas. A. R. P. P. 1883). This range of activities would have been deemed suitable for both men and women and diversified their lives.

There is little evidence about the furnishings at the Hospital, but a comment made by Dr. Coutie to the Royal Commission of 1883 perhaps reflects existing conditions. The new pavilions, he recommended, could be made more homely by the provision of curtains for ward windows, pictures for the walls, and ordinary home furniture, along with cutlery and crockery to eat food with in place of tinware and fingers (Tas. R.C. Report 1883 Q. 80, 82). This would clearly imply that these features were lacking in the Hospital which must have added to the bleakness and strangeness of life there.

The use of verandahs as living and exercise space demonstrates the problematic nature of living space within the Hospital. Certainly the use of verandahs would not have supported a varied range of activities for the men and women, and probably contained a limited range of furnishings. It appears from the documentary evidence that some small spaces may have been used as day rooms in the early years of the Hospital but priority was given to accommodation as the patient population increased and, depending on the year day rooms may or may not have existed. The later additions of purpose-built day rooms for the men's division, women's division and refractory women's ward some 25 years after the Hospital opened must have been a significant improvement. However, it appears from the documentary evidence that only the women's day room was large enough for use for recreations and religious worship. The two quadrangles of the male division appear to have been served by a single day room possibly located in the large room in the rear quadrangle, although it is unclear whether men in Willow Court would have been taken around the buildings to access these, or whether they only used the verandahs.

The 1888 plan shows that the original 1830s paired cells and the 1861 women's Hospital building were still in use in the male division, and that only one male ward and one female ward at this time were provided with corridors. Effectively, all the other ward rooms were only accessible to the attendants from the outside. This meant that supervision and observation, which were key parts of the new treatment regimes, would have been problematic. The original doors may have included inspection panels through which to view the patients inside or alternatively some attendants may have slept in the larger dormitories of the male division, as there were never any attendants' rooms. The Matron indicated to the Royal Commission that the nurses slept, ate and lived with the patients day and night (Tas. R.C. Report 1883 Q. 238, 251). The Superintendent and Assistant Medical Officer never lived within the Hospital except perhaps in the 1830s. There is no evidence about the location of their offices, however, and it is difficult to judge how this affected the supervision of both staff and patients. Certainly the arrangement of the buildings, both externally and internally, did not allow ease of supervision.

Interestingly, if the 1883 plan had been implemented it would have seen the Matron losing her cottage and being given two rooms in the Women's Hospital, while her cottage would have been given over to a nurses home. While this may seem to be a more practical use of space, it would also have indicated a loss of status for the Matron, with a consequent lack of any privacy.

Overall, then, the world of the patient at New Norfolk was extremely confined and often basic. The day for the women was spent on the ward or in the day room; the only other living space was the exercise yard with its high walls. The location of the laundry is not clear for most of the period of time discussed, and it is unclear whether it was in one of the women's exercise yards, maintaining a link to the wards. Its placement outside of the yard would have provided a minor change of scene. The use of the women's day room for activities further limited variation in the women's days. It seems unlikely that the violent women of the refractory ward were taken to entertainments or outside for games or picnics, meaning an even more limited life. The men's world was similarly restricted, with the only variation being work around the Hospital and possibly visits to the women's day room for entertainments. This only changed for the men and women when walking parties, sports or picnics occurred. The life for the attendants seems equally bad, as there was no place during the day, and probably the night, to separate oneself from the patients unless they returned home to sleep. Attempts to maintain patient and ward cleanliness had to be difficult due to the almost complete lack of sanitary provisions.

DISCUSSION

From the available evidence it is clear that, prior to its handing over to the Tasmanian Government, New Norfolk was a custodial institution. There was little provision of living spaces, only a few men appear to have been employed and a patient's day was not broken by any activities, the day being spent in the sleeping room or in a small exercise yard surrounded by high walls. Moral treatment appears to have been limited to religious services, through which the institution could emphasize particular moral focuses or characteristics required by society.

The history of New Norfolk between 1855 and 1890 is more complicated. There is clear evidence that there was a strong awareness of what was needed at New Norfolk to make it a curative Hospital, both in terms of its physical features and in the management regime applied on the part of the New Norfolk Commissioners and the Official Visitors who replaced them in 1886, as well as the Joint Committee members of 1859 and the Royal Commissioners of 1883. Yet the reality of the Hospital as revealed through an analysis of the building history shows that while amusements, work and a range of outdoor activities were introduced to the Hospital from 1859, the buildings remained custodial in nature with little sanitary provision, in poor condition, with only basic internal furnishings and little space for classification. Overall New Norfolk fell far short of Conolly's paternalistic 'ideal' asylum, which focused on providing an environment that supported classification and adaptation to the needs of particular classes, a diversity of spaces for patients to experience, and a high level of cleanliness.

Both South Australia and Tasmania fell short of Conolly's 'ideal' asylum. In the next chapter the institutions of both colonies are considered together and against the British Asylums to determine what factors were influencing the built provisions made.

The 'Ideal' Asylum: A World of Difference | 9

In Chapter Four, the ideas of a range of nineteenth century lunacy reformers were discussed, and models developed from the books and articles of Browne, Jacobi, Conolly, Sankey, Arlidge and Robertson. These authors presented the most detailed specifications for the physical environment of the lunatic asylum, and from their works a range of features were identified that were archaeologically testable against the data sets of documents, photographs, plans, and building histories. From this research it became clear that John Conolly's 'ideal' asylum of 1847 could be used as the core of a comparative model. This work provided the first full description of what an asylum should be, and later British writers were to build on it, with variations in the physical arrangement of rooms and sleeping accommodation. While the data sets generated by the testing of these features against the three case studies of British, South Australian and Tasmanian asylums allowed me to determine which features of the 'ideal' asylum the built asylums had, and from this to build a picture of life in these institutions, it is possible to go beyond this event based archaeology and ask further questions of the generated data sets. These form the highest level of questions as advocated by Cleland (2001: 2, 5, 7), which go beyond the single site or country in this case to identify wider forces at work in the provision of these places. These questions are:

- Can any patterns in the adoption of 'ideal' asylum features be identified in Britain, South Australia and Tasmania that are similar to each other?
- Was the realization of the 'ideal' asylum model responsive to social, cultural and economic circumstances within a country or colony?
- Is it possible to identify particular factors common to both South Australia and Tasmania in influencing the adoption of the 'ideal'

asylum that transcend their different histories as a free and penal colony respectively?

In Chapter Five it was argued that the British county lunatic asylums fulfilled many of the requirements of John Conolly's model. The county asylums came closest to the model in achieving an appropriate environment, with buildings supporting classification and activities; and in providing a healthy environment through the provision of water closets, baths, and an arrangement of galleries which allowed ventilation and light to come in (Table 14). There was however a general lack of recreational spaces. Chapels were provided in most asylums in the sample, but the presence of a large hall for recreations, school rooms and galleries, which acted as additional living spaces, was more infrequent. The provision of a separate dining hall for attendants was variable, and reflected the often poor working conditions of attendants.[1] Was the same pattern of provisions to be found in South Australia and Tasmania?

By using the descriptive framework of John Conolly's 'ideal' asylum model as a base it is possible to generate data sets from widely separated countries that are directly comparable and can be used to answer these questions.

BRITISH ASYLUMS AND AUSTRALIAN INSTITUTIONS: COMMONALITIES OR DIFFERENCES?

A - An Appropriate Site and B - An arrangement that allowed light in and provided for cross ventilation

All three of the Australian asylums had an appropriate site. Only Parkside joined the majority of British asylums in having a building design that allowed light in and free ventilation (Table 14).

C - A Linear Layout and D - It should accommodate no more than 360 to 400 patients

Only Adelaide Asylum could be said to have a linear design. New Norfolk was similar in size to a couple of British asylums, which fulfilled the requirement of having only 360 to 400 patients.

---

[1] Conolly (1847) Chapter Five.

British Asylums and Australian Institutions

Table 14. A Comparision of Conolly's Ideal Aylum Features and the Asylums and Hospitals of Great Britain and Australia

Lunatic Asylum	Date	A	B	C	D	Ea	Eb	Ec	F	G	Ha	Hb	Hc	Hd	Ia	Ib	J	K	L
Cheshire	1827–8	X		X		X	X			X		X				X		X		
Derby	1844	X	X	X	X	X	X	X	X	X			X		X	X	X	X	
Abergavenny	1852		X	X	X	X	X		X				X	X	X	X		X	
Eglinton	1852		X	X		X	X		X	X			X	X	X		X		
Lincolnshire	1852	X	X	X	X	X	X		X	X	X		X	X	X	X	X		
Buckinghamshire	1853	X	X	X	X	X	X		X	X	X	X	X	X	X	X			
Essex	1853	X	X	X		X	X		X	X	X	X	X	X	X	X		X	
Cambridgeshire	1858	X	X	X	X	X	X	X	X			X	X	X	X				
Cumberland	1858	X	X	X	X	X	X	X	X	X	X		X	X	X		X		
Sussex	1859	X	X	X		X	X	X	X		X		X	X	X	X	X		
Bedford	1860	X	X	X		X	X		X				X	X	X				
Bristol	1861	X	X	X		X	X	X		X	X		X	X	X		X		
Surrey	1862					X	X		X				X		X				
Hereford	1871		X	X	X	X	X		X	X	X		X	X	X	X			
Whittingham	1873		X			X	X		X				X		X		X		
Adelaide	1852	X		X		X	X								X				
Parkside	1870	X	X			X	X		X		X		X	X	X	X	X		
New Norfolk	1830	X			X						X		X		X	X	X		

Key

A - An appropriate site with some form of scenery
B - An arrangement of the buildings that allowed light in and cross ventilation, with no building overshadowing another or the airing courts
C - A linear form to the layout
D - It should accommodate no more than 360 to 400 inmates
Ea - A building that offered a range of wards for classification
Eb - Each ward should have its own attendant's rooms
Ec - There should be open areas as opposed to day rooms for patients
F - Each ward should have access to a bathroom, lavatory and water closets
G - Each ward should have a wide gallery furnished as a day room with windows low enough to allow a view outside
Ha - There should be a large recreation room
Hb - School rooms
Hc - Work rooms and workshops
Hd - A chapel for the use of patients

Table 14. A Comparisision of Conolly's Ideal Aylum Features and the Asylums and Hospitals of Great Britain and Australia (continued)

Lunatic Asylum	Date	A	B	C	D	Ea	Eb	Ec	F	G	Ha	Hb	Hc	Hd	Ia	Ib	J	K	L

Ia - The offices should be centrally located
Ib - There should be a means of accessing the various wards without passing through each
J - Attendant's should have their own dining hall
K - Accommodation should primarily be in the form of single rooms with a few dormitories
L - Above all the asylum should be light, cheerful and liberal in the space it offerered

Ea - A building that offered a range of wards for classification, Eb- Each ward should have its own attendant's rooms, and Ec – There should be open areas as opposed to day rooms for patients

Adelaide and Parkside shared with all the British asylums a range of sleeping accommodation that supported classification beyond two classes. However, it should be remembered that Adelaide and Parkside did not share the design features of the British asylum layout that saw wards only marginally connected to each other, increasing the separation of the classes. Both South Australian asylums followed the pattern established in the county asylums of having attendant's rooms on or near the wards. All three institutions reflected the British pattern of not having the open day rooms recommended by Conolly.

F - Each ward should have access to a bathroom, lavatory and water closets and G - Each ward should have a wide gallery furnished as a day room with windows low enough to allow a view outside

Adelaide and New Norfolk, however, went against the British trend of providing water closets and baths on the wards. As indicated earlier, water closet or privy design at Adelaide was problematic and New Norfolk repeated this pattern. The New Norfolk Commissioners were keenly aware of the need for proper bathhouses, awareness not apparent in South Australia. Interestingly, while galleries were a common design feature in England, they are not found in any of the Australian institutions. At New Norfolk, this seems to be a result of the process of conversion of a convict institution into a Hospital for the Insane, as, from the 1850s onwards; the buildings were slowly improved to include some form of galleries. At Adelaide, there appears to have been little thought given to the design of the living spaces possibly due to the small number of patients the asylum was intended to accommodate. Forty to sixty patients spread over four wards with day spaces meant that gallery space was probably not considered important.

Ha - There should be a large recreation room, Hb - School rooms, Hc - Work rooms and workshops, and Hd - A chapel for the use of patients

As with the British asylums, there was no provision of a large recreation hall at the South Australian asylums or New Norfolk, and it is here that the multifunctionality of spaces becomes clear. As indicated previously, a large day room or ward was re-arranged to act as a space for concerts and entertainments at Adelaide. A purpose-built recreation hall was requested for New Norfolk, but was never funded, and a large day room served this purpose instead. The absence of a hall at Parkside is inexplicable, as the Adelaide experience of room/ward conversion must have indicated a need for a dedicated hall.

The general non-provision of school rooms in England was followed in Australia. Workshops and workrooms formed a part of the world of all the British asylums. As indicated previously this labor supported the asylum economy. At New Norfolk there were several workshops and patient labor was used to build and rebuild the Hospital reflecting a similar economic role. Sometime late in the nineteenth century workshops were added to Adelaide beyond the airing courts but the distance from the wards may suggest that patients were not employed in them. At Adelaide there was no female workroom, instead a ward was used. The same occurred at New Norfolk. At Parkside there was one workroom on the female side but no workshops.

As mentioned in Chapter Seven, South Australia prided itself on its freedom of religious worship and the absence of chapels, which was a common feature of British asylums, is explainable in this context. However the use of one of the larger rooms for Divine Service at Adelaide indicates that the patients wished for religious worship. At Parkside the women's dining room served as a chapel and recreation hall from 1881 reflecting a similar need. The un-consecrated nature of most asylum chapels supported their use as multifunctional spaces. The 1836 proposed additions for New Norfolk had included a chapel, however this was never built, and again a room was used for religious services. Considering the funding problems experienced by the New Norfolk Commissioners, funding had to be directed to sleeping accommodation and basic domestic and sanitary provisions before a discretionary building such as a chapel.

Ia - The offices should be centrally located and
Ib - There should be a means of accessing the various wards without passing through each

Centralization of offices was found in all the British asylums as well as the two South Australian asylums. There is virtually no evidence as to the location of the offices at New Norfolk. The larger British asylums had in some cases provided separate communication corridors. The South Australian asylums and New Norfolk were all designed differently. However, in all of them, access through the buildings was difficult and required the staff to go in and outside of buildings simply to traverse the wards. Supervision was consequently more difficult.

J - Attendants should have their own dining hall and K - Accommodation should primarily be in the form of single rooms with a few dormitories

While some British asylums had attendants' dining rooms, of the Australian institutions only Parkside had such rooms. One was proposed for New Norfolk in the 1880s but there is no evidence that one was built. Half the British asylums considered had more single rooms than dormitories and this appears to have been the case with Parkside, though there is no evidence of the exact ratio of single beds to dormitory beds at any of the institutions.

Overall Parkside Asylum came closest to the pattern established in England in terms of Conolly's features. Adelaide and New Norfolk were further removed, and in general the South Australian asylums and the Tasmanian hospital did not share as many of the features of Conolly's models as the British asylums (Table 14).

SOUTH AUSTRALIA AND TASMANIA: SIMILARITIES AND DIFFERENCES

South Australia and Tasmania had very different histories, one as a colony without a convict presence and the other as a convict colony. Interestingly, despite these differing histories, which would suggest differing responses based on the perception of who would be accommodated in an institution for the insane, the Adelaide Asylum and New Norfolk Hospital were to share similarities in their provision of spaces and rooms.

A consideration of Table 14 suggests that the Adelaide Asylum and New Norfolk Hospital shared only one feature in common, that of an appropriate site. However, if the building histories of Adelaide and New Norfolk are compared they reveal similar problems in both places, which were a consequence of their poor designs and their lack of a range of rooms and spaces as recommended in the 'ideal' asylum models. These problems included a lack of sufficient beds and wards to support classification of the patients. Consequently, those recovering from their illnesses were subject to the noises and behavior of those in the full throes of their illness. Both places lacked sufficient day space, and this led to ad hoc solutions. At the Adelaide Asylum, shelter sheds in the yards, with the addition of fireplaces, became fully-fledged day rooms. At New Norfolk, verandahs were used as day rooms and exercise spaces, and wooden buildings may have been used as day rooms at various periods. The absence of galleries reduced the possibilities for living space, and made supervision more difficult.

Similarly the original designs of both the Asylum and Hospital did not support the expansion of the buildings, and they were both to become simply collections of buildings with no coherent arrangement. Their layouts meant that supervisory visits to each ward by the medical officers required them to go in and out of buildings often covering considerable distances. Both Adelaide and New Norfolk lacked proper sanitary provisions such as indoor water closets, lavatories and bathrooms, and little provision was made for activities and employment. Interestingly, both places saw the use of female wards as work rooms, and the use of a female day room for a chapel and recreation hall. This multi-functionality of space reflected a failure on the part of those charged with designing the places to recognize the need for variety within the daily lives of patients as represented by the employment of patients and taking part in concerts, entertainment and dances. It seems likely that economic restraints may have played a part in both colonies, but importantly there were no requests for a recreation hall for Adelaide until the 1880s or for Parkside. The more pressing need at Parkside was for a female dining room. That it was of a size suitable for entertainments and Divine Service was only a secondary factor.

In effect, both Adelaide and New Norfolk only provided sleeping, eating and exercise spaces. There was no consideration of the occupation of patients' minds or the effects of the long periods of time spent in these institutions by some patients. Conolly's model and those of Sankey and Arlidge had all recommended a range of living spaces to provide some level of variation to the daily life of patients. South Australia and Tasmania differed in the respect that, on taking over management, the New Norfolk Commissioners as well as the Joint Commissioners of 1859, had realized the need for additional day spaces and a recreational hall. They requested funding to build these places. In contrast, there were no requests for additional day spaces, workshops or for a substantial period of time, a recreation hall for the Adelaide Asylum. Parkside, opened 18 years later, simply replicated the problem by having extremely limited day space for the number of patients it was to house. There was, however, a billiards room for the men and a work room for the women, which made a small concession to the needs of the patients, while at the same time reflecting the absence of any intention to employ the men. The problems highlighted by the relocation of internal furnishings to allow various rooms at Adelaide to be used for recreational activities does not seem to have produced any effect on the design of Parkside. There is no clear answer why Parkside repeated the failings of Adelaide. A range of factors appear to have affected the development of the Parkside Asylum. The most probable explanation lies with the incompletion of the design for Parkside and the subsequent problems in achieving funding for completing the airing courts with their additional day rooms. New Norfolk was similarly affected by a lack of funding and never achieved the vision held by the New Norfolk Commissioners who wished to have a Hospital equal to the best overseas institutions.

FACTORS INFLUENCING THE BUILT PROVISIONS OF BRITISH ASYLUMS

The closeness of the British asylums to Conolly's model may have been a result of a number of particular factors at work in England, that were present to a far lesser degree in the Australian colonies. These relate, in particular, to the knowledge pool available to the British asylum architects or designers. As was discussed in Chapter Four, the nineteenth century saw a growing emphasis on new modes of treatment in England along with revelations of the treatment of the insane in madhouses and charity hospitals. In response to these new forces, the County Asylum system was established. Those designing the new lunatic asylums could work from details of what was wrong with the present care of the insane as publicized by the various Parliamentary Inquiries. Books such as Browne's, also highlighted what was wrong with the built provisions currently existing and what asylums should be. These sources built upon books such as John Conolly's, and the extensive literature discussing all facets of the lunatic asylum in the *Asylum Journal of Mental Science*. If this was not sufficient, an interested person could go on tours of inspection of asylums and madhouses. This knowledge pool was supplemented by a rise in the development of a professional body of doctors who specialized in the care of the insane, and who, as indicated in Chapter Five, were in some cases involved with the design of county asylums (for example John Bucknill at Devon, Hill at Cambridgeshire, Robertson at Sussex, and Holland at Whittingham) or who could advise on what was required in an asylum. As discussed in Chapter Six there was an increasing uniformity in the construction of lunatic asylums in the mid-nineteenth century, which may have implied some copying of existing designs. Indirectly this may have seen the replication of desirable features in a lunatic asylum. For example Derby Asylum, which was considered by Conolly to be the 'ideal' asylum, had been built relatively early in 1844, at the beginning of an active period of asylum building. Later asylums may have copied aspects of it.

Certainly, the establishment of the Board of Commissioners in Lunacy under the 1845 County Asylums Act (Jones 1993: 89) saw an increasing emphasis being placed on bringing the lunatic asylum up to standard. The Commissioners were charged with monitoring practices relating to lunatics, establishing standards, and visiting lunatics wherever they resided. Importantly in conjunction with the Home Secretary, the Commissioners supervised the construction and management of the new county asylums (Hervey 1985: 103–4).

One means by which the Commissioners in Lunacy were able to establish standards for the construction of lunatic asylums was through the publication of the *Suggestions and Instructions in reference to (1) Sites; (2) Construction and Arrangement of Buildings; and (3) Plans of Lunatic Asylums* in the *Journal of Mental Science* in 1859. The *Suggestions and Instructions*, as published in 1859 and 1871, were wide ranging in their scope. For example with respect to the site they considered the soil; placement of the asylum in relation to towns; orientation; agricultural development; water supply; ventilation and light. In terms of the buildings themselves they considered classification; workers' and imbeciles' cottages; required rooms (limited to day rooms, a library, dining hall and chapel); staff residences; the proportion of single rooms to dormitories; the placement of sleeping rooms, day rooms, chapels, work rooms and workshops, and communication passages; staircases; floor surfaces and fireproofing; along with the provision of bath rooms, slop rooms, infirmaries, airing courts, farm buildings and workshops. What the *Suggestions* did not cover was the exact arrangement of the various parts in relation to each other and to the overall asylum layout.

How much do these *Suggestions and Instructions* reflect the development of ideas about the 'ideal' asylum up to that date? Clearly, at a general level they reflect the reformists' ideas about site location, separation of the sexes, basic classification, ventilation and sanitation. These had been particular concerns of Jacobi and Conolly. There was some suggestion of providing spaces suited to the patients as detailed by Jacobi, in assigning single rooms to the sick, dirty and excited patients. But nothing in the *Suggestions and Instructions* indicates that these patients should be physically separated into different wards. The *Suggestions and Instructions* of 1859 followed Jacobi and Conolly's 'ideal' asylums in having water closets and lavatories on each ward, but only specified that the ward for dirty patients have a bath room. For the other patients there should be general bathrooms conveniently located, rather than on all the wards as recommended by Conolly (*Suggestions and Instructions* 1859: point 23). Following Conolly's ideas the Commissioners recommended that windows should be large and easily opened, and that the asylum should have workshops, women's work rooms, a chapel, central dining hall, and a 'library and reading room, capable of serving for the general purposes of instruction and recreation'(*Suggestions and Instructions* 1859: points 7, 18, 19 and 33).

Variations from Conolly included the recommendation of more dormitories than single rooms and the use of day rooms rather than galleries and alcoves. The proportion of single rooms and dormitories instead reflected the ideas of Sankey and Arlidge, who wrote from the perspective of ten years later and thus from the experience of a greater number of county asylums. Of the possible spaces for recreational activities which the reformers emphasized, the Commissioners only mentioned airing courts, of which they thought two would be sufficient, planted as gardens and with ha-ha walls (sunken in a trench) to allow an unobstructed view. The Commissioners also omitted any reference to rooms for the attendants.

In 1871 the *Suggestions and Instructions* were republished with some amendments. Following the ideas of Sankey, the Commissioners now recommended the placement of all living rooms on the ground floor and sleeping accommodation on the floors above, and that assistant medical officers should have their rooms close to the acute and sick wards (*Suggestions and Instructions* 1871: points 6, 11). Interestingly in specifying the numbers of rooms to be provided for each class the Commissioners were advocating a return to an asylum for 200 patients as recommended by Jacobi in 1841, in sharp contrast to the large asylums being built which had arisen as a result of ongoing additions to existing asylums. This returned the asylum to a manageable size where the patient might receive individual treatment.

Thus, the Commissioners in Lunacy provided another source of information for those designing lunatic asylums, which reflected ideas about the reform of the lunatic asylum environment as expressed by several reformers. Through their Annual Reports, the Board was further able to detail what was wrong with the asylums visited, and what was improved, emphasizing what was required for the care of the insane. Conolly's 'ideal' model had been very much concerned with the provision of a healthy and comfortable environment for the insane which supported supervision, and this made many of his features basic requirements in an asylum.

For the British designer of lunatic asylums there were rich sources of information available to drawn upon, and the accompanying power of the Commissioners in Lunacy in approving plans, was a means by which much could be achieved in asylum design. This in turn may be the reason that the British lunatic asylums came much closer to the 'ideal' requirements of Conolly and the other reformers.

Why did the Adelaide Asylum and New Norfolk Hospital for the Insane, and to a lesser degree Parkside Asylum, fail to come close to the 'ideal' asylum models discussed?

FACTORS INFLUENCING THE BUILT PROVISIONS OF THE ADELAIDE AND PARKSIDE ASYLUMS

While it is possible to identify the factors influencing the closeness of the British asylums to Conolly's model, the emphasis given to each factor's relevance has to be entirely speculative without consultation of the documents relating to each asylum and the work of the Commissioners in Lunacy. By considering the case studies of South Australia and Tasmania, it is possible to be far more specific in identifying factors that influenced the built provisions in each colony, and in assigning a level of importance to each. Four factors have been identified: these are economic constraints, knowledge of overseas treatment of the insane, social perceptions of the insane and treatment regimes.

Economic Constraints

From the history of the built provisions for the insane in South Australia it is possible to identify periods of passive and active responses to the provision of buildings and asylums that may have been linked to economic changes. In the 1830s and early 1840s only limited attention was given to the question of providing for the insane. Without the established system of madhouses and charity hospitals as in England, the colonial authorities were reluctantly forced to provide for the insane, particularly as the desired option of placing individual lunatics with private medical practitioners met with little success (Quartly 1966: 15–16). The first lunatic asylum was a rented house unsuited to the care of lunatics. This seems to have been realized fairly quickly, and South Australia moved into a period of active response to the needs of the insane. Within two years of the realization of the inappropriateness of this building, the Colonial Surgeon had begun the search for a new site for a purpose built lunatic asylum and the Colonial Engineer had prepared a design. Construction began in 1850 and the Adelaide Lunatic Asylum was completed by 1852.

Factors Influencing the Built Provisions of the Adelaide

With economics restraining the size of the asylum and no consideration being given to the growth in the number of lunatics requiring care, it was realized within a few months of opening that the building was going to be insufficient. In September of 1853 the Select Committee on Public Works discovered that the cost of alterations to the Asylum and the addition of new wards would, in fact, be double the original cost of building the asylum. Their recommendation that £10,000 be placed on the Estimates for the construction of a new asylum was quickly followed by the purchase of the Woodforde land in January 1854 and the preparation of plans for a lunatic asylum based on the best of English designs and capable of accommodating 228 patients (S.A. C.S.O. Letters 24/6/2506). Perhaps in response to the huge cost of this proposal (£80,000) and changing economic circumstances, the colonial authorities entered a period of passivity in response to the needs of the insane. The new lunatic asylum plan was shelved and the considerably cheaper option of altering the Adelaide Gaol to accommodate the insane was considered in 1855 (£900). This, in turn, was decided against and expansion of the Adelaide Lunatic Asylum was once more advocated (S.A. C.S.O. Letters 24/6/545) (S.A. S.C. 1856: iii). This appears to have been a response to concerns over the care of the lunatics in the Gaol revealed by the 1856 Select Committee into the Treatment of Lunatics. The Committee itself believed a new lunatic asylum was needed, but the government did not respond to this recommendation, and, in the continuing passive phase, even diverted funds from the expansion of the present asylum, instead favoring the recycling of the public hospital as an annex to the Adelaide Asylum (S.A. S.C. 1856: iii).

It was not until 1864 that the response to the needs of the insane again became active. The Minutes of Evidence of the Commission into the Management of the Lunatic Asylum (1864) again highlighted the need for a new lunatic asylum (S.A S.C. 1864). In response to the Commission, the Government Architect, W. M. Hanson, prepared estimates for a new asylum in 1865. Land for the asylum was purchased at Parkside in 1866 and the new asylum foundations laid in December of that year (Kay 1970: 10; *South Australian Register* May 23rd 1868). Again economics seem to have played a part, with only one of the three pavilion buildings at Parkside being completed. This active phase quickly became a passive phase again, as having built the pavilion, work slowed, and the airing courts so essential for the patient's exercise were not completed. Seven years after first being occupied the front rooms of the Parkside Asylum were still not in use because there was insufficient day space or airing court space.

The active phase re-emerged in 1880 when construction of a series of buildings began, including the original intended second pavilion block for women, the criminal block and a series of cottages, and continued to 1888 (Piddock 2003 Appendix B).

A major contributing factor to the failure to provide the best lunatic asylum possible was the sheer cost of providing one along the best English lines. This situation was worsened by the high cost of materials and labor (S.A. C.S.O. Letters 24/6/2506), and it must be recognized that, as a colony in a "new" land, there were considerable demands on the South Australian Government to provide a wide range of infrastructure for those requiring care within the colony, including single unmarried mothers, destitute adults and children, orphans, reformatory children, criminals and the ordinary sick (see Piddock 1996 Chapter 6). Clearly there is a need for an economic history of South Australia that would allow these phases of activity and passivity to be matched against periods of recession and growth within the economy over the nineteenth century.

The initial intention to build an expensive purpose-built asylum at Woodforde had been quickly turned into a desire to modify the Gaol, to make it a partial lunatic asylum, and finally this gave way to the possibility of making improvements to the poorly designed Adelaide Lunatic Asylum. The difference between a new asylum and the Gaol modifications was profound. Could such a switch be entirely attributed to economic realities? In providing for the insane there was certainly a level of understanding of what should be provided, but how deep was this knowledge? Were class based judgments affecting the provisions within the lunatic asylums?

Knowledge of the Overseas Treatment of the Insane

Effectively, there were three pools of possible information that could have fed into the design of the new lunatic asylums. One was a familiarity on the part of the Colonial Engineer with lunatic asylums in England through his work in an architectural practice, or through architectural journals such as *The Builder*. The second was a familiarity on the part of the Colonial Surgeons and Resident Medical Officers of the treatment regimes of moral management and non-restraint, which had appeared in the early decades of the nineteenth century. The third pool of information was based on a familiarity with the literature of reformers such as John Conolly by South Australians in general.

The available documents do not give any definitive answer as to the level of personal knowledge of asylums amongst those involved in their planning and management. From responses to the various Parliamentary Committees and Commissions held in 1856, 1864, 1869 and 1883, it appears that those directly involved in some way with the care of the insane - from the Colonial Surgeon to the Visitors - actually had limited experience with, or variable knowledge of the care of the insane. For example, the evidence given before the Select Committee of 1856 reveals that the Surgeon working in the Adelaide Asylum, Dr. Thomas, had no direct experience of English lunatic establishments and their use of restraints. Similarly, of the keepers, only Head Keeper Morris had any experience with the treatment of the insane, having worked in the Dublin and Limerick District Asylums of Ireland where restraint was practiced (S.A. S.C. 1856: Q. 461, 631, 639, 670, 724).

Dr. Moore, who in 1858 had introduced non-restraint to Adelaide, was more familiar with English practices. He had visited the Middlesex Asylum at Hanwell and attended lectures by John Conolly: "It is a branch of my profession, to which l have paid some special attention" (S.A. S.C. 1864 Q. 82). Clearly there was no pool of knowledge about the treatment of the insane in the colony in the first years of the Adelaide Asylum's operation. Instead care rested with the personal self-education and interests of the Colonial Surgeon. This argument is supported by the fact that the Master Attendant in the 1860s, who had no experience with lunatics, was in charge of the daily management of the Asylum. This was only balanced by his having worked in the Adelaide Asylum for 14 years (S.A. S.C. 1864 Q. 31, 149). It seems likely that this lack of knowledge may have been the result of the migration process and the size of the colony's population. The growth in the number of asylums in Britain offered those interested in the treatment of lunatics many opportunities for employment. If these men and women did not choose to migrate the considerable distance to the new colonies the possible pool of knowledge became severely limited.

The Minutes of Evidence of the Commission of 1864 showed some knowledge of English asylums among the Adelaide Asylum Visitors. Certainly from his evidence, Mr. Boothby was aware of English trends, and was able to comment on the Ninety-Second Report of the English Lunacy Commissioners. Boothby used the Report to support his argument for a separate place for patients who were likely to recover, noting that it indicated that the incurable could be accommodated more cheaply than the recent and curable cases (S.A. S.C. 1864 Q. 589). The main source of information seems to be books; Boothby recommended that the Commissioners obtain Dr. Conolly's work for themselves to see what he recommended in relation to amusements (S.A. S.C. 1864 Q. 590, 5961). In addition Thomas English and Rev. C. Farr, who also gave evidence before the Commission, both spoke from some knowledge of other asylums through visits (S.A. S.C. 1864 Q. 536, 772).

Earlier in 1859, in debating the best site for a lunatic asylum, several members of the Legislative Council appear to have been familiar with the British practices of placing lunatic asylums in countrified settings away from towns, and the medical authorities' recommendation of exercise, light employment and cheerful recreation for patients (S.A. P.D. 23/8/1859). Yet these examples are only piecemeal, and there is little real evidence of this knowledge being applied in requests to change or modify the Adelaide or Parkside Asylums. The selection of Parkside for the new asylum and its design may have represented the application of this knowledge, even if the full design for the asylum was never completed.

Among the Colonial Architects, Bennett Hays appears to have been familiar with English Asylums, and certainly expressed the wish to build an asylum based on the best English models when the Woodforde site was purchased in 1854 (S.A. C.S.O. Letters 24/6/984). In 1864, the then Colonial Architect, W. Hanson indicated that he had worked for a practice that had designed two or three lunatic asylums in England, and he was familiar with plans published in *The Builder* (which he considered the best source of information) and other unspecified books. Interestingly he favored the radial design, even though by this time that design had fallen from favor in England (S.A. S.C. 1864 Q. 910).

Before work had begun on the design of the Parkside Lunatic Asylum an experienced medical officer, who was familiar with the treatment of the insane, had been employed to advise on the best site and design for the new asylum (S.A. V. & P. 28/7/1864). This position was filled by Arthur Harrison for a year, then by Alexander Paterson of Yarra Bend Asylum, Victoria. However it appears that Paterson's knowledge of lunatic asylums may have been restricted to his four years at Yarra Bend Asylum rather than a working knowledge of British asylums (S.A. S.C. 1869 Q. 2147, 2179).

While it is not possible to argue definitively from this evidence provided in response to the Parliamentary Inquires and that provided by the asylum history, it would suggest only a limited use of this knowledge in any attempts to improve the quality of patients' lives and in creating an improved design for the Parkside Asylum. This limited knowledge is interesting to consider as many of the people involved with the lunatic asylums were recent immigrants from England where lunatic asylums were rapidly becoming a part of the landscape, and where discussion of lunacy and asylums was a common topic of journals such as the *Quarterly Review* (1844, 1857 for example). Could the answer to why the South Australian asylums did not achieve more of the features of the 'ideal' asylum lie with perceptions of the possible nature of the patients?

Social Perceptions of the Insane

While South Australia was not a convict colony, it did retain the class-based social stratification of England that saw a similar division of society into higher, middle and lower classes.

The Adelaide Lunatic Asylum was not intended as an asylum purely for the pauper lunatics like the British county asylums, but to accommodate all patients, including those paying for treatment. The county asylums were not required to provide accommodation suitable for the middle classes; this in turn had affected their overall design. However, under the existing South Australian lunacy law, pauper patients were to be admitted to the asylum before paying patients. At the same time, however, the Colonial Surgeon or Resident Surgeon at the asylum did not have the authority to discharge private patients in order to make way for paupers (S.A. S.C. 1856: Q. 600). The planned Woodforde Asylum included accommodation for 'superior' patients in partially detached buildings at the end of the wings of the main building (S.A. C.S.O. Letters 24/6/2506).

Equally, there was an important perception amongst those working or visiting the asylum that the patients were not the same as those found in British asylums. This had important implications for the choice of treatment regime and how the daily life of the patients was managed, which in turn was manifested in the provisions made within the Asylum or the uses of the existing spaces and rooms. Both Dr. Moore and the Rev. Farr, a Visitor to the asylum, offered the view before the Commission of 1864, that certain activities were not appropriate for the patients. In Dr. Moore's view, the patients of the English asylums were people drawn from the educated or middle classes, while the South Australian patients were drawn primarily from the laboring classes. Hence, putting on balls and providing a more extensive range of reading material was not called for; concerts though would be welcome (S.A. S.C. 1864 Q. 71, 72). Reverend C. Farr, who was familiar with Lincoln Asylum in England, having gone over it several times, offered a similar view, believing that a great deal of lunacy in the colony was caused by alcohol and that these patients had to be kept quiet (S.A. S.C. 1864 Q. 780, 784).

The belief that insanity in the colony was caused by intemperance had been supported by a number of witnesses before the 1856 Select Committee. Dr. Gosse believed that a large portion of the insanity found in the colony was caused by drunkenness, rather than being hereditary, a view supported to a degree by Keeper Morris, who gave equal weight to hereditary causes and intemperance. Dr. Woodforde, another Visitor, believed there was no one cause, but agreed that intemperance and the heat could play a part (S.A. S.C. 1856: Q. 138, 887, 1070–72).

The emphasis placed on intemperance has several implications, suggesting class-based judgments about the groups in society most likely to be afflicted with insanity, and the possible stresses involved in living in a new colony. Equally, the treatment regime offered may have been structured to reflect possible beliefs about the curability of insanity brought on by drunkenness and hereditary weakness. This class-based view continued amongst the colonists of South Australia during Dr. Paterson's residence. As early as 1872, Paterson in his Annual Report to the South Australian Parliament had acknowledged that public opinion believed that insanity was caused by the vices, self-indulgences, and intemperance etc. of the person. Not discounting the role of dissipation in many diseases, he offered a different view. He believed that, in a large number of cases, the malady was unavoidable as it was caused by physical weakness of the brain. This may have been hereditary or caused by circumstances before birth. Any exciting cause, including overwork, deprivation, insufficient food, mental strain or intemperance, would bring on an attack of insanity. The Adelaide and Parkside Asylums, he argued, contained many sober, industrious people who had led quiet peaceful lives, and intemperance resulted from attempts to deal with the encroaching disease (S.A. A.R. 28/3/1872).

There is little evidence that class-based judgments had an effect on the use of space within the South Australian asylums. However, it did affect the life of the patients. In 1864 the better educated patients, for example, were allowed to sit up till ten p.m., generally used No. 2 yard, and were allowed certain comforts. The class-based division of the patients was often subtle, as in John Cavanagh's comment that the females in No. 2 ward did all the sewing while the *coarser* (sic) class did all the washing (S.A. S.C. 1864 Q. 130 191). The main problem with this evidence is that it can only be securely applied to a few years surrounding the Commission, and cannot be applied to the entire period of the asylums operation. If the class-based divisions had only limited impact on the use of spaces within the asylums, they could have had some real impact on the attitudes towards what should be required in an asylum accommodating a large body of laboring people, whose lifestyle may have contributed to the development of insanity.

Treatment Regimes

As treatment regimes, both moral management and non-restraint required a specific environment and a regime of classification, work, recreation, exercise and supervision which gave rise to 'ideal' asylum models. There is little evidence of the practice of moral management and non-restraint before Dr. Moore became Colonial Surgeon in 1858, and was given charge of the Adelaide Lunatic Asylum (see Appendix 2 for full details). While Dr. Gosse, who was Acting Colonial Surgeon from 1856, had expressed the belief that kindness was the only way to treat lunatics, evidence given before the Select Committee appointed to inquire into the Treatment of Lunatics in 1856 indicates that restraint was being practiced and baths used as a punishment for difficult behavior (S.A. S.C. 1856: Q. 40, 50, 52, 97–8, 511–525, 773, 776). Dr. Moore, influenced by his interest in the treatment of lunatics, introduced full non-restraint and possibly moral therapy as well (S.A. S.C. 1864 Q. 6, 20–22, 34–5, 82).

Dr. Moore's regime appears to have continued under Dr. Paterson, who was employed as the Resident Medical Officer for the Adelaide Lunatic Asylum in 1867. He testified before the 1869 Select Committee that the insane could only be managed by moral arguments and inducements; modern treatment forbade coercion (S.A. S.C. 1869 Q. 6, 12). However, Dr. Paterson favored the view that insanity arose from organic causes (as opposed to faulty reasoning) and consequently concluded that, of 220 patients in the Adelaide Asylum, only 20 were curable (S.A. S. C. 1869 Q. 19–22, 259). Consequently moral management may have been a day-to-day means of controlling the patients' behavior rather than a curative regime.

It is difficult to argue for a direct impact of this change in treatment regime from restraint to non-restraint and moral treatment on life within the asylum. Certainly, despite a subsequent period of relatively intense building activity at the Adelaide Asylum and the consideration of the design for a new asylum that culminated with the construction of Parkside, there were no requests for rooms or spaces to provide a more diverse life for the patients reflecting the requirements of moral therapy and non-restraint. These requirements included employment of and activities for the patients. Rather, additions focused on the provision of sleeping accommodation, and when workshops were provided in 1869, they were relatively small and placed outside the exercise areas at the back of the asylum suggesting that the male patients were not often employed in them.

It is difficult to tell the difference between cause and effect at the Adelaide Lunatic Asylum. Was the absence of reasonable living space and dedicated rooms the reason elements of moral management were absent until the 1870s? Or was it a failing within the treatment regime that caused these elements to be missing? There is evidence that the lack of religious services in 1864 was a consequence of a lack of interest among clergymen in attending to the needs of lunatics, rather than the lack of the chapel. The non-employment of the men may have resulted from problems with finding suitable work for them that could be done in the available space, suggesting that the absence of proper rooms was affecting the treatment of the patients (S.A. S.C. 1864 Q. 10–11, 16–17, 76, 772, 774–775). Certainly the lack of classification, an important part of the new treatments, came down to the limited ward space available and the numbers requiring accommodation. It seems likely that decisions about the treatment applied and the absence of the appropriate spaces were both impacting on life within the asylum.

It is clear that despite the introduction of moral treatment, there was no move to provide new rooms that could have improved the quality of life for the patients, and would have in turn brought both Adelaide and Parkside Asylums closer to Conolly's 'ideal' asylum.

Discussion

Clearly, a number of factors were affecting the choice of the original designs for the South Australian asylums and the choices made with respect to additions and modifications to both asylums. Economics would appear to have played a key role, along with a general lack of knowledge of current trends in the treatment of the insane overseas amongst those involved with the asylums. The latter may have been one of the more important reasons for the failure of the Adelaide Asylum to meet the 'ideal' models. The knowledge pool in the colony rested primarily on casual visits to asylums and literature rather than direct experience of the management of the insane or of asylum operations. Not surprisingly Parkside Asylum, which comes closest to the models, was built when there was increased knowledge of the care of the insane amongst those involved with it.

Although the asylums were not specifically built with paupers or the working class in mind, there is evidence that the patients of the asylum were coming from these classes. Whether class-based judgments were affecting the amount of money spent on the lunatic asylums is more difficult to answer. A similar pattern of activity and passivity had occurred with the Destitute Asylum of Adelaide, which had seen promises of a new asylum not realized (Piddock 1996). The absence of a recreation hall at Parkside may be seen in terms of economics, swayed by class-based judgment of what was appropriate for the perceived nature of the patients. This remains conjecture though as there is no hard and fast documentary evidence to support this conclusion. Conolly had still thought these types of discretionary spaces important in an asylum designed for the working class.

FACTORS INFLUENCING THE BUILT PROVISIONS OF NEW NORFOLK

With respect to the South Australian lunatic asylums, a number of factors have been identified that probably influenced the history of the provisions made and affected whether they came close to the 'ideal' model. Did these factors play a similar part in Tasmania?

Economic Constraints

The costs of providing for the insane probably influenced the nature of the provisions made and the choice of whether to remodel New Norfolk or to begin again with a new asylum. The building history of New Norfolk indicates that, on being transferred from the English Government to colonial control, there was a spurt of building activity to bring New Norfolk up to a reasonable standard. Despite the near bankruptcy of the colony, £1,208 8s. was spent on repairs, building new service buildings and making some additions to existing buildings (Townsley 1991: 98–100; NN Correp. 14/9/1858, 2/2/1859). The Commissioners were hopeful that the government would continue to unhesitatingly vote moderate sums to improve New Norfolk (Tas. P.P. No. 1859 No. 10 6/7/1859).

This hope was realized only periodically, with funding not appearing to follow any particular pattern. For example in 1860 £6,000 was included in the Parliamentary Estimates for alterations and the purchase of land. However a request in 1862 for £4,500 for construction of a recreation hall, new bake house and kitchen, and the conversion of the latter to a bathhouse was not met, despite the significant improvements they would have made to the lives of the patients.

The period 1865 to 1871 saw the Commissioners indicate that funding was insufficient to meet the needs of the Hospital (Tas. A.R. P.P. 1862, 1866). Interestingly after many years of requesting funding for a Ladies' Cottage, the Parliament finally provided £1,200 for it in 1867 (Tas. A.R. P.P. 1867, 1872). Concerns about the mixing of free women with convict women may have finally become persuasive enough to force the Parliament to allow this funding even if no more was to be provided. Perhaps reflecting continuing economic problems in the colony, the New Norfolk Commissioners did not ask for additional buildings in the early to mid 1870s, despite the Hospital reaching its upper limit of accommodation (Tas. A.R. P.P. 1873).

When the Cascades Asylum opened in 1877, it did not provide an overflow for the New Norfolk Hospital; rather its sole function was to house the insane convict men formerly kept at the Port Arthur Lunatic Asylum. It did not provide a further asylum for the insane or a solution to the pressures on accommodation at New Norfolk.

That funding continued to be problematic is indicated by the fact that, although plans were prepared and tenders called for a new dormitory for the refractory wards in 1877–78, work was not undertaken till late 1879–1880 (Tas. A.R. P.P. 1878, 1881). Before the Royal Commission of 1882, the New Norfolk Commissioners indicated they had asked for £1,344 for repairs in 1883 which had not been met (Tas. R. C. Report 1883 Q. 22, 25). The realities of funding for New Norfolk are best reflected in the former Superintendent, Dr. Huston's evidence that, while a comprehensive plan had been drawn up for improvements in 1859, along with other suggestions, the funding had not been provided. The only reason given by the Government for not meeting these requests was a want of funds (Tas. R.C. Report 1883 Q. 224).

As a consequence of this lack of consistent funding, work was undertaken in a piecemeal fashion, with the provision of recommended attendants' accommodation, the spacious workshops, and the day rooms for all classes not being achieved in the nineteenth century. These recommendations would have brought New Norfolk far closer to the 'ideal' asylum as recommended by Conolly.

Economic pressures also appear to have affected how building work was conducted at the Hospital, with the conversion of old buildings to new purposes - a cheaper solution than building two new buildings. One example was the conversion of the old kitchen into a bathhouse when a new kitchen was built, and often building materials were recycled, again suggesting the limited funding available (Tas. N.N. Corresp. 9/8/1861, 24/9/1861).

Despite the failings of New Norfolk, as revealed by Bishop Willson's letters and the New Norfolk Commissioners Annual Reports, there were no real attempts to consider the option of a purpose-built lunatic asylum until the Royal Commission of 1882. However attention always focused on the re-modeling of New Norfolk to bring it closer to the standards of England.

From this very limited evidence it appears that New Norfolk was not a financial priority to the colonial authorities, and the level of funding was not sufficient to bring about wholesale changes to the Hospital as recommended by the New Norfolk Commissioners, the Joint Committee of 1859, and Royal Commission of 1883, who wished to see New Norfolk remodeled as a series of cottages and pavilions following the best new practices. There is, again, a need for an economic history that allows one to plot possible ups and downs in the economy that would have influenced funding. A comparative study of other Tasmanian institutions would be useful in further identifying issues in the funding of such places, particularly those with a strong association to convicts.

Social Perceptions of the Insane: The Presence of Convicts

However, the question needs to be asked: did the perceptions of who was being accommodated in New Norfolk also affect the willingness of the Tasmanian Government to spend money on re-modeling the hospital or in providing a new asylum? Was New Norfolk seen as a convict establishment even after transportation finished? Social stratification had begun to appear in Tasmania in the 1840s and 1850s. At the top were the Lt. Governor, the Colonial Officials, landowners, then came a merchant class, followed by free working people, then the emancipist who bore the stigma of their convict past, and lastly the convicts (Townsley 1991: 18–19).

New Norfolk had begun as a convict establishment for the care of invalid and insane convicts. By the time the New Norfolk Commissioners were appointed in 1855 the Hospital was accepting convicts and free people. The Commissioners indicated that there was no separation of accommodation and treatment for those of the 'better' classes, and in the Male division those suffering from temporary and/or partial insanity were:

> ... herded with convicts of the most degraded class, and were thus irritated and injured by contact with men from whose habitual coarse propensities of speech, gesture, and behavior - lunacy had withdrawn every decent restraint (Commissioners quoted in Gowlland 1981: 50).

Similarly in the Female division 'virtuous' women were associated with those of 'notorious careers'. Consequently the Commissioners sought funding for a Gentlemen's Cottage initially. That they wished for a cottage would suggest that the anticipated number of the 'better' classes requiring accommodation was quite small as it would have had only six sleeping apartments of two beds each (Tas. A.R. P.P. 1865). The Ladies' Cottage was opened several years later.

This highly negative view of the convicts was repeated again in the President of the New Norfolk Commissioner's letters of defense against the criticisms of Bishop Willson. E. S. P. Bedford felt that conditions at New Norfolk should be seen in light of the nature of its patients:

> ... It must be borne in mind that a large majority of the Patients heretofore confined in the Asylum have been of the Convict class, the offspring of diseased parents, inheriting in very many cases a defective intellect, brought up from the earliest childhood in misery and vice, and leading in after years a life of

> sensual debauchery and crime, resulting in enfeeblement alike of body and mind - a more hopeless class of subjects it would be almost impossible to collect together in one Institution; (Tas. P.P. 1859 No. 10 6/7/1859).

Despite this vision of the patients of New Norfolk as hopeless cases, as will be discussed below, there was a constant effort by the Commissioners to introduce modern treatment and to provide a curative regime.

This strongly worded statement more than anything suggests class-based judgment about the nature of the patients, which is interesting as the patient statistics indicate that the balance between those described in the Official Statistics of Tasmania as free people and convicts was fairly even (Table 12). The marked reduction in convicts from 1859 to 1865, and then the subsequent rise, may be a product of new definitions of convict, with emancipists formerly referred to as free now being classed with convicts by the Commissioners. This would suggest that one's past marked one permanently in some way. Reynolds in his article 'That Hated Stain': The Aftermath of Transportation in Tasmania' clearly indicates that there was a clear perception of emancipists being linked to crime, disease and poverty, a fact supported by the high numbers of emancipists in the prisons and in pauper establishments (Reynolds 1969: 20, 21, 22). This social division is most clearly indicated by the Official Statistics of Tasmania which indicated that there were 119 free men and 94 free women in New Norfolk in 1860, and only three male and seven women convicts. In contrast the Commissioners Report for that year indicates that there were 75 patients who had arrived free in the colony and 145 convicts under treatment (Tas. A.R. P.P. 1861). This division may have been reinforced by the fact that convicts and former convicts were maintained by the Imperial Government and the free by the Colonial authorities (Tas. A.R. P.P. 1862). It is unclear whether emancipists and their children were still being classed as convicts. A further problem lies in the fact that the documents dealing with New Norfolk do not make it clear whether the convicts and the non-convict working class patients were seen as one and the same, or whether the latter fell into the Commissioners' 'better classes'.

The class-based view of New Norfolk was deeply entrenched as indicated by the following. In a letter to the Colonial Secretary the New Norfolk Commissioners were to:

> ... deprecate most strongly the idea that class distinctions should in any degree enter into the system of management of the Asylum, they cannot but feel that in estimating these requirements justly it is necessary to take into account the former life and previous habits of the present, and probable future patients (Tas. P.P. 1860 No. 13: 2).

Perceptions of class directly affected the lives of the patients, for the Joint Committee Report of 1859 was to comment that the provision of the detached building for men of "refined habits and education" prevented these men from mixing with pauper patients, from having to share the same quality of utensils and tables, or their prison diet (Tas. J.C. Report 1859: 4). A similar argument was used to support the requests for a Ladies' Cottage, as New Norfolk was the only place in Tasmania where the insane could be treated (Tas. A.R. P.P. 1866). This class-based judgement of the greater appreciation of their surrounding by the educated classes was a common one in nineteenth century writings on lunacy (Browne 1837: 182–183 and Conolly 1847: 9). For the Commissioners, the physical separation of the patients was necessary for a cure to be achieved (Tas. A.R. P.P. 1865).

The link between insanity and a convict heritage continued in the minds of the New Norfolk Commissioners who, in 1870–1, stated their belief that the number of insane in the Colony was a direct result of the "former circumstances of a large proportion of its population" which created an abnormally high rate of insanity. With the deaths of the remaining convicts and former convicts, the Commissioners expressed the belief there would be fewer patients needing to be accommodated (Tas. A.R. P.P. 1871). This belief was probably supported partly by the significant drop in the number of prisoners and paupers in the colony with the death of the emancipists (Reynolds 1969: 22). In 1879, however, the Commissioners changed their mind. Referring to discussions in Parliament, which echoed their former views, the Commissioners indicated that this hope was not sustained by experience to the hoped for extent:

> ... Insanity leaves an inheritance which disappears, even under highly favourable moral and physical conditions, only by degrees; and there are not wanting new causes of local origin tending to develop disease, either temporary or permanent, in forms which the Hospital at New Norfolk is designed to meet. (Tas. A.R. P.P. 1880).

Consequently, there was no decrease in the number of insane, but a requirement to meet the needs of all classes of the insane. From this limited evidence it appears that New Norfolk was seen primarily as a convict establishment, even though it also provided accommodation for the 'better' classes. The possibilities of the continuation of the convict taint with respect to emancipists and the children of convicts clearly needs further investigation to clarify its nature. The documents clearly show, as well, a continuing class-based judgement about which classes the patients of New Norfolk would come from. There appears to be some confusion of the terms 'convicts' and 'working class' within the documents relating to the Hospital, with the terms used interchangeably. This may in fact reflect the internal divisions and perceptions of the nature of the classes in Tasmanian society although this needs further investigation. Reynolds' article does not cover this question in any detail, but he does indicate the lack of male franchise for half the male population before 1884. This arose from a fear of emancipists achieving political power (Reynolds 1969: 23–4). It is highly possible that there was no working class as such in Tasmanian society, rather divisions based on wealthy among the free settlers creating upper and middle classes, and below this an emancipist class after transportation ceased.

Knowledge of the Overseas Treatment of the Insane

The New Norfolk Commissioners often referred to the best overseas institutions in their Reports, but what level of knowledge existed in the colony of overseas treatment regimes? The Commissioners' knowledge of recent trends in the treatment of lunacy may have come from books and articles. In 1864 they had decided to purchase both of John Conolly's books, reflecting a knowledge of some of the literature in the field.[2] In addition the Annual Report for 1871 had indicated that the Commissioners had sought returns and reports of Hospitals for the Insane in other parts of Australia, as well as overseas, as a means of comparing their own curative, financial and general management arrangements (Tas. A.R. P.P. 1872). In terms of personal experience, Bishop Robert Willson was the most experienced person in the colony, having spent seven years (1830–1842) on the board of management of the Nottinghamshire County Lunatic Asylum in England at a time when they were instituting new treatment practices. He was also licensed to privately care for lunatics (Southwood 1973: 140).

The Joint Committee of 1859 demonstrated some awareness of English experiences and recommendations regarding the provisions required in a lunatic asylum, in this case of the ratio of land per patient, but it is unclear where this knowledge came from (Tas. J.C. 1859: 3). The architect, Mr. Hunter, in evidence to the Committee, again, shows the influence of the journal *The Builder* as an important source of information. Hunter recommended that a new asylum for 200 could be built for £30,000 using the plan of the Cumberland and Westmoreland Lunatic Asylum in *The Builder* as a base. The presence of the plan in such an "authoritative journal", Hunter believed, indicated that it would feature those modern improvements expected

---

[2] John Conolly (1847) *The Construction and Government of Lunatic Asylums and Hospitals for the Insane* and John Conolly (1856) *Treatment of The Insane Without Mechanical Restraints*.

Factors Influencing the Built Provisions of New Norfolk

in a newly constructed institution and make it an 'ideal' model (Tas. J.C. Report 1859: 7). While in evidence before the Royal Commission of 1882, three decades later, Dr. Macfarlane, the Superintendent, described a pavilion asylum that would meet Sankey's first, second, fifth and seventh requirements and all but one of Robertson's requirements, suggesting knowledge of ideas about asylum design (Tas. R.C. Report 1883 Q. 38).

Unfortunately, the available evidence gives only a limited perspective on the experience of the treatment of the insane among the medical staff involved with New Norfolk. There is no evidence about the experience of Dr. Huston, the Medical Superintendent for 25 years. His successor, Dr. Macfarlane, indicated before the Royal Commission of 1882 that his knowledge came from reading, as did his assistant Dr Coutie. Only the Lady Superintendent, Mrs. Bland, had any direct experience of the treatment of the insane, having spent seven and a half years as Matron at Gladesville Lunatic Asylum in New South Wales. Dr. John Coverdale, who had charge of the Cascades Asylum, had no experience of the treatment of the insane, but had worked at a variety of institutions within the colony (Tas. R.C. Report 1883: Q. 36, 70, 258). Of the 19 medical men interviewed, some had visited asylums and all had read articles in medical journals. Given this evidence it appears likely that Dr. Macfarlane and Dr. Coutie's recommendations for a pavilion and cottage system for the reform of New Norfolk were based on their readings, possibly including such authors as Arlidge, Sankey, and Robertson. Overall there was little direct experience of the treatment of the insane and the requirements of a good asylum among those involved with New Norfolk.

Treatment Regimes

If New Norfolk was a convict establishment accommodating a fair number of insane convicts who were seen as largely incurable, how did this affect the treatment regime practiced and what implications did this have for treatment regimes linked to the requirements of the 'ideal' asylum and its use of space?

From the evidence of the treatment regime at New Norfolk (for full details see Appendix 3), it is clear that any perception of the patients as being convicts or working class did not affect the attempts to introduce the most effective treatment regime possible, again reflecting the best of overseas experience. If there were class distinctions in the management, it seems rather to have affected the furnishings and the tasks given to the patients rather than the actual treatment regime. From the opening of the Hospital it appears that moral treatment was used as a reasoning tool along with some form of restraint. The Colonial Surgeon saw the treatment regime as being curative and argued that patients should be as little harassed in body and mind as possible (Tas. C.S.O. Letters 7th Feb. 1832 pg. 141–2). From the very beginning, however, it was realised that the lack of space hindered the recovery of the patients, as they could not be separated into groups based on their mental state (i.e. acute, convalescent) (Tas. C.S.O. Letters 1/811/17340).

The New Norfolk Commissioners, on taking charge, felt that this former regime was not curative: the patients had little room for exercise, and there were no religious services or amusements, although some patients appear to have been employed. The Commissioners were not, however, to effect an immediate change as indicated by the Joint Commissioners, who found with respect to the men, that there were no books, newspapers, music, pictures, sport or pleasurable occupations undertaken despite the fact that all these "are universally dwelt on in England as forming an essential part of a curative system" (Tas. J.C. Report 1859: 5). The women were probably experiencing the same conditions. It seems likely that priority had been given to transforming the buildings, new funding must have been provided allowing for the purchase amusements, as in their Annual Report for 1859, the Commissioners indicated that books, draughts, dominoes and magic lantern shows were now part of the lives of the patients (Tas. A.R. P.P. 1860). The range of activities were to be further expanded with dances, music nights, visiting entertainments, summer walks and picnics outside of the asylum walls, along with regular Divine Services being part of hospital life in 1864. Pictures, birds and other animals had also been introduced and the grounds planted with flowers and grass (Tas. A.R. P.P. 1865). The Commissioners spared no effort to:

> ... conform the Institution, as closely as circumstances and the means within enabled them to do, to the example of kindred institutions in Europe in which improvement has been carried farthest. (Tas. A.R. P.P. 1865).

In this range of activities the Commissioners were following the recommendations of the lunacy reformers who saw activities and employment as both a reformative tool and a means of distracting the thoughts along healthy and normal channels (Tas. R.C. Report 1883 Q. 69). Moral treatment recommended the employment of patients, and at New Norfolk there was a class-based division of work tasks. Miss Laland indicated in 1883 that the penal class did the washing and the other women sewed clothes and linen (Tas. R.C. Report 1883 Q. 252). The men had been employed from the earliest days in manual work around the Hospital, and they in addition made boots and clothing (Tas. A.R. P.P. 1870). One tenet of moral treatment - classification - was always to present an insoluble problem while the Hospital retained its current layout and design. The lack of specific rooms and spaces, however, did not prevent the New Norfolk Commissioners and Medical Officer from achieving as much of a curative regime as possible. The lack of funding meant that the requested dedicated spaces, such as a recreation hall, chapel and day rooms, were never provided. There absence did not, however, arise from any failing to request funding for the provision of these places by the Commissioners.

Discussion

When considered together, the building history, the treatment regimes, and the attitudes towards the inmates, they paint a complex and tangled picture. The funding of improvements at New Norfolk on the change from Imperial to Colonial control would suggest that the need to provide an appropriate environment for the insane weighed more heavily than any perception of the inmates as predominantly convict. Later funding may or may not have become more problematic, possibly in response to economic conditions within the colony, or in response to the continuing view of New Norfolk as a convict establishment. However, any perception of the inmates as being drawn from the convict or lower classes did not affect the desire of the Commissioners to make the New Norfolk Hospital as good as the best overseas institutions, or to pursue a curative regime with as varied a life as possible for the inmates. From the perspective of the New Norfolk Commissioners, the only effect of the perceived role of the Hospital as a convict establishment seems to have come in the provision of the Ladies' and Gentlemen's cottages, with their more home-like surroundings and possibly better diet, for those considered to be of a better class. Whether the Tasmanian Government and people saw New Norfolk in the same way as the New Norfolk Commissioners is not clear due to a lack of primary documentation.

Certainly the nature of the inmates did not affect the Commissioners efforts to reform the buildings of New Norfolk and to impose a curative regime, nor did it affect the recommendations of the Joint Committee of 1859 and Royal Commission of 1882. However the Joint Committee and the Royal Commission identified serious problems with the buildings of New Norfolk that had arisen from a lack of appropriate funding over a long period, and ultimately perceptions of the nature of the inmates may have affected the decision not to build a new purpose-built asylum. Particularly as the anticipated drop in the number of the insane with the death of the convict class would have made such expenditure unnecessary and the rebuilding of New Norfolk more logical and probably less expensive. Equally a perception that the insane would slowly disappear from society with the death of the convicts may have led to the limited efforts to improve the New Norfolk buildings in the late 1870s and 1880s, as despite all efforts, it remained a poorly designed place lacking real living space and sufficient wards for all classes of patient.

CONCLUSION

At the beginning of this chapter three questions were asked:

- Can any patterns in the adoption of 'ideal' asylum features be identified in Britain, South Australia and Tasmania that are similar to each other?
- Was the realization of the 'ideal' asylum model responsive to social, cultural and economic circumstances within a country or colony?
- Is it possible to identify particular factors common to both South Australia and Tasmania in influencing the adoption of the 'ideal' asylum that transcend their different histories as a free and penal colony respectively?

From a consideration of the various plans and data sets there appears to have been no particular pattern to the adoption of the 'ideal' asylum requirements that were universal. As indicated, the factors affecting the possible adoption of the 'ideal' asylum were different in Britain and the Australian colonies, and these led to different choices in the adoption or copying of features that matched the models. However there was a pattern that seems to be common to all institutions. This pattern related to the rooms provided and their use. In both the British asylums and the Australian institutions there was a multifunctionality of rooms, rooms were not simply used for their designated function but to meet the changing needs of the asylum over time. In South Australia and Tasmania, for instance, dining halls served as recreation halls and chapels, and wards could become work rooms for women. In general dedicated discretionary spaces, such as recreational halls and school rooms, were a low priority, however British asylums generally provided chapels.

In answer to the second and third questions, the adoption of the 'ideal' asylum features can be directly related to social, economic and cultural forces at work within the colony. In South Australia, the most influential factors appear to be economic constraints and a lack of

Conclusion

knowledge of overseas trends in the treatment of the insane. The social perceptions of the patients appear to have most directly affected the range of activities available for them. However it cannot be ruled out as influencing the level of funding made available for providing for the insane, there is simply not enough evidence to argue a case. In Tasmania, the most important factor again appears to have been economic constraints, but here the perceptions of whom was to be accommodated can almost certainly be directly related to the funding provided for the care of the insane. The insane were generally convicts, who it was believed would eventually 'die out' thus reducing the number of insane requiring accommodation. In both colonies there was a pattern of discussion of what was required in providing for the insane. This discussion centered on better built provisions. In South Australia the focus was on the construction of a new asylum, and in Tasmania on the remodeling of New Norfolk. While this discussion occurred repeatedly, in both colonies there was a failure to realize these improvements and the insane were left in buildings with significant failings and with a life that was extremely limited in both its activities and the rooms and spaces that contained it.

While South Australia and Tasmania chose different paths with the provision of purpose-built asylums and the re-modeling of New Norfolk, in both places the ups and downs within the economy and the level of funding provided over several decades had the most direct impact on provisions made for the insane. A lack of funding meant institutions in both places lacked sufficient spaces and rooms to support either a curative regime or a reasonable standard of living for the patients and staff living within them. The two colonies shared in common a lack of direct experience in the treatment and management of the insane by those directly charged with their care. In Tasmania only Bishop Willson had any experience and the medical staff relied on reading to maintain their knowledge. A similar situation occurred in South Australia. This was in sharp contrast to the extensive knowledge base to be found in Britain, and must have directly impacted on the design and management of both the design of the institutions provided and on the experience of the patients within them. While there is evidence that *The Builder* was considered an important source of information about new lunatic asylum designs, a plan in a journal does not provide any information about the interaction of spaces or the reasons for their provision. In this situation it becomes easy to omit spaces and rooms that might be seen as luxuries or unnecessary without realizing the impact on the lives of patients. The plans in *The Builder* represented a growing body of experience in Britain in the construction of lunatic asylums and of the intellectual world of ideas about the treatment of the insane that led to the articles and books on what an asylum should be. Further there was no guarantee that these plans were in fact the best in asylum design, rather than simply records of asylums constructed. However as discussed, the British Asylums included in *The Builder* included those which came closer to meeting Conolly's 'ideal' asylum. Because the South Australian and Tasmanian institutions did not copy any of these British designs, they lacked some of the necessary features to support patient management and to provide an appropriate environment. For example, there were insufficient wards to support a range of classification, no bathrooms were provided and there were no functional water closets on each ward (Adelaide Asylum's water closets were removed as they were poorly designed). The ward arrangements within the buildings did not support easy supervision or passage through the various wards as did the W-shape adopted for many British asylums, and there was no provision of workshops for the employment of male patients.

10 Conclusion: Archaeology and Lunatic Asylums

Charles Cleland (2001: 2) argues that historical archaeology has become focussed too much on event based archaeology and not on wider cultural questions. This book has taken up this challenge and has sought, not just to explain the visible remains on the landscape - the buildings of the Parkside Lunatic Asylum and the New Norfolk Hospital for the Insane, but to understand both the forces at work within society shaping these buildings and what life was like within them for the unvoiced.

In general a gap exists in lunacy studies where the buildings of the lunatic asylum are given little importance in the overall consideration of the role of the lunatic asylum in the nineteenth century. Similarly there was little recognition of the asylums as more than collections of buildings. In this book it has been shown that the lunatic asylum buildings played a fundamental role in the treatment of the insane, which in turn led lunacy reformers to describe what the lunatic asylum should be.

The asylum was not simply a collection of floors, walls and spaces; it was imbued with meaning for the patient and society as a whole. In this book it has been argued that buildings can be considered a form of communication, and can allow us access to a range of beliefs, attitudes and practices about the insane that may not find ready expression in documents. This communication can be accessed by considering the rhetoric about the lunatic asylum and the reality of the built environment.

ARCHAEOLOGY AND INSTITUTIONS

By their nature, institutions present unique problems for archaeologist. One difficulty is the continuing use of these buildings today. Many lunatic asylums are still in use as psychiatric hospitals, and are not open to excavation and survey. Institutions which are open to excavation may present further problems in the assignment of artefacts to particular groups as demonstrated by Sherene Baugher in her study of the New York Almshouse (2001: 186–7). Unlike houses, shops, hotels and so forth, artefact collections may be small due to the use of solid concrete floors, restrictions on the possession of personal items, different waste disposal practices of the institution or the recycling of material goods through other institutions also present problems, which become more apparent when dealing with large scale nineteenth century institutions such as lunatic asylums. Some asylums had their own dinner services and uniforms for patients and staff. The variable periods of time spent by individual patients in the asylum makes the linking of particular items to known residents almost impossible. This does not, however, prevent us from undertaking archaeological studies of these places. In fact by not excavating it is possible to open up new areas of research. By not limiting questions to how these artefacts came to be here or how these walls were built, it is possible to widen the concept of material culture beyond excavated artefacts.

In this book buildings are seen as material culture, and the plans and photographs of them are expressions of this material culture, records in fact, and are accessible when the buildings themselves are not. By generating various data sets composed of plans, photographs and building histories, which detailed room uses and building modifications, it was possible to recreate the material world of the institutions in the colonies of South Australia and Tasmania. To some these data sets cannot be considered archaeological. However, archaeology is very much about a way of seeing and asking questions, not simply a set of physical techniques for data collection. It goes beyond a simple physical description of features to the actual use of these spaces and the human interaction with them. Thus this study asks questions about the Adelaide, Parkside and New Norfolk institutions as material culture even though they are not available for excavation.

The methodology developed was based on Leone and Potter's (1988: 13–14) description of the application of Binford's middle range theory to historical archaeology, with the focus being on three elements: the independence of the archaeological and documentary records; the concept of ambiguity or discrepancy; and the use of descriptive grids. The concept of ambiguity or discrepancy relates to the testing of a descriptive grid against material culture. The discrepancies are generated by what is expected to be found and what is found. This in turn generates new questions that seek to explain these discrepancies.

By using a descriptive framework of what the lunatic asylum should be as written about by Browne, Jacobi, Conolly, Sankey and Robertson and testing it against the plans of lunatic asylums in Britain, it was possible to understand the relationship between the world of ideas and their actual use. Through an understanding of what was and was not adopted of the 'ideal' models, it was possible to understand life within the asylums and attitudes towards the insane.

The comparison against a range of British lunatic asylum plans covering the period of the 'ideal' asylum models revealed that Browne's model was developed in response to what was not occurring in British asylums, in other words there was little correspondence between the asylums and his model. From 1845 to 1870 the county asylums came close to fulfilling most of Conolly's requirements to varying degrees. Interestingly the spaces most commonly absent were those that weren't essential to providing a healthy, reasonable living environment. The spaces found less frequently were those that I have called discretionary. They were not essential but rather provided a diversification of day to day life for the patients. These included recreation halls, school rooms and female workrooms. Faced with financial constraints in building an asylum they were the least important and could be omitted. The continued absence of these types of spaces from some asylums and the belief that they were still needed can be seen in the recommendation for the inclusion of libraries and dining rooms in the 1850s descriptions of Sankey and Arlidge. The 'ideal' models of Sankey and Robertson, however, that argued for a re-organisation of the day and night spaces of the asylum were not realised in the sample plans.

By considering the asylums as a group it became clear that there was a pattern to asylum design in Britain. Prior to 1845 when the building of county asylums became compulsory, there had been considerable experimentation with layouts and internal arrangements. After 1845 there was an overall uniformity to the designs that saw the adoption of the W-shape with its linear wards for most asylums. The experimentation did not return until after 1870, when the problems of accommodating an ever increasing and large resident asylum population meant that the original W-shape was continually extended with additional linear wards until they became unworkable.

Clearly by using plans it was possible to identify the presence or absence of rooms and spaces, but this does not tell us about changes over time to room use which may have brought the asylums closer to the 'ideal' models or further from them. Through the case studies of South Australia and Tasmania it was possible to understand in much greater depth the relationship of the ideals to the reality of the built environment and why certain elements were or were not adopted. A comparison of the Adelaide and Parkside Asylums in South Australia to the descriptive framework of the 'ideal' revealed a limited range of matches to all of the models. In fact the Adelaide Asylum was revealed to be poorly designed, with few of the characteristics that would have created a reasonable and healthy environment for both patients and staff. Later additions to the original asylum only brought it slightly closer to Conolly's requirements. Parkside Asylum, opened 18 years later, proved to be similarly deficient in many respects, though it had more matches to Conolly's model. In general, both South Australian asylums had fewer matches to Conolly's model than the British asylums. A similar situation existed in Tasmania. The New Norfolk Hospital for the Insane similarly fell far short of the 'ideal' models, providing only the most basic accommodation and sanitation. Of all the models the feature most commonly met was that of an appropriate site. This in fact may be more reflective of the availability of land within the colonies or the need to place such institutions reasonably close to towns, due to questions of access to public transport and the cost of supplies hauled over large distances in a colonial setting. In both colonies the poor designs of these institutions directly affected the quality of life for the patients, and the Adelaide Asylum and the New Norfolk Hospitals became ad hoc collections of buildings that hindered effective supervision by staff.

LIFE WITHIN THE ASYLUM

Life within institutions is often seen in terms of concepts of dominance/resistance and paternalism. Primarily because of their nature as places where various groups of people were cared for, and where these people were exposed to a reformative regime informed by particular values held by society, archaeologists have sought in the archaeological record responses to the imposed life of these institutions (Prangnell 1999 and Casella 2001). While the lunatic asylum falls within the realm of paternalism with its organised spaces and movement through these spaces, which saw access to quieter wards and landscaped rather than plain airing courts as rewards for appropriate behaviour and self restraint, responses to this paternalism are far more difficult to detect. The problem arises of discriminating between deliberate actions on the part of the patient from those arising from uncontrolled mental illness, which alters behaviour and invests new meaning in simple objects. When is the possession of rocks, pieces of material, and feathers a resistance to a life that allows few personal items? (Casella 2001: 60, 64) or when is it simply a collection of pretty found objects? Clearly such an approach is not effective for understanding life within a lunatic asylum. In this study an alternative approach was taken using the descriptive framework of what lunatic asylums should be to understand life within these places. The 'ideal' asylum models as detailed were not simply descriptions of rooms but were concerned with the provision of a range of spaces that would support moral treatment and non-restraint. At the heart of these regimes, as was shown in Chapter Four, was the organisation of patients into groups based on their mental state, the provision of a range of activities, both leisure and work based, free access to airing courts for exercise, religious consolation, observation and individual treatment of the patient's mental illness.

John Conolly's model extended beyond the provision of wards for classification, day spaces, airing courts, and work areas, to consider features of non-restraint as he envisaged it. These included keeping the wards and patients clean, and providing an environment that offered intellectual stimulation through windows low enough to offer a view of the outside world and a diversity of spaces and furnishings to break the monotony of life. These features were combined with others that supported the effective management of the patients, to provide a description of the best possible asylum environment.

The comparison of the material culture of the South Australian and Tasmania institutions to the descriptive framework revealed that these places provided a limited and constrained life for the patients, which fell short of the ideal world of the asylum as envisaged by Conolly and others. The focus was on the provision of wards, day spaces, and exercise areas. There was little consideration of the provision of discretionary spaces within the institutions. There were no dedicated recreation halls, chapels, workshops, or school rooms, which would have provided variation within the daily routine through a change of scenery. Instead, importantly for the archaeologist, this study has revealed a multifunctionality of room use, not just in Australia but also in Britain. It has become clear that room and space indications on plans do not provide accurate indications of room use; rather they indicate intended room use on the part of the architect. Only by creating histories of room uses over time from plans and documents is it possible to understand the multifunctionality of spaces within the lunatic asylum, which saw laundry rooms become recreation halls, and recreation halls become wards in Britain. In the Australian institutions offices and wards doubled as recreation halls, while women's day rooms became work rooms. At New Norfolk and Parkside Asylum the same solution was reached in response to limited funding, which affected the provision of dedicated rooms with a women's day room serving the multiple purposes of day room, chapel and recreation hall.

Within the world of the asylum the range of activities undertaken appeared to depend on the interests of the superintendent and attendants, and on the flexibility of spaces and the portability of their furnishings, which allowed some areas to serve as recreation spaces for dances and musical entertainments.

The designs further affected both the imposition of the new treatment regimes of moral therapy and non-restraint. The link between the asylum environment and the treatment regime is most clearly demonstrated at New Norfolk, where non-restraint could not be introduced until the buildings were physically modified in 1860, despite the acknowledged benefits of non-restraint to patient management and lives, which had been recognised from the 1830s. As Conolly had argued there was no evidence that the insane lacked any awareness of their surroundings, yet the Australian institutions, like those in Britain, provided what must have been a basic and unwelcoming environment. It is clear from the documentary evidence that while efforts were made to provide a place for the insane where they might be cured, a sense of social duty did not extend to the provision of furnishings, curtains, painted walls, cutlery, and amusements. Here again we have the difference between the rhetoric of provision and the reality of the asylum. This difference is most interesting in relation to New Norfolk where, it has been argued, there was a reasonable level of awareness of what should be provided in a curative asylum along the best European lines, although the reality was one of wooden, vermin-ridden buildings still in use after 50 years.

As Lu Ann De Cunzo (1995) has demonstrated, the world of an asylum could be filled with symbolic meaning, and passage through the world of the Magdalen Asylum in Philadelphia, which had a ritual component. Lunatic asylums encompassed similar ideas of symbolic meaning and ritual movement through space. Within the world of the lunatic asylum as envisaged by the advocates of moral treatment, forward movement through classified wards indicated that one was achieving greater self control and controlling the thoughts that had led to the mental illness in the first place (Hill 1838: 39–40). Any lapses saw the patient moved back to the early admission wards. For Jacobi, this classification saw a minimum of five divisions (Jacobi 1841: 57). Despite these ideas of ritualised movement with its associations with rewards and punishment, the physical provisions of the British county asylums and the Australian institutions in terms of wards would suggest that these ideas were not put into practice, and classification was probably based on refractory and convalescent criteria; with separate provision made for the physically ill. The overcrowding was such that at Adelaide and New Norfolk even the basic of classifications were broken down, with the need to provide beds where physically possible overriding classifications. Here then is a sharp contrast between the world of ideas about the treatment of the insane and its physical expression in the buildings of the asylum in the early nineteenth century and the reality of the lunatic asylums as built.

A GENDERED EXPERIENCE

While the mirror imaging of the two sides of the British lunatic asylums may suggest that life for men and women was the same, a consideration of the rooms provided for each and the documentary evidence proves this was not the case. While men were provided with workshops and access to outdoor activities, the world of the asylum for women was dominated by a cult of domesticity which saw their lives constrained to employment in the laundries and in sewing. The usefulness of women's work to the asylum economy was such that reformers were concerned that women were tied to their work, whether in the laundry or the day room, and were not taken out to exercise. For Arlidge employment of the patients, that saw a life little different from outside employment, found its worst expression in the development of worker's wards. Here the patient lived and ate above their work places. The asylum's emphasis on self sufficiency had resulted in a life little different from the stresses that had caused the initial illness. The use of day rooms as work rooms for women, rather than their separate provision as recommended by Conolly, meant that some women spent their entire day on the ward, with pleasurable activities taking place in the work areas. This increased the sheer monotony of daily life. By the 1850s the British asylums saw a significant rise in the number of permanent residents, if 10 or 20 years or more were to be spent in the asylum, a greater variety of spaces became necessary.

In the world of the asylum women were passive onlookers, who would visit the gardens but not work in them, watched men playing sports but had to be persuaded to go for walks. It may be wrong to assume that women did not play some part in this passivity, as it seems likely life experiences outside of the asylum, either within middle class society or from a working class life, affected decisions made by women as to what activities they would take part in.

The different experiences of men and women within the South Australian asylums found greater physical expression than in the British asylums. Different provisions were made with respect to airing courts and their landscaping, and in the placement of the laundry in the airing court at Adelaide. The different experiences of men and women are reflected in the provision of a work room for the women and a billiards room for the men at Parkside Asylum. Men were generally not employed and had greater access to a range of outdoor spaces.

There is no clear evidence of why the men could not be employed beyond outdoor work in South Australia, except a belief that the men were from a labouring class that did not have many skills. Tasmania presented a slightly different picture with no evidence of different working lives for the men and women. Both sexes were employed in sewing, and the placement of the washhouses suggests that men possibly were employed in laundering.

AN ARTIFICIAL WORLD

The lunatic asylum was a totally artificial world. Its arrangements of wards, day rooms, airing courts, administrative offices, domestic areas and work rooms were designed to support patient management and the treatment regimes applied. Archaeological studies have shown that human beings often have very different views of the uses of their household spaces and often divide their spaces into public and private, work and non-work areas (Kent 1984: 61–2, 104–5: Pearson and Richards 1994: 7). The ward designs, often featuring dormitories and large galleries, meant there was little personal privacy for those aware of their surroundings. In the airing court, ward, or work area they were constantly observed and surrounded by other patients. Lunatic asylum management placed heavy emphasis on observation and even gardens had to be designed to allow the patients to be observed at all times. There was no separation of the public and private space for patients, and movement through the spaces of the asylums were strictly contained. With the use of day rooms as work rooms and the development of worker wards there was little separation of work and non-work areas. As Arlidge (1859: 201, 204–5) had pointed out the world of the asylum was as far as possible from that of the home, and he had advocated the provision of a range of rooms for day time activities that would reflect the middle class world. However there is no evidence that this idea was taken up, and considering the overall lack of discretionary spaces found in the asylums studied, it seems likely that this suggestion would have fallen on deaf ears. Interestingly there appears to have been some efforts to maintain class divisions within the Australian asylums with different furnishings provided for the better off in the Adelaide Asylum, and separate buildings at New Norfolk. Overall, the worlds of the Adelaide Asylum and the New Norfolk Hospital for the Insane were custodial, with the Parkside Asylum offering a life only slightly less so.

THE TWENTIETH CENTURY

The rooms and spaces of nineteenth century lunatic asylums have been replicated in the designs of modern psychiatric hospitals which are often built around the core of nineteenth century lunatic asylums and added to throughout the decades until today. The limitations of the modern hospital environment may have reinforced the public view of the mental hospital as a custodial place. The hospitals are composed of single rooms and dormitories of generally two to four beds, a dining room, an activity room, and usually some form of lounge where videos are played or religious services held. The main variation today is the separation of the different classes of patient into separate buildings. A redevelopment and diversification of the mental hospital spaces may in fact return the hospital to a comfortable place for those, who through their illness do not fit within the mainstream of society, and can be seen as a 'dangerous' threat to the general public because their behaviour does not fit into what we perceive as 'comfortable' and 'appropriate' when outside of our homes. The mentally ill are gradually being deprived of the care of the hospital but are given nothing in its place.

In this study it has been argued that, while there was a range of reformist nineteenth century works describing the 'ideal' lunatic asylum, the actually constructed lunatic asylums exhibit a wider range of designs which reflected the knowledge of reforms in the treatment of the insane, the treatment regime applied, and various social and economic factors. In fact, the reality of the lunatic asylums was far more complex than its extant and visible remains on the landscape would suggest.

Appendix 1
The Location of Illustrations of Lunatic Asylums discussed in Chapter 6

1. Bethlem Hospital. Jonathon Andrews et. al. *The History of Bethlem* (1997) p240
2. Bevans' seven armed radial asylum. T. Markus *Buildings and Power: Freedom and Control in the Origin of Model Building Types* (1993) p137, Fig 5.40
3. Watson and Pritchett's West Riding Asylum at Wakefield. T. Markus *Buildings and Power: Freedom and Control in the Origin of Model Building Types*. (1993) p140
4. Middlesex County Asylum at Hanwell. Vieda Skultans *English Madness. Ideas on Insanity 1580–1880*. (1979) p103
5. Devon Lunatic Asylum by C. Fowler. *The Builder* 25/7/1846 and Devon Lunatic Asylum by C. Fowler from Andrew Scull et. al *Masters of Bedlam. The Transformation of the Mad-Doctoring Trade*. (1996) p191
6. Derby Lunatic Asylum from John Conolly *The Construction and Government of Lunatic Asylums and Hospitals for the Insane*. 1847
7. Asylum for the Counties of Monmouth, Herford, Breneck, Radnor (Abergavenny). *The Builder* Vol. 10 No. 483, 1852 p297
8. Eglinton Lunatic Asylum (ground floor). *The Builder* Nov 27th 1852 p754
9. Lincolnshire Lunatic Asylum. Edward Palmer "Description of the Lincolnshire County Asylum" *The Asylum Journal* Vol. 1 No. 5 1859 p72
10. Buckinghamshire Lunatic Asylum from John Crammer *Asylum History. Buckinghamshire County Pauper Lunatic Asylum-St. John's*. (1990)
11. Essex County Asylum. *The Builder* May 16 1857 and Frederick Norton Manning *New South Wales Report on Lunatic Asylums*. Appendix G. (1868)
12. Bristol Lunatic Asylum. *The Sixteenth Report Of The Commissioners in Lunacy to the Lord Chancellor* July 1862 Appendix F.
13. The Cambridgeshire Isle of Ely and Borough of Cambridge Lunatic Asylum. *The Sixteenth Report Of The Commissioners in Lunacy to the Lord Chancellor* July 1862 Appendix F.
14. Cumberland and Westmoreland Lunatic Asylum. *The Builder* May 1st, 1858 p294–5
15. Sussex Lunatic Asylum from C. Lockhardt Robertson 'A Descriptive Notice of the Sussex Lunatic Asylum, Hayward's Heath.' *The Journal of Mental Science* Vol. VI No. 33 April 1860: 282
16. The Bedford, Hertford and Huntingdon Lunatic Asylum at Arlsey. *The Sixteenth Report Of The Commissioners in Lunacy to the Lord Chancellor* July 1862 Appendix F.
17. The Bedford, Hertford and Huntingdon Lunatic Asylum at Arlsey. *The Sixteenth Report Of The Commissioners in Lunacy to the Lord Chancellor* July 1862 Appendix F.
18. Carmarthen Lunatic Asylum. *The Builder* Aug 22nd 1863 pp602–3
19. Surrey County Asylum. Frederick Norton Manning *New South Wales Report on Lunatic Asylums*. Appendix G. (1868)

20. Cheshire Asylum. Frederick Norton Manning *New South Wales Report on Lunatic Asylums*. Appendix G. (1868)
21. City and County Asylum, Hereford. Jeremy Taylor *Hospital and Asylum Architecture in England 1840–1914. Building For Health Care*. (1991) p145
22. The County Asylum, Whittingham 1873. George T. Hine 'Asylums and Asylum Planning.' (1901)

Appendix 2
Treatment Regimes in South Australia

Insights into the treatment of the insane in the South Australian lunatic asylums during the early years are few. It is possible to draw some conclusions from various comments made by the Visitors to the Adelaide Lunatic Asylum and from the evidence presented before the Select Committees and Commissions of the South Australian Parliament. Unfortunately the Committees and Commissions rarely asked directly about the treatment regime being practised. Rather information comes as a result of questions respecting the possible ill-treatment of patients. Despite this the various Minutes of Evidence remain one of the most important sources of information regarding the treatment of the inmates, attitudes towards the insane amongst South Australians and familiarity with overseas practices as well as trends in provisions for the insane.

From the evidence presented to the Select Committee appointed to inquire into the Treatment of Lunatics in 1856, it appears that the initial treatment regime was based on custodial care and restraint. Despite moral therapy having been practised for several decades in England and elsewhere, and the non-restraint movement gathering momentum, there is no evidence of them being practised in the early years of the Adelaide Asylum's existence. This may have been a consequence of the Colonial Surgeon, James Nash's lack of experience with the treatment of lunatics. The first evidence of attempts to introduce partial non-restraint came with Dr. Gosse's time as Acting Colonial Surgeon around 1856. Dr. Gosse, however, did not reside at the Lunatic Asylum, and while he testified before the Select Committee that kindness was the most effective form of treatment and restraint was never used as punishment, in evidence Keepers Nash and Morris admitted that the plunge bath was used as punishment for difficult patients (S.A. S.C. 1856: Q. 40, 50, 52, 97–8, 511–525, 773, 776). The evidence would suggest that there was a marked gap between the desired treatment and the actual treatment of the lunatics.

As indicated in the Select Committee Minutes of Evidence life for inmates was dominated by monotony with no amusements beyond board games, cards, and reading for the men, the women lacked even these. Employment was restricted to the women who worked in the laundry and kitchen. The garden which may have provided work for the men was not secured by walls (S.A. S.C. 1856 Q. 91, 93, 126–7). This again argues for the non-application of moral management as there were no attempts to make life for the inmates more bearable or to bring them to back to sanity by moral arguments. Rather economics were more important to Gosse than the employment of an extra keeper to employ the men (S.A. S.C. 1856: Q. 130). Religious services were not held. Morris was to further testify that the treatment regime, which included the use of restraints and baths, was similar to that he had experienced in Ireland, with the exception being that no classification was achievable at the Adelaide Asylum due to overcrowding. Certainly the more extensive classification used by Hill and others could not be practised as Adelaide in effect had only two wards for each sex, and Morris's evidence seems to indicate that even the separation of new cases from convalescent patients was not occurring (S.A. S.C. 1856: Q. 796, 1048). It appears that the asylum was primarily a custodial institution with some implied efforts towards a non-restraint system, rather than a curative institution as envisaged as part of moral treatment. This is supported by the use of the Gaol as a lunatic asylum.

It was Dr, Moore, the Colonial Surgeon from 1858, who introduced full non-restraint and possibly some form of moral therapy to the Adelaide Asylum. As indicated in his evidence to the Select Commissioners in 1864 he had a special interest in the treatment of lunatics: "It is a branch of my profession, to which I have paid some special attention" and he had attended lectures by John Conolly, the non-restraint reformer (S.A. S.C. 1864 Q. 82). He had gone as far as to dismiss an attendant who would not work under the non-restraint system and had met with some resistance among other attendants on introducing non-restraint (S.A. S.C. 1864 Q. 6, 20–22, 34–5). The Master Attendant who had worked at the Asylum for 14 years, found that the new system was more successful and less troublesome, reflecting the English experience (S.A. S.C. 1864 Q. 31, 149). Happily Dr. Moore reported that the cure rate stood at over 50 percent (S.A. S.C. 1864 Q. 92).

Under Dr. Gosse there had been little attempt to employ the inmates or introduce other aspects of moral treatment. Dr. Moore appears to have made greater efforts as he believed work was useful in itself rather than for any economic value it may have had. Dr. Moore indicated clearly that he wished for more employment of the patients, particularly for those unable to do housework or outdoor work in 1864.

Appendix 2 Treatment Regimes in South Australia

Of 110 male patients only twenty were capable of outdoor work. It appears that mat-making and sewing bags had been done in the past but supplies of materials had not been regular. Many patients could not be encouraged to do anything and none were forced to work. (S.A. S.C. 1864 Q. 10, 11, 16, 17, 76). Activities appear to have been limited to chess, draughts, and bagatelle. Silk worm farming occupied patients for six weeks at a time. Caged birds and rabbits had also been bought into the wards to brighten them (S.A. S.C. 1864 Q. 77, 80).

As with the earlier Select Committee the evidence was primarily about the men, and the references to games seems to apply to them, for Dr. Gosse and Dr. Bayer, another Visitor, had noted that the women had no amusements apart from hard physical labour in the washhouse and some knitting and sewing, and only a small yard to walk in (S.A. S.C. 1864 Q. 305, 349). The separation of the sexes meant that the women could not go into the main garden at the same time as the men. Consequently Sunday afternoon was the only time they could go into the garden, and this had come to be seen as a privilege (S.A. S.C. 1864 Q. 458–459).

The Adelaide Lunatic Asylum's regime seemed to be severely lacking in variety in its day to day life and the lack of grounds and the shortcomings of the buildings were playing a part in this failure. The other failing repeatedly mentioned was the lack of classification (S.A. S.C. 1864 Q. 327, 384). This had implications not just limited to the disturbance of convalescent patients by refractory ones. There was the question of the plan of treatment. The encouragement of patients recovering from their sanity had to be limited if the attendants were occupied by refractory cases. Similarly extra comforts and indulgences in amusements and furniture for convalescents could not be followed through with if day space was extremely limited. As Boothby indicated:

> ... what is wanted is to induce a cheerful spirit amongst the patients; they should always have some sort of occupation; their safe custody should not be the only matter considered (S.A. S.C. 1864 Q. 591).

Even religious instruction which may have helped lift the spirits of the inmates was not being attended to as no ministers were visiting the asylum regularly (S.A. S.C. 1864 Q. 5). While there was no specific chapel, a room capable of holding forty to fifty was set apart for religious services and patients were given prayer books and Bibles (S.A. S.C. 1864 Q. 60, 201). Reverend Farr believed that there should be a designated clergyman for the Asylum, if not a resident minister. Farr, quoting Dr. Charlesworth of Lincoln Asylum, indicated that religious instruction could help induce new associations leading away from the erroneous thinking that led to insanity (S.A. S.C. 1864 Q. 772, 774–5).

Overall the evidence given before the Commission seems to indicate that attempts to achieve a better life for the inmates were being made, but only in a piecemeal way with no plan of management, which would suggest the full application of the treatment regimes suggested by non-restraint reformers. This is supported by the lack of a Resident Medical Officer due to no accommodation being available for him, Dr. Moore, the Colonial Surgeon, visited every second day (S.A. S.C. 1864 Q. 1–3, 31). The Resident Officer would certainly have been able to maintain a perpetual influence over the patients and the management of the asylum (S.A. S.C. 1864 Q. 288–295, 334, 394–5, 523–4, 576, 579–581).

This scheme of moral management appears to have continued under Dr. Paterson initially. In evidence before the 1869 Select Committee he indicated that the insane could only be managed by moral arguments and inducements; modern treatment forbade coercion (S.A. S.C. 1869 Q. 6, 12). Refractory patients were locked up only when they disturbed the whole yard, assaulted another patient, or disturbed the quiet of three or four patients. Seclusion was a tool to prevent violence and a part of the medical treatment (S.A. S.C. 1869 Q. 18). But while Dr. Paterson appears to have been practising moral management, its curative aims were tempered by his belief that the majority of the inmates of the Lunatic Asylum were hopelessly insane (S.A. S.C. 1869: 19–22, 259). Dr. Paterson certainly from the evidence given had attempted to bring life closer to the ideals of moral management and non-restraint practises, which were very much about making life more bearable and distracting the thoughts of the inmates. In terms of amusements for the men there was bagatelle, cricket, walking expeditions, newspapers, books, backgammon, and so forth. For the women, Paterson found it was more difficult to find amusements. They had walking expeditions, the *Illustrated News*, and 'a great deal of needlework'. Again the borders between amusements and work were blurred; if he wanted to give a bazaar female patients would be employed to make goods (S.A. S.C. 1869 Q. 27).

The class attitudes that informed some of the attitudes towards activities appear to have changed with Dr. Paterson's appointment as he indicates that dances were now being held, along with concerts, theatrical entertainments, 'Christy Minstrels', and other entertainments. These were attended by all but the sickest inmates (S.A. S.C. 1869 Q. 27, 29). The range of activities now more closely followed those recommended in England to alleviate the boredom of an enclosed life within the asylum. Paterson indicates that nothing was as beneficial to the patient as entertainments, apart from work. Several women had shown improvements after attending entertainments (S.A. S.C. 1869 Q. 45–47). The retirement time of patients also had been extended with

Appendix 2 Treatment Regimes in South Australia

patients now staying up to 8 p.m. and visits by Ministers of religion had recommenced (S.A. S.C. 1869 Q. 76, 203–211).

Paterson indicated that he liked to keep the inmates as much at work as possible. The women were employed in doing all the washing and in making all the clothes for the establishment apart from the stockings. Interestingly the tailor, who lived in the Asylum, worked with only two male patients; presumably he was not allowed contact with the women (S.A. S.C. 1869 Q. 1507). The employment of the men was not detailed but the Asylum employed a gardener to attend the vegetable gardens and the general grounds, and the men would have assisted him. All the artisans employed lived in the Asylum and were expected to take a turn at ward duty (S.A. S.C. 1869 Q. 216, 219, 221–2). James Watson, the Head Attendant, indicated some of the activities used to occupy the patients included hair picking, hat and mat making, although the latter was not economic. Hair picking involved separating the hairs matted in wet mattress (S.A. S.C. 1869 Q. 292).

By the 1880s Dr. Paterson's belief in the organic causes of insanity had become more entrenched and his focus had shifted to providing an environment where these physical causes could be treated. He believed insanity was both the product of the disordered function of the brain and organic and physical changes to the brain. The former, the cause of temporary insanity was curable, the latter less so (S.A. Comm. 1884 Q. 486–488). Paterson indicates that many of the newly arriving cases had suffered from too much labour and not enough food. They began to recover after resting and being given good food (S.A. Comm. 1884 Q. 696). This would suggest that physical stress was an important contributing factor in causing insanity in the colony. Paterson firmly believed that cured patients were as good as before if the disease was of a functional nature, organic disease was another matter (S.A. Comm. 1884 Q. 581–3, 648). Clearly moral arguments would have less sway in bringing a person back to sanity if the cause was not some failing of the personality or habits but arose from an organic cause. While moral management had gained favour with many, possible organic causes for insanity had not lost favour with writers on lunacy in England and the growing emphasis on hereditary weaknesses in the second half of the nineteenth century was fuelling a shift in perceptions of insanity (Skultans 1975 for overview). In practice Paterson emphasising rest, proper nutrition and later on work as the curative regime for many cases (S.A. Comm. 1884 Q. 696).

The activities and work tasks listed before the Select Committee of 1864 continued into the 1880s. The women continued to do the washing for the asylum, making all their underclothing and the shirts for the men as well as mattress making and knitting. While the men were employed digging and working in the garden, teasing hair, making new mattresses, and in repairing and cleaning old ones, kitchen and store work. Both sexes did household work. There were fortnightly dances and once a week patients from both Adelaide and Parkside went out in the omnibus (S.A. Comm. 1884 Q. 525, 6085–6090). There was no indication that work had become more regular, particularly as these were basically the same irregular activities as pursued in the 1860s. The major difference was the trips outside of the asylum. Amusements included cards, bagatelle, dominoes, chess, backgammon, dancing, football and cricket for the men (S.A. Comm. 1884 Q. 629). Religious services had become a regular event as these induced habits of regularity and order (S.A. Comm. 1884 Q. 534–5).

There was no training of the inmates in trades; rather those with specific skills were employed in them, for example carpentry. Paterson indicates that most were pick and shovel men (S.A. Comm. 1884 Q. 630–1). Similarly neither asylum had a library despite a government grant of £100 per annum for amusements (S.A. Comm. 1884 Q. 681–3).

Unless a patient had knowledge of the few games provided, asylum life was in effect characterised by monotony both in terms of amusements and work. Little had changed from the first Select Committee in 1854. Classification and improvements to life within the Asylum had only been marginally improved upon, with the majority of patients seeming to have spent their day in the airing court rather than the main building (S.A. Comm. 1884 Q. 3124). Dr. Paterson's evidence before the 1884 Commission was to also indicate the continuing relationship between Adelaide and Parkside Lunatic Asylum. While Adelaide was intended to be a curative asylum and Parkside the chronic asylum, there were still a large number of chronic patients' resident at Adelaide, and acute and chronic cases were still being mixed in the wards. Paterson desired an admitting ward separate from the acute ward at one of the asylums as this would facilitate better care (S.A. Comm. 1884 Q. 497–500). Interestingly there was no policy dictating the removal of chronic patients to Parkside, when room was required patients were moved. This would suggest that Parkside was considered as an annex of Adelaide rather than a chronic asylum with a particular role, such as that envisaged for the chronic asylum in England, of providing lower cost accommodation for the chronic or incurable patients. As in England many of the chronic cases were simply those suffering from senile decay rather than being purely insane, and imbeciles (S.A. Comm. 1884 Q. 814).

The treatment regime at the South Australian lunatic asylums then effectively mirrors changes in the treatment of lunatics that was occurring in England. Beginning with a custodial period, followed by a period of moral therapy with its possibilities there was then a shift to the belief in the organic and hereditary causes of insanity. Similarly there was a shift from restraint to non-restraint. In England these changes had been accompanied by a focus on the living environment of the insane, to providing initially a curative environment where the building is used to support the curative process through classification and rewards of better rooms and galleries. Here through authors, such as John Connolly, the idea of an 'ideal asylum' was developed, where the patient was occupied, kept comfortable with a reasonable standard of living, and the building design supported the effective supervision and management of the inmates.

From the establishment of the first Colonial Lunatic Asylum in 1846 to 1890 the treatment of the lunatics in the colony was to run the full gamut from restraint to non-restraint, from moral management to a curative regime that focussed on the lunatics' health.

Appendix 3
Treatment Regimes in Tasmania

Evidence about the treatment regimes practised at New Norfolk Hospital as with that for South Australia is piecemeal. The New Norfolk Hospital was established in 1830–1 when the non-restraint movement was beginning to gain momentum in England. Robert Gardiner Hill's book *Total Abolition of Personal Restraint in the Treatment of the Insane* was to be published in 1838.

The earliest remarks indicate that restraint was being used possibly in combination with moral discipline as a curative regime (Tas. C.S.O. Letters 21st Nov 1831 pg. 137–8). The Colonial Surgeon, J. Scott in 1832 offered the view that the removal of lunatics to the asylum should be as easy as possible: "the early placing of such patients under proper treatment with as little harassment as possible to both body and mind increases the chance of recovery." (Tas. C.S.O. Letters 7th Feb 1832 pg. 141–2). However the buildings even at this early stage were a problem, Dr. Officer, who was in charge of New Norfolk, in a letter to the Colonial Surgeon dated 27th June 1836 indicated the need for additional buildings, particularly as it was impossible to achieve any classification among the lunatics based on their malady or constitution of mind: "under such circumstances, the chance of recovery is greatly lessened and their domestic comforts (a most necessary part in their treatment), sadly diminished" (Tas. C.S.O. Letters 1/811/17340). Despite these remarks the general view of New Norfolk Hospital was of a place of imprisonment rather than cure, where imprisonment caused mental derangement, and of a convict establishment where visitors were not welcome as they might reveal what went on behind the walls (Editorial *Colonial Times and Tasmanian* of December 10th 1847).

On being appointed in 1855 the New Norfolk Commissioners found little evidence of a curative regime being practised, coercion and restraint were common. Moral management had included classification, the employment of inmates, amusements and exercise as part of the treatment regime. The Commissioners found that only the men required as labourers were ever taken outside of the high walls of the exercise yards. No amusements had been tried and religious ministrations, which soothed the mind, occurred only once a week (quoted in Gowlland 1981: 50). Yet despite the recognition of these failings, the Joint Committee of 1859 found little improvement. With respect to the men, the Committee found that there were no books, newspapers, music, pictures, sport or pleasurable occupations undertaken despite the fact that all these: "are universally dwelt on in England as forming an essential part of a curative system" (Tas. J.C. Report 1859: 5). The women probably were experiencing the same conditions. It seems likely that limited finances saw most of the available money being devoted to building repairs. Things were to improve possibly in response to the Joint Committee Report; the Commissioners were to indicate in their Annual Report for 1859 that amusements now included books, draughts, dominoes, and a magic lantern which the Commissioners wished to add to. Restraint was being used to a limited extant and all patients able to work were employed. The men were employed in gardening, wood cutting, carpentry, blacksmithing, painting and glazing, repairing shoes and clothes, and making new clothes. The women were employed in washing, needlework and domestic duties. The Commissioners noted there was no proper place for Divine Service and a chapel might be built in future (Tas. A. R. P.P. 1860).

The use of restraint up until 1860 appears to have been a direct consequence of the unsuitability of the buildings for their purpose, for in 1861, the New Commissioners were to indicate that physical changes to the Hospital had directly affected the patients, who were now improved in conduct and demeanour, and mechanical restraint had been abolished (Tas. A.R. P.P. 1861).

The New Norfolk Commissioners in their Annual Reports clearly state that they were directly responsible for the new treatment regime which over the last few years had enlarged freedom, created comfortable conditions and allowed all possible safe relaxations. This in turn had had a direct effect on the calmness and cheerfulness of the patients. The Commissioners indicated that the Superintendent and Medical Officer, Dr. Huston, had seconded every proposal for the amelioration of the Hospital that the Commissioners had made, as well as treating the patients with tact, discretion, and kindness (Tas. A.R. P.P. 1864). Whereas in Adelaide the Visitors were ineffective having little real power, the opposite was true in Tasmania where the management of New Norfolk was placed in the hands of the Board of Commissioners over the Medical Superintendent in the 1858 Act regulating the care and treatment of the insane (22 Victoria No. 23). In 1865 they indicated that they visited New Norfolk as a group once

Appendix 3 Treatment Regimes in Tasmania

a month and as individuals in-between ensuring their management was effective (Tas. A.R. P.P. 1865).

Reflecting an active interest in their work the Commissioners decided to purchase John Conolly's book on the treatment of the insane without mechanical restraint and the earlier work on the construction and management of the insane in 1864. Clearly the Commissioners were familiar with the literature available in England (Tas. N.N. Corresp. 15/4/1864).

In 1863 the Commissioners reviewed their progress. On taking office they found the Hospital was composed of several small buildings, badly constructed, ill ventilated, dark and dismal. The yards were small and surrounded by high walls. There was no classification and the temporarily insane were mixed with harden cases. Virtuous women were mixed with those of a notorious career. There had been no amusements as part of a curative treatment and no spaces for them. Religion was not used in a formal way, and patients were never taken beyond the walls. Restraint was the principle mode of treatment. Under the guidance of the Commissioners there were now airy and spacious apartments, verandas, open grounds, flower gardens and grass plots. There was a commodious cottage for the better class of gentlemen. Amusements had been introduced: dances, music nights, visiting entertainments were utilized, and summer walks and picnics held outside the walls reducing the feeling of captivity among the inmates and helping in their physical and mental recovery. Books, pictures, domesticated birds and other animals had been introduced for the patients to care for. Drafts and dominoes were readily available along with a bagatelle board for the paying patients. Regular Divine Service occurred. These beneficial changes in no way induced them:

> ... to relax no exertion to conform the Institution, as closely as circumstances and the means within enabled them to do, to the example of kindred institutions in Europe in which improvement has been carried farthest (Tas. A.R. P.P. 1865).

The day to day practice of the humanising system of treatment clearly indicated that harsh measures were unnecessary, and general quietude and contentment prevailed. Even in the refractory ward acts of violence were rare. The Medical Officer soothed and reasoned with the patient, with seclusion the last resort (Tas. A.R. P.P. 1865). Clearly the Hospital at New Norfolk was operating fairly closely to the curative regime advocated by authors such as John Conolly.

By the late 1860s the employment of the inmates was fulfilling the double role of curative agent and economic benefit. General repairs required around the Hospital were done by the men. The return of articles of clothing &c. made and repaired indicates that both men and women were employed in these tasks including making coats, trousers and footwear (Tas. A.R. P.P. 1870). The work activities for men at the New Norfolk Hospital were strikingly different from those at the South Australian Asylums where male employment was limited to a great extent to gardening and only a handful were employed in tailoring and boot work. While it would be easy to attribute this to some difference in the perceptions of class differences or backgrounds this cannot be proved from the available evidence. The South Australian males were seen as primarily manual workers but there is nothing that indicates that the Tasmanian men were significantly different. It is possible the Commissioners were more willing to undertake the training of the men in the necessary skills to work. On a percentage basis the women made the most new clothes and linen, while the men did most of the repairs to items.

In 1880 the Commissioners again indicated that the treatment regime was based on: "moral influence and persuasion on the part of the employees". While this may have been assumed previously there had only been references to the best of European treatments (Tas. A.R. P.P. 1881). On October 1st 1880 Dr. Huston retired as Superintendent of New Norfolk after 25 years in this position. The Assistant Medical Officer, Dr. Macfarlane assumed the role of Superintendent.

Reviewing life for the patients in 1883, the Commissioners indicated the activities available to the patients included dances, theatrical performances, concerts, cricket, lawn tennis, croquet, rounders, draughts, chess, cards and bagatelle, country walks, and drives; while part of the farm had been turned into a vegetable and fruit garden. The Commissioners, however, felt the need for a library (Tas. A.R. P.P. 1884). The patients were generally employed, this was seen as: "valuable adjuncts to both their physical and mental condition." (Tas. A.R. P.P. 1883).

Dr. Macfarlane was to describe the treatment regime practised to the Royal Commission of 1883. He indicated that he employed both moral and medicinal methods: "Moral treatment, including work, recreation, restraint and discipline. Medicinal treatment, embracing the use of sedatives, alternatives, narcotics, tonics and stimulants." Restraints were applied as needed and include camisoles, sleeves or canvas mittens, along with the use of seclusion in a room or yard. These were used to the minimum (Tas. R.C. 1883 Q. 31–2, 104). Dr. Coutie, the Assistant Medical Officer, was to define moral treatment as the diversion of the patient's thoughts from their morbid inclinations and into more healthy and normal channels, through work and amusements

(Tas. R.C. 1883 Q. 69). Prayers were read daily and religious services held (Tas. R.C. 1883 Q. 60). Classification, one of the principle tenets of moral treatment, was by no means complete. The women were not classified beyond the violent cases in the refractory division. (Tas. R.C. 1883 Q. 15). Dr. Coutie felt that the lack of classification was affecting the recovery of patients but the present buildings did not allow any opportunities to do things differently (Tas. R.C. 1883 Q. 93–4).

Dr. Huston, who had been Superintendent at New Norfolk, appears to indicate that he too had practiced moral therapy in the form of domestic discipline, employment and recreation, and seclusion with minor restraint (Tas. R.C. 1883 Q. 202, 219). There were few questions about the possible ill-treatment of the patients, though C. R. Smales, the Clerk for 27 years at New Norfolk had known the Medical Officer summarily dismiss attendants accused of mistreatment, and even take them to the Police Court if required (Tas. R.C. 1883 Q. 136).

In terms of work the men were employed in doing the foul linen, which was probably heavier than the normal clothes, and in helping the tradesmen/attendants who included a plumber, bricklayer, farmer and wood-yard man (Tas. R.C. 1883 Q. 8, 45). While Miss Laland indicates that there was a class based division of women's labour, with the penal class doing the washing. When these people no longer entered the Hospital there would be no one to do the washing. She thought the better class of women could use knitting machines to make hosiery (Tas. R.C. 1883 Q. 252). The labour of the patients was worth more than a £1,000 a year (Tas. R.C. 1883 Q. 46).

From the evidence above it appears that the treatment regime at New Norfolk was based consistently on moral management and minimal restraint from the mid to late 1850s when the Hospital was given over to the charge of the Colonial Government and the New Norfolk Commissioners were appointed. The biggest problem with applying this treatment regime lay in the problem of achieving classification due to the small number of buildings comprising the Hospital and their overall design. It appears from the evidence that the inmates were employed most of the time and that exercise was permitted, but restrained by the size of the grounds. Recreational activities certainly appeared to have been a part of inmate's lives from the Commissioners appointment in 1855.

Abbreviations

ENGLAND

Art. 111. - Article 111. 'Response to Several Committee Reports with Regard to Lunacy.' *Quarterly Review*. 1857 January and April. Vol. 101, No. 202, p353–393.

Art. 5 - Article V. 'Report of the Metropolitan Commissioners in Lunacy to the Lord Chancellor. *Quarterly Review,* Vol. LXXIV. June & October 1844, No. CXLVIII. p416–447.

11th Report Comm. in Lunacy - *Eleventh Report of the Commissioners in Lunacy to the Lord Chancellor*. July 1857. Including Appendix on Cold and Warm Baths in Asylums, Hospitals, and Licensed Houses.

16th Report. Comm. in Lunacy - *Sixteenth Report Of The Commissioners in Lunacy to the Lord Chancellor*. July 1862. Appendix E Copies Of Entries Made In The Visitor's Books of County & Borough Asylums by the Commissioners

SOUTH AUSTRALIA

S.A. A.R. - Annual Reports of the Medical Superintendent of the Adelaide and Parkside Lunatic Asylums published in the Government Gazette of South Australia

S.A. Comm. 1884 - *Report of the Commission appointed to report upon the Adelaide and Parkside Lunatic Asylums*. Parliamentary Papers of South Australia

S.A. C.S.O. Letters - South Australian Colonial Secretary's Letters

S.A. G.G. - Government Gazette of South Australia

S.A. P.D. - Debates of the South Australian Parliament

S.A. P.P. 1859 - *Report on Public Works (of the Province for the half year ended 31st Dec. 1858)*. Parliamentary Papers of South Australia. No. 31

S.A. P.P. 1885 - *Report on Certain Clauses of the Lunacy Commission Report*. Parliamentary Papers of South Australia. No. 60

S.A. S.C. 1856 - *Report of the Select Committee of the Legislative Council of South Australia appointed to inquire into the Treatment of Lunatics*. Parliamentary Papers of South Australia

S.A. S.C. 1864 - *Report on Lunatic Asylum by Commission appointed to inquire into and report on the Management etc,. of the Lunatic Asylum and Hospital*. Parliamentary Papers Of South Australia

S.A. S.C. 1869 - *Report of the Select Committee of the House of Assembly Appointed to Inquire into the Management of Lunatic Asylum [sic]*. Parliamentary Papers of South Australia

S.A. Visitors - Visitors Book to the Adelaide and Parkside Lunatic Asylums, South Australia

S.A. V.& P - Votes and Proceedings of the South Australian Parliament.

TASMANIA

Tas. A.R. P.P. - *Annual Reports of the Commissioners for the Hospital for the Insane at New Norfolk*. Papers of the Legislative Council of Tasmania

Tas. Comm. Min. Book - New Norfolk Commissioner's Minute Book

Tas. C.S.O. Letters - Colonial Secretary's Letters

Tas. J.C. Report 1859 - Report of the Joint Committee on the Accommodation of the Hospital for the Insane. Papers of the Legislative Council of Tasmania

Tas. N.N. Corresp. - New Norfolk Hospital Correspondence

Tas. Official Visitors Report P. P. 1886 - *Hospital for the Insane, New Norfolk: Interim Report of Official Visitors*. Papers of the Legislative Council of Tasmania

Abbreviations

Tas. P.P. 1859 - *Hospital for the Insane, New Norfolk Return to an order of the Council.* Bishop Willson Correspondence. Papers of the Legislative Council of Tasmania. No. 10

Tas. P.P. 1860 - *Correspondence Relative to the Site and Accommodation of the Hospital for the Insane, New Norfolk.* Papers of the Legislative Council of Tasmania. No. 12

Tas. R.C. Report 1883 - *Royal Commission on the State of the Lunatic Asylums in Tasmania. Report of the Commissioners 1883.* Papers of the Legislative Council of Tasmania

References

Allderidge, P.
    1985 Bedlam: fact or fantasy. In W. F. Bynum, R. Porter, & M. Shepherd (Eds.) *The Anatomy of Madness. Vol. 2 Institutions and Society* (pp. 17–33). London: Routledge.

Allen, J.
    1847 *South Australia As It Is & How To Get To It*. London, Public Library of South Australia facsimile editions, No 91. 1963.

Anderson, T. B. & R. G. Moore
    1988 Meaning and the Built Environment. A Symbolic Analysis of a 19th-Century Urban Site. In M. P. Leone, & P. B. Potter Jr. (Eds), *The Recovery of Meaning* (pp. 379–406). Washington: Smithsonian Institution Press.

Andrews, J., Briggs, A., Porter, Tucker, P. & Waddington, K.
    1997 *The History of Bethlem*. London: Routledge.

Andrews, J. & Digby, A. (Eds.)
    2004 *Sex and Seclusion, Class and Custody. Perspectives on Gender and Class in the History of British and Irish Psychiatry*. New York: Rodopi.

Annual Reports of the Medical Superintendent of the Adelaide and Parkside Lunatic Asylums. In *Government Gazette of South Australia*. (S.A. A.R.). Adelaide: Government Printer.

Anonymous
    1862 Description of a Proposed New Lunatic Asylum for 650 Patients on the Separate-Block System, for the County of Surrey. *The Journal of Mental Science* 7 (40), 600–608.

Arlidge, J. T.
    1858 On the Construction of Public Lunatic Asylums. *The Asylum Journal of Mental Science, IV, 24*, 185–204.

Arlidge, J. T.
    1859 *On the State of Lunacy and the Legal Provision for the Insane, with Observations on the Construction and Organization of Asylums*. London: John Churchill.

Armstrong, D. V.
    2001 Attaining the Full Potential of Historical Archaeology. *Historical Archaeology, 35, 2*, 9–13.

Article 111.
    1857 Response to Several Committee Reports with Regard to Lunacy. *Quarterly Review. 101, 202*, 353–393.

Article 5.
- 1844 Report of the Metropolitan Commissioners in Lunacy to the Lord Chancellor. *Quarterly Review, LXXIV, CXLVIII*, 416–447.

Bartlett, P.
- 1999 The asylum and the Poor Law: the productive alliance. In J. Melling & B. Forsythe (Eds.). *Insanity, Institutions and Society, 1800–1914*. (pp48–67). London: Routledge.

Baugher, S.
- 2001 Visible Charity: The Archaeology, Material Culture, and Landscape Design of New York City's Municipal Almshouse Complex, 1736–1797. *International Journal of Historical Archaeology*, 5, 2, 175–202.

Beaudry, M. C.
- 1996 Reinventing Historical Archaeology. In L. A. De Cunzo & B. L. Herman (Eds) *Historical Archaeology and the Study of American Culture* (pp. 473–497). Knoxville: Winterthur.

Bostock, J.
- 1968 *The Dawn of Australian Psychiatry*. Sydney: Australian Medical Association Mervyn Archudell Medical Monograph No. 4.

Brand, I.
- 1998 *Penal Peninsula. Tasmania's Port Arthur and its Outstations 1827–1898*. Launceston: Regal Press.

Bristol Lunatic Asylum competition.
- 1857 March 21 *The Builder*

Brockbank, E.
- 1934 *A Short History of the Cheadle Royal from its Foundation in 1766*. Manchester: Sherratt and Hughes.

Browne, W. A. F.
- 1837 *What Asylums were, are and ought to be*. Edinburgh.

Burdett, H. C.
- 1891–3 *Hospitals and Asylums of the World: Their Origin, History, Construction, Administration, Management, and Legislation*. London: J. & A. Churchill.

Burke, H.
- 1999 *Meaning and Ideology in Historical Archaeology. Style, Social Identity and Capitalism in an Australian Town*. New York: Kluwer Academic/Plenum Publishers.

Burrows, G. M.
- 1828 *Commentaries on the Causes, Forms, Symptoms and Treatment of Insanity*. London: Thomas and George Underwood. Arno Press Reprint 1976.

Bynum Jr., W. F.
- 1981 Rationales for Therapy in British Psychiatry, 1790–1835. In A. Scull (Ed.) *Madhouses, Mad-Doctors and Madmen* (pp35–57). Pennsylvania:University of Pennsylvania Press.

Casella, E.
- 1996 'One or two globular lamps made of glass': Archaeology and the cultural landscapes of Tasmanian convictism. In S. Ulm, I. Lilley & A Ross (Eds) *Australian Archaeology '95: Proceedings of the 1995 Australian Archaeological Association Conference*. (pp257–264). *Tempus* Vol. 6.

Casella, E. C.
- 2001 To Watch or Restrain: Female Convict Prisons in 19th-Century Tasmania. *International Journal of Historical Archaeology*, 5 (1), 45–72.

References

Cleland, C.
  2001   Historical Archaeology Adrift? *Historical Archaeology*, 35 (2), 1–8.

Clouston, T. S.
  1879   An Asylum, or Hospital-Home, for Two Hundred Patients: constructed on the principle of adaptation of various parts of the needs and mental states of inhabitants; with Plans, &c. *The Journal of Mental Science*, Oct, 368–388.

Colonial Secretary's Letters Received and Sent, GRG. 24/6 and 24/4 (S.A. C.S.O. Letters). Held State Archives of South Australia.

Colonial Secretary's Letters 1/83/1838. Held by the State Archives of Tasmania

Colonial Times and Tasmanian

Commissioners in Lunacy (Scotland)
  1859   Suggestions and Instructions in reference to (1.) - Sites; (2)- Construction and Arrangement of Buildings; (3)- Plans of Lunatic Asylum. *Journal of Mental Science*, V (30) July, 478–481.

Commissioners in Lunacy
  1857   *Eleventh Report of the Commissioners in Lunacy to the Lord Chancellor*.

Commissioners in Lunacy
  1862   *Sixteenth Report of the Commissioners in Lunacy to the Lord Chancellor*. Appendix E Copies of Entries Made in the Visitor's Books of County & Borough Asylums by the Commissioners.

Commissioners in Lunacy (England)
  1871   Suggestions and Instructions. *Journal of Mental Science*, LXXVL (76) Jan., 627–631.

Conolly, J.
  1847   *The Construction and Government of Lunatic Asylums and Hospitals for the Insane*. London: Dawsons of Pall Mall. Reprint 1968

Conolly, J.
  1856   *Treatment of the Insane Without Mechanical Restraints*. Folkstone: Dawsons of Pall Mall.

Cooter, R.
  1981   Phrenology and British Alienists, ca. 1825–1845. In A. Scull (ed.) *Madhouses, Mad-doctors and Madmen*. (pp 58–100). Philadelphia: University of Pennsylvania Press.

Crammer, J.
  1990   *Asylum History. Buckinghamshire County Pauper Lunatic Asylum-St. John's*. London: Gaskell.

Crowther, M. A.
  1981   *The Workhouse System 1834–1929*. London: Batsford

De Cunzo, L. A
  1995   Reform, Respite, Ritual: An Archaeology of Institutions; The Magdalen Society of Philadelphia, 1800–1850. *Historical Archaeology*, 29 (3). Single issue devoted to the one topic.

De Cunzo, L. A
  2001a On Reforming the "Fallen" and Beyond: Transforming Continuity at the Magdalen Society of Philadelphia, 1845–1916. *International Journal of Historical Archaeology*, 5 (1), 19–43.

De Cunzo, L. A.
  2001b Comments on Historical Archaeology Adrift/ a Forum. *Historical Archaeology*, 35 (2), 14–19.

De Cunzo, L. A.
  2006   Exploring the Institution: Reform, Confinement, Social Change. In M. Hall & S. W. Silliman (Eds.), *Historical Archaeology* (pp167–189). Malden: Blackwell Publishing.

Delle, J. A.
   1998   *An Archaeology of Social Space. Analyzing Coffee Plantations in Jamaica's Blue Mountains*. New York: Plenum Press.

Description of a Proposed New Lunatic Asylum for 650 Patients on the Separate-Block System, for the County of Surrey. (1862) *The Journal of Mental Science*, VII, (40), 600–608.

Digby, A.
   1985   *Madness, Morality and Medicine. A Study of the York Retreat 1796–1914*. Cambridge: Cambridge University Press.

Donelly, M.
   1983   *Managing the Mind*. London: Tavistock Publications.

Driver, F.
   1993   *Power and Pauperism. The Workhouse System 1834–1884*. Studies in Historical Geography. Cambridge: Cambridge University Press.

Editorial
   1844   Report of the Metropolitan Commissioners in Lunacy to the Lord Chancellor. *Quarterly Review*, LXXIV, CXLVIII, 416–447.

Editorial
   1857   Response to Several Committee Reports with Regard to Lunacy. *Quarterly Review*, 101, 202, 353–393.

Editorial Lunatic Asylums.
   1866   June 3rd *The Builder*

Feister, L. M.
   1991   The Orphanage at Schuyler Mansion. *Northeast Historical Archaeology*, 20, 27–36

Finnegan, F
   2001   *Do Penance or Perish. A Study of Magadelan Asylums in Ireland*. Kilkenny: Congrave Press.

Forsythe, B., Melling, J. & Adair, R.
   1999   Politics of lunacy: central state regulation and the Devon Pauper Lunatic Asylum, 1845–1914. In J. Melling, & B. Forsythe (Eds.), *Insanity, Institutions and Society, 1800–1914* (pp. 68–92). London: Routledge.

Foucault, M.
   1979   *Discipline and Punish: The Birth of the Prison*. Trans. Alan Sheridan, New York: Vintage.

Garton, S.
   1991   Palaces for the Unfortunate: Lunatic Asylums in New South Wales 1880–1940. *Journal of the Royal Historical Society*, 76 (4), 297–312.

Geller, J. L. & Harris, M.
   1994   *Women of the Asylum. Voices from Behind the Walls, 1840–1945*. New York: Anchor Books, Doubleday.

Gowlland, R. W.
   1981   *Troubled Asylum*. Tasmania: Society for the Study of Intellectual Disability.

Government Gazette of South Australia (S.A. G.G.)
   1834 onwards   Adelaide: Government Printer.

Greene, R.
   1880   A Public Asylum, Designed for 414 Beds, capable of Extension to 600. *The Journal of Mental Science*, XXVI (*114*): July: 233–244.

Greenwood, R. S.
   2001   Historical Archaeology Adrift?: Comments from CRM/West' *Historical Archaeology*, 35 (2): 25–27.

References

Halliday, A.
  1828 *A General View of the Present State of Lunatics and Lunatic Asylums*. London.
Hardesty, D. L.
  2001 Comments on "Historical Archaeology Adrift." *Historical Archaeology. 35* (2): 23–24.
Harrison, B.
  1966 Philanthropy and the Victorians. *Victorian Studies, 9* (4): 353–74.
Hervey, N.
  1985 A Slavish Bowing Down: the Lunacy Commission and the Psychiatric Profession 1845–1860. In W. F. Bynum, R. Porter & M. Shepherd (Eds), *The Anatomy of Madness Vol. 2 Institutions and Society* (pp. 98–131). London: Routledge.
Hill, B.
  1994 *Women, Work & Sexual Politics in Eighteenth-Century England*. Montreal: McGill-Queen's University Press.
Hill, R. G.
  1838 *Total Abolition of Personal Restraint in the Treatment of the Insane*. London.
Hilliard, D. & Hunt, A. D.
  1986 Religion. In E. Richards (Ed.) *The Flinders History of South Australia. Social History*. (pp. 194–234). Netley: Wakefield Press.
Hine, G. T.
  1901 Asylums and Asylum Planning. *Journal of the Royal Institute of British Architects, VIII*, 3rd series, (8): 161–180.
Hunter, R. & MacAlpine, I.
  1974 *Psychiatry for the Poor. 1851 Colney Hatch Asylum - Friern Hospital 1973*. Folkstone: Dawsons of Pall Mall.
Isaac, R.
  1992 Imagination and Material Culture: The Enlightenment on a Mid-18th-Century Virginia Plantation. In A. E. Yentschen & M. C. Beaudry (Eds.) *The Art and Mystery of Historical Archaeology* (pp. 401–423). Boca Raton: CRC Press.
Jackman, M. R.
  1994 *The Velvet Glove: Paternalism and conflict in gender, class, and race relations*. Berkeley: University of California Press.
Jacobi, M.
  1841 *On the Construction and Management of Hospitals for the Insane*. Translated by John Kitching. London: John Churchill.
Jensen, E. & Jensen, R.
  1980 *Colonial Architecture in South Australia*. Adelaide: Rigby.
Jones, K.
  1993 *Asylums and After*. London: The Athlone Press.
Kay, H. T.
  1970 *1870–1970 Commemorating the Centenary of Glenside Hospital*. Adelaide: Griffin Press.
Kent, S.
  1984 *Analysing Activity Areas. An Ethnoarchaeological Study of the Use of Space*. Albuquerque: University of New Mexico Press.
Kerr, J. S.
  1984 *Designs for Convicts*. Sydney: Library of Australian History.
King, A.
  1966 Hospital Planning: Revised Thoughts on the Origin of the Pavilion Principle in England. *Medical History, 10*: 360–73.

Knott, J.
  1986 *Popular Opposition to the 1834 Poor Law*. London: Croom Helm.
Leone, M.
  1984 Interpreting ideology in historical archaeology: using the rules of perspective in the William Paca Garden in Annapolis, Maryland. In D. Miller & C. Tilley (Eds.) *Ideology, Power and Prehistory* (pp25–35). Cambridge: Cambridge University Press.
Leone, M & Crosby, C. A.
  1987 Epilogue: Middle-range Theory in Historical Archaeology. In S. Spencer-Wood (Ed.) *Consumer Choice in Historical Archaeology* (pp. 397–410) New York: Plenum.
Leone, M. & Potter, Jr., Parker
  1988 Introduction. Issues in Historical Archaeology. In M. P. Leone and P. Potter, Jr (Eds.) *The Recovery of Meaning* (pp. 1–22). Washington: Smithsonian Institution Press.
Lucas, G.
  1999 The archaeology of the workhouse; the changing uses of the workhouse buildings at St. Mary's, Southampton. In S. Tarlow and S. West (Eds.) *The Familiar Past? Archaeologies of later historical Britain* (pp. 125–139). London: Routledge.
Lunatic Asylums and Treatment of the Insane.
  1859 Nov 5 *The Builder*, p722.
MacKenzie, C.
  1988 Social Factors in the Admission, Discharge, and Continuing Stay of Patients at Ticehurst Asylum, 1845–1917 (pp146–174). In W. F. Bynum, R. Porter & M. Shepherd *The Anatomy of Madness. Vol. 2 Institutions and Society*. London: Routledge.
Main, J. M.
  1986 Men of Capital. In E. Richards (Ed.) *The Flinders History of South Australia. Social History* (pp.105–113). Netley: Wakefield Press.
Manning, F. N.
  1868–9 *Report on Lunatic Asylums*. Parliamentary Papers of New South Wales, Legislative Assembly Vol. 3.
Markus, T. A.
  1993 *Buildings and Power: Freedom and Control in the Origin of Model Building Types*. London: Routledge.
Marland, H.
  1999 'Destined to a perfect recovery': the confinement of puerperal insanity in the nineteenth century. In J. Melling & B. Forsythe (Eds.), *Insanity, Institutions and Society, 1800–1914*. (pp137–156). London: Routledge.
Nance, C.
  1982 Making a Better Society? Immigration to South Australia 1836–1871. In R. Nicol & B. Samuels (Eds.), Insights into South Australian History (pp28–36). Volume 1. Adelaide: Historical Society of South Australia.
Norfolk Hospital Correspondence Book HSD 45/1. Held by the State Archives of Tasmania
Norval M. & Rothman, D.
  1998 *The Oxford History of Prisons*. New York: Oxford University Press.
Observations on the Structure of Hospitals for the Treatment of Lunatics.
  1809 Edinburgh. No author given or Publisher given.
Palmer, E.
  1859 Description of the Lincolnshire County Asylum. *The Asylum Journal of Mental Science, 1* (5), 72–75
Parry-Jones, W. L.
  1972 *The Trade in Lunacy*. London: Routledge & Kegan Paul.
Pearson, M. P. & Richards, C.
  1994 Architecture and Order: Spatial Representation and Archaeology. In M. P. Pearson & C. Richard (Eds.), *Architecture and Order. Approaches to Social Space* (pp.38–72). London: Routledge.

References

Perkin, J.
1995 *Victorian Women.* New York: New York University.

Philo, C.
1989 "Enough to drive one mad": the organization of space in 19th-century lunatic asylums. In J. Wolch & M. Deer (Eds.), *The Power of Geography: How Territory Shapes Social Life* (pp258–290). Boston: Unwin Hyman.

Piddock, S.
1996 *Accommodating the Destitute. An Historical and Archaeological Consideration of the Destitute Asylum of Adelaide.* Unpublished Master of Arts Thesis submitted to Flinders University of South Australia.

Piddock, S.
1999 *A Space Of Their Own: Institutions and Gendered Space.* Unpublished Paper presented at the 5th Women in Archaeology Conference, Sydney.

Piddock, S.
2001 "An Irregular and Inconvenient Pile of Buildings": The Destitute Asylum of Adelaide, South Australia and the English Workhouse. *International Journal of Historical Archaeology, 5, 1,* 73–95.

Piddock, S.
2003 *A Space of Their Own: Nineteenth Century Lunatic Asylums in England, South Australia and Tasmania.* . Unpublished Doctoral Thesis submitted to Flinders University of South Australia.

Pike, D.
1967 *Paradise of Dissent. South Australia 1829–1857* (2nd ed.). London: Melbourne University Press.

Pinel, P. H.
1806 *A Treatise on Insanity.* Translated by D. Davis, M.D., New York: Hafner Publishing Company. Reprint 1962.

Porter, R.
1981–2 Was there a moral therapy in the eighteenth century? *Lychos,* 12–26.

Porter, R.
1987 *Mind Forg'd Manacles.* London: The Athlone Press.

Prangnell, J. M.
1999 *'Intended solely for their greater comfort and happiness': Historical archaeology, paternalism and the Peel Island Lazaret.* (Doctoral Thesis, University of Queensland, 1999).

Quartly, M.
1966 South Australian Lunatics and Their Custodians, 1836 – 1846. *Australian Journal of Social Issues. 2,* 13–31.

Reports of Lunatic Asylums published during
1857 & 1858 *The Journal of Mental Science.* (Jan 1859). No. 28, Vol. V, 157–200.

Reynolds, H.
1969 'That Hated Stain': The Aftermath of Transportation in Tasmania.' *Historical Studies, 14,* (53), 19–31

Ripa, Y.
1990 *Women and Madness.* Cambridge: Polity Press.

Robertson, C. L.
1860 A Descriptive Notice of the Sussex Lunatic Asylum, Hayward's Heath. *The Journal of Mental Science, VI,* (33), 247–283.

Robertson, C. L.
1863 On the want of a Middle Class Asylum in Sussex, with Suggestions how it may be established. *The Journal of Mental Science, VIII, 44,* 465–482.

Robertson, C. L.
1867 Pavilion Asylums. *The Journal of Mental Science, XII, 60,* 467–475.

Rosenau, H.
  1970 *Social Purpose in Architecture: Paris and London Compared, 1760–1800.* London: Studio Vista.
Russell, R.
  1988 The lunacy profession and its staff in the second half of the nineteenth century, with special reference to the West Riding Lunatic Asylum. In W. F. Bynum, R. Porter, & M. Shepherd *The Anatomy of Madness. Vol. 3 The Asylum and its Psychiatry* (pp. 273–315). London: Routledge.
Salt, A.
  1984 *These Outcast Women. The Parramatta Female Factory 1821–1848.* Sydney: Hale & Iremonger.
Sankey, W. H. O.
  1856 Do the Public Asylums of England, as present constructed, afford the greatest facilities for the care and treatment of the Insane? *The Asylum Journal of Mental Science, II,* 466–479.
Saunders, J.
  1988 Quarantining the Weak-minded: psychiatric definitions of degeneracy and the late-Victorian asylum. In W. F. Bynum, R. Porter & M. Shepard (Eds.), *The Anatomy of Madness. Vol. 3 The Asylum and its Psychiatry* (pp. 273–296). London: Routledge.
Schuyler, R.
  1988 Archaeological Remains, Documents, and Anthropology: a Call for a New Culture History. *Historical Archaeology, 22,* (1), 36–42.
Scott, E.
  1991 A Feminist Approach to Historical Archaeology: Eighteenth-Century Fur Trade at Michilimackinac. *Historical Archaeology, 25,* (4), 42–53
Scott, E. (Ed.)
  1994 *Those of Little Note: Gender, Race and Class in Historical Archaeology.* Tucson: University of Arizona Press.
Scull, A.
  1979 *Museums of Madness. The Social Organization of Insanity in Nineteenth-Century England.* London: Allan Lane, Penguin Books.
Scull, A.
  1981 Moral Treatment Reconsidered: Some Sociological Comments on an Episode in the History of British Psychiatry. In A. Scull (Ed.) *Madhouses, Mad-doctors and Madmen.* (pp. 105–118). Philadelphia: University of Pennsylvania Press.
Scull, A.
  1993 Museums of Madness Revisited. *Social History of Medicine,* 6 (1), 3–23.
Scull, A., MacKenzie C. & Hervey, N.
  1996 *Masters of Bedlam. The Transformation of the Mad-Doctoring Trade.* New Jersey: Princeton University Press.
Shlomowitz, E. A.
  1990 *The Treatment of Mental Illness in South Australia, 1852–1884. From Care to Custody* (Doctoral Thesis, Flinders University of South Australia 1990).
Showalter, E.
  1981 Victorian Women and Insanity. In A. Scull (ed.) *Madhouses, Mad-doctors and Madmen* (pp. 313–336). Philadelphia: University of Pennsylvania Press.
Skultans, V.
  1975 *Madness and Morals. Ideas on Insanity in the Nineteenth Century.* London: Routledge & Kegan Paul.

References 253

Skultans, V.
    1979 *English Madness. Ideas on Insanity 1580–1880*. London: Routledge & Kegan Paul.
Stark, W.
    1807 *Remarks on the Construction of Public Hospitals for the Cure of Mental Derangement*. Edinburgh.
South Australian Parliament. *Debates of the South Australian Parliament*. Adelaide: Government Printer.
South Australia Parliament
    1856 Report of the Select Committee of the Legislative Council of South Australia appointed to inquire into the Treatment of Lunatics. *Parliamentary Papers of South Australia*, No. 119. Adelaide: Government Printer.
South Australia Parliament
    1857–8 Report on Public Works (of the Province to June 30th 1857. *Parliamentary Papers of South Australia*, No. 102. Adelaide: Government Printer.
South Australia Parliament
    1864 Report on Lunatic Asylum by Commission appointed to inquire into and report on the Management etc. of the Lunatic Asylum and Hospital. *Parliamentary Papers of South Australia* No. 30. Adelaide: Government Printer.
South Australia Parliament
    1865 Cost of Erecting Certain Buildings. *Parliamentary Papers of South Australia*, No. 130. Adelaide: Government Printer.
South Australia Parliament
    1869–70 Report of the Select Committee of the House of Assembly Appointed to Inquire into the Management of Lunatic Asylum [sic]. *Parliamentary Papers of South Australia*, 2 (68). Adelaide: Government Printer.
South Australia Parliament
    1884 Report of the Commission appointed to report upon the Adelaide and Parkside Lunatic Asylums. *Parliamentary Papers of South Australia*, No. 136. Adelaide: Government Printer.
South Australia Parliament
    1885 Report on Certain Clauses of the Lunacy Commission Report. *Parliamentary Papers of South Australia*, No. 60. Adelaide: Government Printer.
South Australia Parliament
    1834+ *Votes and Proceedings of the South Australian Parliament*. Adelaide: Government Printer.
Southwood, W. T.
    1973 Bishop R. W. Willson's Work for the Insane in Tasmania. *Tasmanian Historical Research Association Papers and Proceedings*, 140–153.
Spencer-Wood, S. M.
    1994 Diversity in 19th Century Domestic Reform: Relationships Among Classes and Ethnic Groups. In E. Scott (Ed.) *Those of Little Note: Gender, Race, and Class in Historical Archaeology* (pp.175–208). Tuscon: University of Arizona Press.
Spencer-Wood, S. M.
    2001 Introduction and Historical Context to the Archaeology of Seventeenth and Eighteenth Century Almshouses. *International Journal of Historical Archaeology*, 5 (2), 115–122.
Spencer-Wood, S. M. & Baugher, S.
    2001 Introduction and Historical Context for the Archaeology of Institutions of Reform. Part 1: Asylums. *International Journal of Historical Archaeology*, 5 (2), 3–17
Stark, W.
    1807 *Remarks on the Construction of Public Hospitals for the Cure of Mental Derangement*. Edinburgh.

THE BUILDER

Editorial Lunatic Asylums,
 July 25th 1846, pp349–355
Asylums under erection,
 25 Sept 1847, p388
Editorial arrangement of lunatic asylums,
 Dec 11th 1847, pp 585–586
Plan of the Asylum for the counties of Monmouth, Hereford, Breneck, Radnor, Vol. 10, No. 483 1852, p297–299
Plan of the Eglinton Lunatic Asylum,
 Nov 27th 1852, pp754–755
Sussex County Lunatic Asylum competition,
 February 2nd 1856
Asserted failure of the Colney Hatch County Lunatic Asylum,
 Dec. 6th 1856, p660
New Hospital at Adelaide, South Australia,
 Feb. 7th 1857
Bristol Lunatic Asylum competition,
 March 21st 1857
Plan and illustration of Essex Asylum,
 May 16th 1857, pp.273–275
Dorset Lunatic Asylum,
 July 11th 1857
Letter - condition of Colney Hatch Lunatic Asylum,
 25th July 1857
Lunatic Asylums and Treatment of the Insane including an illustration and plan of Cumberland and Westmoreland Asylum,
 May 1st 1858, pp293–295
Lunatic Asylums and Treatment of the Insane,
 May 29th 1858, p371–372
Lunatic Asylums and Treatment of the Insane,
 Sept 4th 1858, pp. 597–599
Lunatic Asylums and Treatment of the Insane,
 Nov 5th 1859, pp721–723
Lunatic Asylums in Scotland,
 Jan 7th 1860, pp3–5
Editorial on the construction and arrangement of lunatic asylums
 May 4th 1861, p299
Plan and illustration of Carmarthen Lunatic Asylum,
 Aug 22rd 1863, pp602–605
Editorial Lunatic Asylums,
 June 23rd 1866, pp 457–458
Berkshire, Reading, and Newbury Lunatic Asylum,
 April 2nd 1870, pp264–265
Editorial concerning lunatic asylums
 June 25th 1870, pp499–500
Opening of Macclesfield New County Asylum,
 June 3rd 1871, p424
The enlarging of Worcester Lunatic Asylum,
 July 8th 1871, p532

References

The South Australian Register. Microfilm held by the State Library of South Australia.
Tasmanian Parliament
    1858   22 Victoria No 23 An Act for the Regulation of the Care and Treatment of the Insane, and for the Appointment, Maintenance, Regulation of Hospitals for the Insane. *Parliamentary Papers of the Legislative Council of Tasmania*. Hobart: Government Printer.
Tasmanian Parliament. *Parliamentary Papers of the Legislative Council of Tasmania*. Hobart: Government Printer.
Tasmanian Parliament
    1856   onwards Annual Reports of the Commissioners for the Hospital for the Insane at New Norfolk. *Parliamentary Papers of the Legislative Council*. Hobart: Government Printer.
Tasmanian Parliament
    1859   Hospital for the Insane, New Norfolk. Return to an order of the Council. *Parliamentary Papers of the Legislative Council* (Bishop Willson Correspondence), No. 10. Hobart: Government Printer.
Tasmanian Parliament
    1859   Report of the Joint Committee on the Accommodation of the Hospital for the Insane. *Parliamentary Papers of the Legislative Council*, No. 91. Hobart: Government Printer.
Tasmanian Parliament
    1860   Correspondence Relative to the Site and Accommodation of the Hospital for the Insane, New Norfolk. *Parliamentary Papers of the Legislative Council*, No. 12. Hobart: Government Printer.
Tasmanian Parliament
    1883   Royal Commission on the State of the Lunatic Asylums in Tasmania. Report of the Commissioners 1883. *Parliamentary Papers of Legislative Council*. Hobart: Government Printer.
Tasmanian Parliament
    1886   Hospital for the Insane, New Norfolk: Interim Report of Official Visitors. *Parliamentary Papers of Legislative Council*, No. 48. Hobart: Government Printer.
Taylor, J.
    1991   *Hospital and Asylum Architecture in England 1840–1914. Building For Health Care*. London: Mansfield Publishing Ltd..
The Hobart Town Courier.
Toller, E.
    1865   Suggestions for a Cottage Asylum. *The Journal of Mental Science*, X (51), 342–349.
Townsley, W. A.
    1991   *Tasmania From Colony to Statehood 1830–1945*. Hobart: St. David's Park Publishing.
Tuke, S.
    1813   *Description of The Retreat*. London: Reprint by Dawsons Of Pall Mall 1964.
    Visitors Book to the Adelaide and Parkside Lunatic Asylums, Vols. 1 and 2. State Archives of South Australia GRG 34/97. Unpublished Books
Walton, J. K.
    1981   The Treatment of Pauper Lunatics in Victorian England: The Case of Lancashire Lunatic Asylum 1816–1870. In A. Scull (Ed.) *Madhouses, Mad Doctors and Madmen* (pp. 166–197). Pennsylvania: University of Pennsylvania Press.
Walton, J. K.
    1985   Casting Out and Bringing Back in Victorian England: Pauper Lunatics, 1840–70. In W. F. Bynum, R. Porter, & M. Shepherd (Eds.), *The Anatomy of Madness. Vol. 2 Institutions and Society* (pp. 132–146). London: Routledge.

Waselkov, G. A.
   2001   Historical Archaeology, with Sails Set and Tacking into the Wind. *Historical Archaeology*, *35*, (2), 20–22.

Welter, B.
   1966   The Cult of True Womanhood 1820–1860. *American Quarterly*, *18*, (2, Part 1), 151–174.

West, S.
   1999   Social Space and the English county house. In S. Tarlow & S. West. (Eds.) *The Familiar Past? Archaeologies of later historical Britain* (pp.103–122). London: Routledge.

Wood, M. E.
   1987   *The writing on the wall: Autobiographies in American mental institutions, 1868–1890*. (Doctoral dissertation, Stanford University, 1987). *U.M.I Dissertation Services*.

Index

A

Abergavenny Asylum, 82, 84, 85, 87, 88, 89, 98, 185

Activities, 10, 16, 17, 39, 40, 42, 43, 51, 52, 54, 55, 57, 58, 62, 64, 65, 66, 68, 74, 78, 80, 91, 98, 100, 101, 102, 104, 106, 130, 136, 141, 142, 145, 146, 147, 154, 157, 171, 174, 176, 178, 179, 180, 181, 182, 184, 190, 191, 193, 198, 200, 201, 210, 213, 219, 220, 221, 222, 228, 229, 230, 235, 236, 237, 238

Acute patients, 72, 73, 76, 123, 128, 135, 139, 140, 193, 232

Adelaide Gaol, 108, 111, 112, 113, 123, 146, 195, 196, 228

Adelaide Lunatic Asylum, 19, 34, 108, 109, 110, 111, 112, 113, 115, 120, 123, 125, 126, 128, 129, 130, 131, 132, 133, 135, 138, 139, 140, 141, 142, 143, 144, 145, 146, 147, 163, 184, 185, 187, 188, 189, 190, 191, 194, 195, 196, 197, 198, 199, 200, 201, 202, 214, 216, 217, 218, 220, 221, 222, 223, 227, 228, 229, 230, 231, 232, 233, 236, 239

Administrative Blocks/Offices, 70, 72, 74, 88, 102, 105, 117, 123, 125, 128, 136, 138, 140, 161, 222

Airing courts, 42, 51, 53, 55, 56, 61, 62, 63, 64, 66, 68, 69, 72, 75, 79, 80, 84, 91, 92, 94, 95, 100, 101, 102, 103, 104, 113, 120, 121, 123, 125, 126, 129, 133, 136, 138, 139, 140, 142, 144, 145, 156, 161, 174, 177, 188, 191, 192, 193, 195, 219, 221, 222, 232

Alcohol (and insanity), 199, 200

Allderidge, P., 44

Allen, J., 107

Almshouses, 7, 9, 10, 216

Amusements *see* Activities

Anderson, T. B., 18

Andrews, J., 23

Annual Reports (South Australia), 34, 123, 130, 143, 145, 200

Annual Reports (New Norfolk), 35, 158, 160, 163, 164, 169, 174, 176, 177, 178, 179, 180, 203, 204, 205, 206, 207, 208, 210, 236, 237, 238

Arlidge, J. T., 30, 46, 64, 67, 68, 69, 71, 75, 77, 79, 92, 95, 96, 97, 101, 102, 136, 183, 190, 193, 209, 217, 221, 222

Armstrong, D. V., 26

Article III, 103, 104, 198

Article VI, 46, 51, 198

Attendants, 41, 54, 55, 56, 60, 61, 65, 66, 68, 73, 74, 80, 82, 86, 102, 104, 106, 112, 113, 138, 143, 145, 179, 181, 184, 193, 219

 rooms for, 61, 62, 63, 64, 71, 72, 82, 83, 86, 88, 91, 92, 93, 96, 113, 117, 120, 128, 129, 131, 135, 143, 157, 160, 166, 171, 173, 177, 181, 187, 189, 204

B

Bartlett, P., 23

Baths, 52, 56, 57, 58, 61, 62, 63, 69, 70, 71, 72, 80, 81, 82, 83, 86, 92, 96, 109, 113, 129, 130, 132, 143, 146, 157, 160, 164, 166, 171, 173, 174, 177, 184, 187, 190, 191, 201, 214, 228

Bathhouse, 166, 171, 178, 203, 204

Baugher, S., 9, 10, 17, 216

Beaudry, M. C., 22, 24, 28

Bedford, E. S. P., 156, 164, 205

Bedford, Hertford and Huntingdon (Three Counties) Lunatic Asylum, 45, 82, 84, 86-87, 88, 89, 92, 95, 96, 101, 185

Bedrooms, *see* sleeping rooms

Bethlem Hospital, 20, 44, 71, 77, 78, 79, 80, 81, 96, 97, 135

Bevan, James, 78

257

Billiards room, 65, 69, 117, 141, 145, 190, 221
Bishop Willson, *see* Willson, Bishop
Bland, Miss. 209
Block asylums/system *see* Pavilion asylums
Board of Commissioners (Tasmania), 154, 155, 156, 163, 236, 237
Bodmin Asylum, 45
Bostock, J., 33
Botanic Gardens, 112, 145,
Brand, I., 160
Brandon, D., 92
Britain, 1, 3, 4, 5, 6, 16, 20, 22, 23, 25, 31, 32, 33, 46, 57, 67, 76, 77, 91, 98, 99, 104, 106, 107, 117, 129, 130, 133, 135, 136, 140, 141, 143, 146, 149, 150, 155, 156, 157, 160, 179, 182, 183, 184, 187, 188, 189, 191, 193, 194, 195, 196, 197, 198, 199, 204, 212, 213, 214, 216, 217, 218, 219, 220, 221, 227, 228, 230, 231, 232, 233, 236, 237
Bristol Lunatic Asylum, 82, 84, 86, 89, 92, 185
Brockbank, E
Browne, W. A. F., 1, 17, 22, 29, 41, 42, 44, 52, 55, 56, 57, 58, 59, 60, 63, 64, 67, 78, 80, 132, 133, 174, 183, 191, 207, 216
Buckinghamshire Lunatic Asylum, 82, 84, 85, 86, 87, 89, 92, 94, 98, 100, 185
Buildings as artifacts, 24, 215
Built environment, 8, 14, 17, 18, 20, 22, 55, 60, 101, 108, 139, 157, 215, 217
Burdett, H. C., 30, 75
Burke, H., 17, 18
Burrows, G. M., 43, 104
Bynum Jr., W. F., 23,

C

Cambridgeshire Asylum, 82, 84, 85, 86, 87, 89, 91, 94, 99, 100, 101, 106, 185, 191
Carmarthen County Asylum, 82, 88, 89, 92
Cascades Asylum, 34, 150, 160, 161, 165, 166, 167, 203, 209
Casella, E., 12, 13, 17, 50, 218

Causes of insanity *see* Insanity
Cells *see also* sleeping cells, 13, 15, 20, 23, 56
Ceramics, 9, 10, 14
Chapel(s), 12, 59, 61, 63, 64, 66, 71, 72, 74, 80, 82, 83, 87, 92, 93, 95, 98, 99, 101, 130, 131, 133, 135, 136, 140, 141, 152, 155, 172, 184, 187, 188, 192, 193, 201, 210, 219, 229, 236
Cheshire Asylum, 46, 82, 83, 87, 88, 89, 93, 185
Chronic asylums, 73, 232
Chronic patients, 60, 71, 72, 73, 76, 96, 123, 128, 140, 232
Class *see* Social class
Classification, 16, 17, 40, 50, 52, 54, 59, 66, 68, 69, 72, 74, 75, 78, 79, 84, 85, 94, 128, 133, 136, 138, 139, 140, 150, 156, 157, 169, 170-171, 182, 187, 189, 190, 192, 200, 214, 219, 220, 223, 228, 229, 232, 239
   of patients, 34, 41, 42, 51, 55, 56, 57, 58, 61, 68-69, 76, 81, 101, 129, 154, 156, 160, 161, 166, 176, 177, 202, 210, 235, 237
   and the provision of rooms, 54, 72, 74, 112
Cleland, C., 24, 25, 26, 27, 108, 183, 215
Clouston, T. S., 30, 75, 104
Colney Hatch Asylum, 100, 103, 104
Colonial Architect (South Australia), 34, 112, 115, 133, 164, 195, 198
Colonial Secretary's Letters (South Australia), 34, 108, 109, 111, 112, 126, 130, 133, 146, 195, 196, 198, 199
Colonial Secretary's Letters (Tasmania), 35, 150, 164, 176, 210, 235
Colonial Surgeon (South Australia), 108, 194, 196, 197, 199, 200, 227, 228, 230
Colonial Surgeon (Tasmania), 235
Commissioners in Lunacy (England), 46, 70, 95, 96, 98, 99, 100, 101, 102, 106, 192, 193, 194, 197
Commissioners in Lunacy (Scotland), 102
Conolly, John, 20, 31, 37, 42, 43, 49, 57, 59, 60, 61, 62, 63, 64, 65, 67, 69, 71, 72, 73, 76, 77, 79, 81, 83, 84, 86, 87, 88, 89, 90, 91, 92, 93, 94, 95, 97,

98, 99, 100, 101, 102, 103, 104, 105, 106, 126, 128, 129, 130, 132, 133, 141, 142, 143, 147, 149, 156, 167, 169, 172, 173, 174, 175, 182, 183, 184, 187, 189, 190, 191, 192, 193, 194, 196, 197, 202, 204, 207, 208, 214, 216, 217, 218, 219, 220, 221, 228, 233, 237
Convalescent patients, 51, 54, 56, 59, 61, 84, 104, 128, 135, 139, 140, 228, 229
Convicts, 12, 21, 33, 107, 108, 149, 150, 154, 156, 167, 171, 176, 178, 189, 198, 203, 204, 205, 206, 207, 209, 210, 211, 212, 213
Convict Establishment, 235
Cooter, R., 23
Cottage asylums, 73, 74
Cottages, 73, 74, 75, 76, 96, 123, 136, 160, 161, 175, 178, 192, 196, 204, 209
  Ladies', 160, 163, 164, 171, 178, 180, 203, 205, 207, 211
  Gentlemen's, 155, 160, 163, 164, 171, 178, 180, 205, 211
County and City Lunatic Asylum at Worcester, 91
County Asylum at Macclesfield, 91
County asylums, 20, 23, 30, 43, 45, 46, 47, 49, 54, 60, 61, 62, 64, 69, 70, 71, 72, 73, 75, 78, 83, 92, 93, 94, 95, 97, 98, 99, 101, 105, 136, 184, 187, 191, 192, 193, 199, 217, 220
Coutie, Dr., 180, 209, 238, 239
Coverdale, Dr. John, 209
Crammer, J., 84
Criminal lunatics, 123, 165, 166, 167
Criminal ward, 123, 125, 196
Crowther, M. A., 7
Cumberland and Westmoreland Asylum, 82, 84, 86, 89, 157, 185, 208
Curative asylum/institution, 2, 16, 17, 28, 37, 43, 46, 47, 49, 53, 54, 57, 73, 76, 101, 105, 155, 156, 157, 160, 220, 228, 232
Curative environment, 57, 59, 75, 78, 105, 133, 161, 233
Curative regime, 2, 65, 73, 75, 106, 169, 179, 201, 205, 210, 211, 213, 231, 233, 235, 236, 237

D

Dances, 136, 141, 179, 190, 220, 237, 238
Day rooms/spaces, 50, 51, 53, 54, 61, 62, 63, 64, 65, 66, 67, 68, 69, 71, 72, 74, 79, 80, 81, 82, 85, 86, 87, 91, 92, 93, 94, 95, 96, 97, 99, 102, 105, 106, 109,111, 113, 117, 119, 120, 123, 126, 129, 130, 131, 132, 136, 138, 140, 142, 143, 144, 145, 146, 157, 160, 163, 166, 169, 171, 172, 173, 174, 176, 177, 179, 180, 181, 187, 188, 189, 190, 191, 192, 193, 195, 204, 210, 217, 219, 221, 222, 229
De Cunzo, L. A., 7, 8, 13, 14, 15, 16, 17, 18, 26, 50, 220
Delle, J. A.
Derby County Asylum, 63, 71, 81, 82, 83, 84, 87, 89, 97, 130, 185, 191
Descriptive framework/grids, 27, 28, 29, 31, 32, 49, 106, 184, 216, 217, 218, 219
Destitute Asylum, 16, 18, 108, 111, 113, 202
Devon County Asylum, 79, 93, 191
Dick, Dr., 163
Digby, A., 23, 39, 40, 53, 67
Dining halls/rooms, 53, 54, 61, 63, 64, 66, 67, 69, 71, 76, 82, 83, 91, 92, 93, 94, 95, 96, 97, 98, 101, 104, 113, 117, 120, 123, 130, 133, 135, 136, 140, 143, 146, 164, 171, 172, 173, 184, 188, 189, 190, 192, 193, 212, 217, 223
Discretionary spaces, 91, 97, 99, 136, 138, 141, 144, 217, 219, 222
Documents, use of, 5, 8, 9, 14, 18, 24, 25, 26, 27, 28, 36, 98, 164
Donelly, M.
Dormitories, 12, 13, 45, 54, 55, 56, 61, 63, 64, 66, 67, 69, 71, 72, 76, 80, 81, 82, 85, 87, 88, 91, 92, 95, 96, 97, 106, 109, 113, 116, 119, 120, 121, 128, 129, 130, 132, 135, 140, 143, 144-145, 157, 160, 164, 166, 172, 173, 177, 179, 181, 189, 192, 193, 204, 222, 223
Driver, F., 7
Dublin Asylum, 197

E

East Sussex Asylum at Hellingly, 97
Economics and asylums, 23, 188, 191, 195, 196, 202, 203, 204, 228, 237
Edinburgh Lunatic Asylum, 29, 51
Eglinton County Asylum, 82, 85, 86, 89, 185
Emancipists, 206, 207, 208
Employment in Asylums, 42, 55, 201, 221, 222, 228, 238, 239
   curative role of, 210, 237
England, see Britain
English County Asylum Acts, 45, 46, 60, 75, 83, 96, 97, 192
Entertainments
Epileptics, 67, 69, 74, 139, 178
Essex County Asylum, 71, 82, 84, 85, 87, 89, 92, 93, 94, 96, 117, 185
Evangelical Movement, 44
Excavation, 8, 9, 12, 13, 14, 17, 18, 22, 26, 27, 216
Exercise yards/areas, 51, 54, 55, 59, 81, 109, 112, 125, 126, 140, 142, 143, 145, 154, 157, 160, 166, 169, 171, 174, 175, 176, 177, 180, 181, 182, 190, 235-236, 237

F

Farr, Reverend C., 197, 199, 229
Faunal assemblages, 10
Feister, L. M., 10
Female Factories, 7, 12, 13, 160, 166, 167
Female Refractory Building
Feminist archaeology, 8, 14
Finnegan, F., 7
Forsythe, B. 23
Foucault, M., 15, 22
Funding of asylums
Furnishings *see* Interior furnishings

G

Galleries, 23, 54, 55, 56, 61, 63, 64, 65, 68, 71, 80, 81, 82, 83, 86, 92, 94, 98, 99, 102, 103, 104, 106, 119, 120, 130, 136, 142, 143, 172, 174, 184, 187, 190, 193, 222, 233
Gardens, 15, 17, 40, 41, 42, 54, 55, 58, 59, 60, 62, 65, 66, 74, 81, 100, 101, 104, 112, 126, 133, 135, 139, 140, 145, 154, 156, 157, 161, 177, 180, 193, 221, 222, 228, 229, 231, 237, 238

Garton, S.,
Geller, J. L., 27
Gentlemen's Cottage (see cottages)
Gender, 8, 17, 23, 95, 99, 101
   provisions for different sexes, 59, 66, 72, 74, 102, 103, 128, 142, 154, 229, 230, 231, 232
Gender roles, 101-102, 103, 104, 144, 145, 221, 236
Glasgow Asylum, 50, 51, 53
Gloucester County Asylum, 45, 73
Gosse, Dr., 199, 201, 227, 228, 229
Gowlland, R. W., 33, 34, 154, 155, 163, 176, 205, 236
Government Gazette, 34, 112, 113
Great Britain *see* Britain
Greene, R., 30, 75
Greenwood, R. S., 26

H

Hants County Asylum, 102
Hardesty, D. L., 27
Harrison, B., 44
Hereford County and City Asylum, 82, 89, 93, 94, 185
Hervey, N., 98, 192
Hill, B., 104
Hill, R. G., 1, 16, 37, 38, 41, 42, 52, 54, 55, 156, 220, 228, 235
Hilliard, D., 142
Hine, G. T., 30, 75, 97
Historical archaeology, 1, 5, 8, 22, 24, 26, 28, 29, 183, 215, 216, 218
History and archaeology, 5, 22, 23-24, 27, 28
Hobart, 149, 150, 156, 157, 163, 167, 174
Hobart Gaol, 155, 176
Huston, Dr., 204, 206, 236, 238, 239
Hunter, R., 23, 103, 104

I

Ideal Asylum, 4, 5, 6, 21, 28, 31, 32, 36, 38, 45, 46, 47, 49, 50, 51, 56, 57, 58, 59, 63, 64, 65, 66, 69, 75, 76, 77, 78, 80, 81, 83, 88, 92, 94, 95, 97, 99, 101, 106, 108, 126, 133, 135, 136, 138, 143, 149, 157, 164, 165, 166, 167, 173, 174, 175, 182, 183, 184, 189, 192, 193, 194, 198, 200, 202, 203, 204, 209, 212, 214, 216, 217, 218, 219, 223, 233

Index

Incurable patients, 51
Infirmaries/Infirmary wards, 54, 61, 66, 69, 71, 75, 86, 93, 95, 96, 109, 128, 133, 135, 157, 192
Insanity, 232
   and heredity, 199, 200, 233
   organic causes of, 199, 200, 233
   and religion, 229
   social causes of, 199, 200, 207, 231
Institutional archaeology, 6, 8, 9, 17, 18
Interior Furnishings, 31, 34, 59, 99, 100, 101, 106, 142, 180, 190, 209, 219, 220
Invalid Establishment, 150
Isaac, R., 26

J

Jacobi, M, 30, 57, 58, 59, 60, 64, 65, 67, 77, 94, 95, 101, 132, 133, 135, 174, 183, 192, 193, 216, 220
Joint Committee (Tasmania), 204, 206, 207, 208, 209, 210, 211, 236
Jones, K., 38, 44, 45, 46, 192

K

Kay, H. T., 33, 195
Kendall, H. E., 92
Kent, S., 222
Kerr, J. S., 21
King, A., 70
Kitchen, 15, 52, 58, 61, 62, 63, 66, 67, 71, 73, 74, 88, 93, 96, 102, 103, 109, 111, 117, 138, 140, 151, 152, 154, 155, 160, 161, 164, 178, 203, 204, 228, 232
Knott, J., 50

L

Ladies' cottage (see cottages)
Laland, Miss, 171, 174, 210, 239
Lancaster Asylum, 45, 99
Laundry/laundries, 52, 58, 61, 62, 71, 72, 74, 75, 79, 87, 92, 93, 96, 98, 102, 103, 109, 111, 123, 133, 136, 138, 139, 140, 142, 143, 144, 145, 155, 157, 161, 163, 179, 181, 219, 221, 228
Lavatories, 61, 62, 63, 69, 70, 82, 86, 109, 119, 123, 129, 130, 160, 164, 166, 171, 187, 190, 192

Leicester Asylum, 46
Leone, M., 17
Leone, M. & Crosby, C. A., 27, 28
Leone, M. & Potter, Jr., Parker, 27, 28
Leper colonies/Lazarets, 7, 11
Libraries, 69, 91, 95, 101, 106, 125, 192, 193, 217, 232, 238
Limerick District Asylum, 197
Lincoln Asylum, 41, 45, 54, 199, 229
Lincolnshire County Asylum, 82, 84, 85, 86, 89, 91, 94, 185
Linear asylums, 60, 70, 76, 81, 85, 133
Linear arrangements, 81, 82, 83, 84, 93, 94, 96, 97, 109, 128, 130, 133, 135, 136, 172, 184, 217
Living spaces, 27, 64, 69, 97, 130, 143, 172, 176, 177, 180, 182, 184, 187, 190, 201
London Asylum, 78, 80
London County Asylum, Canehill, 97
Lucas, G., 16
Lunatic asylums in general, 1, 5, 18, 19, 23, 28, 30, 37, 67, 73, 97, 156, 192, 215
Lying-in Wards, 104

M

Macfarlane, Dr., 160, 179, 209, 238
MacKenzie, C., 23
Madhouses, 20, 38, 40, 43, 44, 47, 49, 50, 191, 194
Magadelen Asylums, 7, 14, 15, 220
Manning, F. N., 32, 84, 94, 96, 163
Markus, T. A., 22, 23
Marland, H., 23
Material culture, 5, 8, 9, 10, 11, 12, 13, 14, 17, 18, 20, 26, 27, 28, 29, 34, 139, 216, 219
Matron's Cottage, 160, 163, 175, 177, 181
Matron's rooms, 88, 109, 117, 119, 173
Medical Superintendent (*see* Superintendent)
Middle class, 9, 15, 69, 83, 135, 199, 208, 221, 222
Middle-range theory, 24, 27, 28, 216
Middlesex Asylum at Hanwell, 42, 60, 61, 64, 79, 80, 99, 101, 104, 197
Montrose Asylum, 42
Moore, Dr., 142, 146, 197, 199, 200, 228, 230

Moral architecture, 15
Moral environments, 7, 52,
Moral management/therapy/treatment, 2, 19, 37, 38, 40, 42, 43, 45, 46, 47, 49, 50, 51, 52, 53, 55, 57, 58, 62, 65, 74, 102, 105, 132, 138, 141, 146, 147, 176, 177, 179, 182, 196, 201, 202, 205, 210, 219, 220, 227, 228, 230, 231, 233, 235, 238, 239
Morris, N., 7
Multi-function rooms/spaces, 123, 130, 131, 138, 142, 179, 190, 212, 219
Music Room, 64, 65, 83, 106

N

Nance, C., 107
Nash, James (*see also* Colonial Surgeon), 108, 111, 227
New Norfolk Commissioners, 35, 155, 158, 160, 163, 164, 167, 169, 171, 172, 174, 176, 178, 180, 182, 187, 188, 190, 191, 203, 204, 205, 206, 207, 208, 210, 211, 235, 238, 239
New Norfolk Hospital for the Insane, 33, 34, 150, 152, 154, 155, 156, 157, 158, 160, 161, 163, 164, 167, 169, 171, 172, 173, 174, 175, 176, 177, 178, 179, 180, 181, 182, 184, 185, 187, 188, 189, 190, 191, 194, 203, 204, 205, 206, 207, 209, 210, 211, 212, 213, 215, 216, 218, 219, 220, 222, 235, 236, 237, 238, 239
Non-Restraint, 2, 6, 37, 38, 40, 41, 42, 43, 46, 47, 49, 51, 54, 55, 60, 62, 78, 132, 139, 141, 146, 147, 156, 174, 177, 196, 197, 201, 210, 219, 220, 227, 228, 230, 233, 235, 236, 237, 238, 239
Norfolk Asylum, 45
Norfolk Hospital Correspondence Book, 35, 155, 203, 204, 237
Nottingham County and Borough Asylum, 45, 98, 100, 155, 208

O

Observations, 29, 51, 52
Officer, Dr. R., 150, 235
Offices, 61, 62, 63, 64, 65, 68, 73, 74, 79, 88, 93, 95, 121, 130, 131, 133, 147, 151, 161, 173, 181, 188
Orphanages, 7, 10, 11

P

Panopticon, 50, 58
Palmer, E., 86, 91
Parkside Asylum, 22, 108, 116, 120, 121, 122, 123, 125, 126, 128, 129, 130, 131, 132, 133, 135, 136, 138, 139, 140, 141, 142, 143, 144, 145, 146, 147, 184, 185, 187, 188, 189, 190, 191, 194, 195, 198, 200, 201, 202, 215, 216, 217, 218, 219, 221, 222, 232
Paternalism, 8, 10, 11, 15, 18, 147, 218
Paterson, Dr. A., 141, 142, 144, 147, 163, 198, 200, 201, 230, 231, 232
Paupers, 45, 46, 69, 83, 94, 199, 202, 206, 207
Pavilion asylums, 69, 70, 71, 72, 73, 93, 94, 97, 128, 156, 209
Pavilion Blocks, 72, 76, 79, 116, 123, 131, 135, 136, 140, 143, 160, 161, 175, 180, 195, 204,
Pearson, M. P. & Richards, C., 222
Perkin, J., 102
Philo, C., 23
Piddock, S., 8, 17, 18, 46, 108, 128, 133, 155, 157, 160, 163, 196, 202
Pike, D., 21
Pinel, P. H., 2, 38, 39
Port Arthur Lunatic Asylum, 150, 160, 165, 166, 167, 204
Porter, R., 20, 23, 39, 40, 43
Prangnell, J. M., 11, 12, 218
Privies (*see also* water closets), 152
Purpose-built asylums, 73, 108, 115, 149, 156, 194, 196, 204, 211, 213

Q

Quakers/Quakerism, 39, 52
Quarterly, M, 33, 194

R

Radial asylums, 50, 78, 79, 97, 198
Reception rooms, 61, 69, 74
Recreation room/hall, 61, 63, 64, 66, 69, 72, 74, 81, 82, 83, 87, 91, 93, 94, 95, 97, 98, 99, 100, 101, 102, 104, 105, 106, 123, 125, 130, 133, 135, 136, 141, 146, 147, 163, 166, 172, 174, 184, 187, 188, 190, 202, 203, 211, 212, 217, 219

Index

Reid, R., 29, 51, 52
Refractory patients, 53, 61, 69, 79, 84, 109, 113, 135, 140, 166, 169, 171, 174, 229, 230
Refractory blocks/wards, 61, 63, 64, 72, 91, 155, 161, 163, 172, 177, 179-180, 181, 204
Religious consolation/services, 42, 43, 131, 139, 141, 142, 174, 176, 177, 178, 179, 180, 182, 188, 190, 201, 210, 219, 228, 229, 231, 232, 236, 237, 239
Resident Surgeon/medical officer, 112, 115, 117, 119, 123, 136, 162, 173, 190, 193, 194, 198, 207, 211, 230, 236, 237, 238, 239
Resistance, 8, 13, 218
Restraint *see* non-restraint
Reynolds, H., 206, 207, 208
Ripa, Y., 23
Ritual, 8, 14, 15, 16, 18, 220
Robertson, C. L., 30, 70, 71, 72, 77, 84, 85, 91, 93, 94, 105, 133, 135, 136, 175, 183, 191, 209, 216, 217
Rosenau, H., 23
Royal Commission (Tasmania), 160, 161, 163, 164, 167, 169, 171, 174, 178, 179, 180, 181, 182, 204, 209, 211, 238, 239
Russell, R., 23

S

Salt, A., 12
Sankey, W. H. O., 30, 64, 65, 66, 67, 68, 69, 71, 72, 77, 94, 95, 96, 101, 104, 133, 135, 136, 174, 175, 183, 190, 193, 209, 217
Saunders, J., 23
School rooms, 61, 63, 64, 69, 82, 83, 87, 91, 92, 97, 101, 130, 141, 172, 184, 187, 188, 217, 219
Schuyler, R., 23
Scott, E., 26
Scull, A., 20, 22, 23, 37, 38, 43, 46, 70, 73, 90
Seigburg Asylum, 57, 58
Select Committees (England), 44, 45
Select Committees/Commission, 27, 34, 111, 112, 113, 115, 123, 125, 126, 128, 130, 131, 132-133, 155, 139, 140, 141, 142, 144, 145, 146, 195, 196, 197, 198, 199, 200, 210, 202, 227, 228, 229, 230, 231, 323
Select Committee (Tasmania), 35, 157, 158, 163, 171, 173, 174, 175, 176, 177, 179, 182, 190
Shlomowitz, E. A., 33
Showalter, E., 25, 104, 105
Single rooms, 50, 54, 56, 61, 63, 64, 65, 69, 71, 72, 80, 85, 88, 91, 96, 97, 111, 112, 113, 117, 125, 128, 132, 160, 173, 189, 192, 193, 223
Sites for asylums, 55, 56, 58, 59, 60, 80, 82, 113, 115, 126, 133, 156, 167, 192, 197-198
Sitting rooms, 16, 54, 67, 68, 69, 96, 160, 164
Size of asylums, 45, 46, 51, 54, 57, 59, 60, 63, 70, 79, 85, 90, 128, 169, 184, 193, 195
Skultans, V., 1, 22, 23, 39, 40, 41, 104, 231
Sleeping cells/rooms, 62, 65, 66, 67, 68, 71, 72, 74, 78, 79, 85, 87, 95, 109, 119, 120, 123, 126, 128, 129, 139, 140, 145, 151, 152, 154, 155, 156, 157, 160, 163, 166, 169, 172, 173, 174, 175, 176, 177, 181, 182, 188, 193, 201, 205
Social class/rank, 51, 52, 54, 58, 59, 106, 144, 149, 154, 155, 156, 174, 175, 178, 179, 196, 198, 200, 202, 205, 206, 207, 209, 210, 213, 222, 230, 237, 238, 239
South Australia, 1, 3, 6, 21, 22, 32, 34, 36, 98, 106, 107, 108, 133, 136, 138, 141, 142, 149, 182, 183, 184, 187, 188, 189, 190, 194, 196, 201, 203, 212, 213, 214, 216, 217, 218, 219, 221, 222, 227, 235, 238
South Australian Government, 111, 112, 113, 196
South Australian Visitors, 108, 109, 113, 123, 145, 146, 192, 227, 236
Southwood, W. T., 34, 155, 208
Spencer-Wood, S. M., 8, 26
Spencer-Wood, S. M. & Baugher, S., 7
Stafford Asylum, 45
Stark, W., 29, 50, 51, 78
St. Luke's Hospital, 67, 71

Superintendent, 18, 50, 51, 55, 59, 71, 73, 74, 81, 91, 93, 94, 105, 138, 144, 147, 160, 181, 198, 209, 219, 236, 238, 239
  rooms for, 135, 144, 151, 152, 160
Surrey County Asylum, 30, 46, 70, 71, 82, 88, 89, 91, 96, 185, 191
Sussex County Asylum, 82, 84, 86, 87, 88, 89, 91, 92, 95, 135, 185
Symbolism, 14, 15, 17, 220

T

Tasmania (*see also* Van Dieman's Land), 1, 3, 6, 12, 21, 33, 36, 98, 106, 107, 108, 149, 150, 155, 160, 182, 183, 184, 189, 190, 194, 203, 204, 205, 207, 208, 211, 212, 213, 214, 216, 217, 219, 222, 236, 238
Tasmanian Government, 176, 182
Taylor, J., 23, 32, 33, 92, 93, 105
The Builder, 32, 84, 86, 91, 196, 198, 208, 213, 214
The Retreat, 39, 40, 49, 50, 52, 53, 54, 105
Third Lancashire County Asylum at Whittingham *see* Whittingham Asylum
Thomas, Dr., 197
Toller, E., 30, 73, 74, 96
Total institutions, 7
Townsley, W. A., 149, 150, 155, 203, 205
Treatment regimes, 19, 20, 23, 34, 37, 38, 39, 40, 41, 42, 49, 138, 141, 144, 149, 177, 181, 196, 199, 200, 201, 202, 208, 209, 210, 211, 220, 222, 223, 228, 230, 232, 233, 235, 236, 237, 238, 239
Tuke, S., 38, 39, 40, 52, 53, 54, 55, 58, 67, 101

V

Van Dieman's Land, 21, 107, 149, 150
Ventilation, 20, 51, 56, 57, 58, 59, 61, 63, 66, 70, 76, 80, 82, 84, 85, 126, 132, 136, 155, 166, 169, 184, 192, 237
Verandahs, 157, 160, 169, 176, 177, 180, 237
Visitors *see* South Australian Visitors
Visitors Book, 34, 111, 113, 130, 139
Visitors, Official (Tasmania) 163, 178, 182

W

Walton, J. K., 23
Wards, 23, 42, 43, 45, 50, 51, 54, 60, 61, 62, 63, 64, 65, 66, 67, 68, 69, 71, 72, 78, 79, 81, 82, 83, 84, 86, 88, 92, 93, 94, 95, 96, 99, 100, 101, 102, 103, 104, 105, 106, 109, 111, 112, 113, 121, 126, 128, 129, 130, 131, 135, 136, 138, 139, 140, 141, 142, 143, 144, 145, 146, 151, 152, 155, 171, 172, 173, 181, 187, 188, 189, 190, 192, 195, 202, 212, 214, 218, 219, 220, 221, 222, 228, 229, 231, 232
Waselkov, G. A., 26
Washhouse, 72, 93, 151, 152, 163, 179, 180, 222, 229
Water closets, 52, 56, 58, 61, 63, 69, 70, 71, 80, 81, 82, 83, 86, 91, 92, 96, 109, 119, 129, 130, 132, 133, 143, 152, 164, 166, 171, 173, 178, 184, 187, 190, 192, 214
Welter, B., 104
West Riding Asylum, 45, 79, 80, 81, 91
West, S., 100
Whittingham Asylum, 82, 89, 93, 94, 95, 185, 191
Willson, Bishop, W., 34, 155, 156, 157, 164, 167, 178, 204, 205, 208, 213
Willow Court (*see also* New Norfolk Hospital), 152, 163, 164, 180
Women's Hospital, 169, 178, 180, 181
Women in asylums, 27
Wood, M. E., 27
Woodforde Asylum, 112, 115, 133, 195, 196, 198, 199
Woodforde, Dr., 199
Worcester County Asylum, 99
Working class, 69, 202, 208, 209, 221
Workrooms, 15, 59, 63, 64, 68, 71, 75, 82, 83, 87, 91, 102, 117, 131, 132, 133, 140, 141, 142, 146, 172, 173, 179, 180, 187, 188, 190, 192, 193, 212, 217, 221, 222

Workshops, 58, 61, 62, 63, 64, 66, 68, 71, 72, 74, 82, 83, 87, 92, 93, 102, 103, 131, 136, 140, 141, 142, 143, 145, 146, 157, 172, 174, 177, 179, 187, 188, 190, 192, 193, 201, 204, 214, 219, 221

Workhouses, 7, 10, 12, 15, 16, 17, 18, 23, 46, 50, 67, 73, 104, 105

Y

Yarra Bend Asylum, 198

Made in the USA
Monee, IL
17 January 2021

e4db50e9-553d-4990-b298-d47f63c89746R01